Textbook of
Urinalysis and
Body Fluids

Textbook of
Urinalysis and Body Fluids
A CLINICAL APPROACH

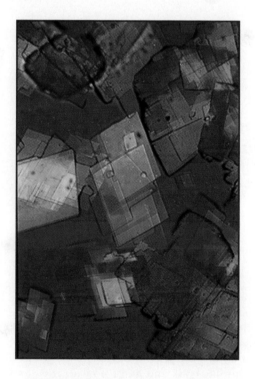

Landy J. McBride, PhD, MT(ASCP)

Professor and Chair
Department of Clinical Sciences
California State University
Bakersfield, California

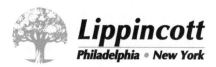

Lippincott
Philadelphia • *New York*

Acquisitions Editor: Larry McGrew
Assistant Editor: Holly Chapman
Project Editor: Jahmae Harris and Roberta Spivek
Production Manager: Helen Ewan
Production Coordinator: Patricia McCloskey
Design Coordinator: Doug Smock

9   8   7   6   5   4   3   2   1

Library of Congress Cataloging-in-Publications Data

McBride, L. J. (Landy James), 1931–
    Textbook of urinalysis and body fluids : a clinical approach/
Landy J. McBride.
        p. cm.
    Includes bibliographical references and index.
    ISBN 0-397-55231-9 (paper : alk. paper)
    1. Body fluids—Analysis. 2. Urine—Analysis. 3. Body fluids—
Analysis—Case studies. 4. Urine—Analysis—Case studies.
I. Title.
    [DNLM: 1. Urinalysis—methods. 2. Body Fluids—physiology.
QY 185 M478t 1997]
RB52.M25 1997
616.07´566—dc21
DNLM/DLC
for Library of Congress   97-38213
                                                    CIP

Care has been taken to confirm the accuracy of the information presented and to describe generally accepted practices. However, the authors, editors, and publisher are not responsible for errors or omissions or for any consequences from application of the information in this book and make no warranty, express or implied, with respect to the contents of the publication.

The authors, editors and publisher have exerted every effort to ensure that drug selection and dosage set forth in this text are in accordance with current recommendations and practice at the time of publication. However, in view of ongoing research, changes in government regulations, and the constant flow of information relating to drug reactions, the reader is urged to check the package insert for each drug for any change in indications and dosage and for added warnings and precautions. This is particularly important when the recommended agent is a new or infrequently employed drug.

Some drugs and medical devices presented in this publication have Food and Drug Administration (FDA) clearance for limited use in restricted research settings. It is the responsibility of the health care provider to ascertain the FDA status of each drug or device planned for use in their clinical practice.

This book is dedicated to my entire family for their patience and understanding during its preparation: my wife Lydia; our daughter Mara Clarke and her husband Richard; our daughter Erin Reed and her husband Roger; and our grandsons, Taylor and Brandon Reed. With much love to all.

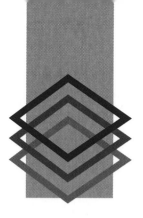

Acknowledgments

I am indebted to California State University, Bakersfield, for providing the three-month sabbatical during which this project was initiated.

Special thanks are due several individuals on the staff at Lippincott–Raven Publishers: Andrew Allen, former executive editor for sharing my vision and giving me the opportunity to work on this book; Larry McGrew and Holly Collins-Chapman for their expert assistance and being patient when I missed deadlines; and the entire production staff, especially those involved in re-drawing several of the figures.

Mary Correia and Wood Hubbard (Specialized Photographic Services) provided extraordinary support in developing all of the photomicrographic film and preparing duplicate slides for the book. Many thanks to you both.

This project would not have been possible without the assistance and cooperation of so many of the staff in the Clinical Laboratory at Kern Medical Center, Bakersfield, California. Thank you for saving specimens for me, obtaining medical records, helping me when I had problems with the laboratory computer (YES!), sharing your bench space and knowledge, and providing helpful discussions on cytotechnology. I am truly grateful to you all.

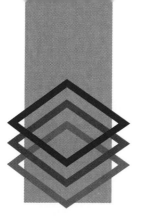

Preface

My original idea for this book was to prepare a simple collection of clinical studies in urinalysis and body fluids. When Lippincott–Raven Publishers indicated their desire to have a Urinalysis and Body Fluids textbook, it was decided that the book would be a combination—a textbook but with case studies occupying a prominent place in the book's organization.

After several years of teaching urinalysis and body fluids to our preclinical and clinical-year medical technology students I am convinced that the use of case studies is one of the best ways to convey clinical information and at the same time to make this material "come alive" to the students. The major chapters of this book begin with a case study to set the stage for the material which follows. These chapters also incorporate illustrative case studies as well as case histories with study questions to bridge the gap between textbook material and the real patients we all seek to serve in our clinical laboratory work. In addition to students of clinical laboratory science (MLTs and MTs), it is hoped that the book will be useful to students of other allied health professions, nursing, and medicine.

It is important to note that for my studies, I obtained the urine and body fluid specimens from the laboratory staff after they had conducted their own analyses. For the photomicrographs of urine sediment I used traditional microscope slides and coverslips because this method gave me more flexibility and better optical control. Thus, for a given patient the urinalysis (from the laboratory computer) might have indicated many WBC's in the sediment whereas I might have been interested in another type of cell in the specimen or a cast, etc. Therefore, the photomicrographs may not necessarily reflect the urinalysis information taken from the computer or represent what was observed in the original examination. My purpose was to screen the specimens and record only their most significant and illustrative aspects.

The book is organized along traditional lines although I have attempted to incorporate more pathophysiology and less "how to do it" information. There are already several excellent textbooks available which treat laboratory methods and procedures in detail. The attempt here is to provide a "case-oriented" textbook which combines basic information on urinalysis and body fluids with emphasis on case studies and case histories/study questions. It is my sincere hope that we have achieved this, and that the text will be useful in teaching the subject of urinalysis and body fluids as well as serving as a resource for clinical laboratory scientists.

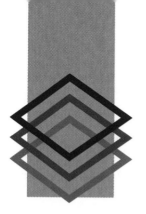

Contents

16

Bronchial Washings and Bronchoalveolar Lavage 257

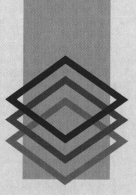

1 Quality Assurance and Safety in the Clinical Laboratory

The aim of this chapter is to review briefly and in a general way quality assurance and safety in the clinical laboratory. Specific aspects of quality assurance and safety in the urinalysis/body fluids section of the clinical laboratory will be taken up in more detail in the succeeding chapters.

ABBREVIATIONS USED IN THIS ABBREVIATIONS USED IN THIS CHAPTER

ACGIH = American Conference of Governmental Industrial Hygienists

AIDS = acquired immunodeficiency syndrome

BSI = body substance isolation

CAP = College of American Pathologists

CDC = Centers for Disease Control and Prevention

CHP = chemical hygiene plan

CQI = continuous quality improvement

DOT = Department of Transportation

EPA = Environmental Protection Agency

HBV = hepatitis B virus

HIV = human immunodeficiency virus

JCAHO = Joint Commission for Accreditation of Healthcare Organizations

MSDS = Material Safety Data Sheets

NCCLS = National Committee for Clinical Laboratory Standards

NFPA = National Fire Protection Association

NIOSH = National Institute of Occupational Safety and Health

NRC = Nuclear Regulatory Commission

OSHA = Occupational Safety and Health Administration

PM = preventive maintenance

QA = quality assurance

QC = quality control

RIA = radioimmunoassay

TQM = total quality management

Quality Assurance in the Clinical Laboratory

Quality may be thought of as satisfaction of the needs and expectations of users or customers.[15] Quality has two aspects: first, an objective reality that is constant and measurable, and second, a subjective aspect closely tied to utility or value. Quantitative physical measurements are the usual standards by which quality is judged, so that quality may also be defined as conformance to requirements.

Total Quality Management

As pointed out by Westgard and Klee, the systems used by healthcare organizations to monitor and ensure quality are evolving in response to public and private pressures to contain costs and improve quality.[15] When faced with these same pressures, other industries have implemented what is known as total quality management (TQM), sometimes also referred to as continuous quality improvement (CQI). TQM provides a management philosophy for organizational development together with a management process to improve the quality of all aspects of work. An example of this approach is reported in an article by Batalden and Stoltz.[2] They demonstrated that the continual improvement of healthcare, with minimal waste and greatest synergy, requires underlying knowledge; leadership that fosters learning, tools and methods; and strategies for daily work applications. Yablonsky[16] presented case studies of healthcare institutions where TQM was implemented to solve problems such as the need to reduce turnaround time and the choice of a laboratory information system.

Quality Assurance

The attainment of quality goals in a service laboratory requires a comprehensive quality assurance (QA) program. Quality assurance, a broad array of plans, policies, and procedures, provides the laboratory with the administrative structure needed to achieve quality goals. Defined another way, quality assurance is the process of delivering the best possible service to the patient and physician. Quality assurance encompasses monitoring and controlling the competence of personnel; monitoring the quality of materials, methods, reagents, and instruments; and reporting test results reliably. Laboratory QA is a system to prevent and control errors that occur from the time a test is ordered until the time it is interpreted. Quality assurance is the total system designed to ensure the quality of results, while quality control (QC) refers to the procedures that must be completed before a particular batch of results is reported. QC is discussed later in this chapter.

A QA program involves just about everything and everybody in the clinical laboratory, and has several essential elements. These include commitment to QA, facilities and resources, technical competence, technical procedures, and a mechanism to solve problems.

Good technical procedures or processes are necessary to provide high-quality laboratory services. Although the technical processes are the general responsibility of the laboratory, problems arise before and after the analysis of patient specimens. To monitor and control these errors, it is helpful to see the system as a series of processes that can be divided into three groups: preanalytical, analytical, and postanalytical.

PREANALYTICAL PROCESSES

Preanalytical processes include patient preparation, test requests, and specimen acquisition and handling. Problems connected with test requests might include these circumstances:

- The test is inappropriate
- Handwriting is illegible
- Patient is not correctly identified
- Special requirements are not specified

Patient preparation involves fasting, posture, preparation of collection site, diurnal variations in analytes, physical activity, and medications.[7] Examples of specimen acquisition and handling errors include:

- Use of an incorrect tube or container
- Incorrect patient identification
- Inadequate volume
- Invalid specimen (e.g., one that is hemolyzed)
- Specimen collected at the wrong time
- Improper transport conditions

ANALYTICAL PROCESSES

Analytical processes include the analytical methodology, standardization and calibration procedures; documentation of analytical protocols and procedures; and the monitoring of critical equipment and materials. Potential errors include:

- Incorrect calibration of instruments
- Specimen "mix-up"
- Incorrect volume of specimen
- Presence of interfering substances or a precision problem with an instrument

One of the important ways the laboratory monitors errors in this area is through internal and external QC programs, as discussed later. In addition to internal and external QC programs, analytical QA includes:

- Proper handling and use of reagents (e.g., label with lot number, date prepared, preparer's initials)
- Calibrating pipetting devices
- Using instrument preventive maintenance (PM)
- Monitoring the accuracy of balances and thermometers
- Monitoring the accuracy of centrifuge speed settings and timing devices
- Periodic assurance that procedure manuals are complete and up-to-date
- Constant assurance that safety procedures are followed

These processes are usually monitored by means of function sheets or checklists initialed by the laboratorian as the functions are performed.

POSTANALYTICAL PROCESSES

Postanalytical processes involve procedures and policies that affect test reporting and test interpretation. Errors in test reporting include:

- Incorrect patient identification
- Failure to post the report on the patient's chart
- Illegible report
- Delayed report
- Transcription error

Errors or problems with test interpretation can involve:

- Failure to recognize interfering substances
- Specificity of test not understood

- Precision limitations not recognized
- Inappropriate analytic sensitivity
- Lack of previous values for comparison

Quality Control

QC is an integral part of the analytical phase of a QA program and is sometimes confused with QA. The term "QC" may refer to those techniques and procedures that monitor performance parameters or to the process of monitoring the accuracy and precision of a laboratory test with control samples.[14,15] These quantitative techniques and procedures serve to monitor particular systems for errors, to estimate the magnitude of the errors, and to call attention to signs that quality has deteriorated. Quality control processes have both internal and external components.

INTERNAL QC

Internal QC involves the analysis of patient specimens alongside control samples. The results are evaluated statistically to determine if the analytical run is acceptable so that patient results can be reported. Internal QC differs from external QC in several ways. Internal QC monitors a test method's precision and analytical bias. The preparation of the control materials and the interpretation of test results are handled in the laboratory. A control sample is a special specimen inserted into the testing process and treated as if it were a patient's sample by being exposed to the same conditions as the patient's sample (e.g., incubation time, temperature, agitation). Characteristics of a good control include the following:

- Close similarity to the patient sample, reacting in the same manner
- Analyte concentrations at medically significant levels
- Stability under storage for a long period of time before and after preparation
- Low vial-to-vial variability
- Being ready to use or requiring a minimum of preparation; being readily available for emergency use
- Availability in large quantities
- Reasonable price

Note that controls are not calibrators or standards.

Calibrators and standards are used to adjust or standardize instruments; they define a "standard curve" for analysis.

For quantitative procedures (predominantly clinical chemistry), monitoring the results obtained with control specimens to detect random and systematic error is done by visual methods using Shewhart or Levey-Jennings charts, or by multirule methods that rely on rule violations to indicate that an error has occurred. Manufactured controls are often supplied at three levels—low (or negative, if appropriate), normal, and high (to monitor the method in the upper range of its sensitivity). For qualitative (bipolar) and semiquantitative procedures, there is no entirely satisfactory statistical evaluation.

As another approach to QC, various protocols using patient samples have been proposed.[14] Several of these methods can be applied to both qualitative and quantitative test procedures. The more common methods include absurd value checks, duplicate analysis and delta checks, average of normal patients, moving averages, and the use of physiologic relationships such as calculation of anion gaps, acid–base balance, and so forth.

EXTERNAL QC

External QC is the process of assaying unknown samples sent to the laboratory from an outside agency. The results are evaluated by the agency that supplied the samples by using an established value for the outside sample derived by laboratories within a peer group. The most common external QC systems are proficiency testing programs. The College of American Pathologists (CAP) Survey Program is one of the best known and is representative of most proficiency surveys.[14] The program includes basic, comprehensive, and specialty surveys in chemistry, hematology, microbiology, blood bank, serology, nuclear medicine, anatomic pathology and cytology, and histology. The CAP and similar surveys are designed to accomplish the following goals:

- Assess the current state of the art of laboratory medicine
- Provide information to help laboratory directors select the best methods and reagents
- Satisfy most regulatory requirements and accrediting agencies
- Provide a voluntary educational peer comparison program that allows a laboratory to compare its performance with its peers

Safety in the Clinical Laboratory

Regulations and Safety Requirements for Clinical Laboratories

Many federal, state, and local laws regulate safe practices to protect employees, the community, and the environment. In 1970, Congress enacted the Occupational Safety and Health Act (PL 91-596) and established the Occupational Safety and Health Administration (OSHA) within the Department of Labor. OSHA has the authority to establish regulations, conduct on-site inspections of workplaces to determine compliance with mandatory safety standards, and assess fines if it finds noncompliance with the regulations. OSHA has promulgated regulations that specifically affect clinical laboratories, which are discussed later in this section.

The Medical Waste Tracking Act was passed into law in 1988. This regulation requires the Environmental Protection Agency (EPA) to establish a program to track medical waste from generation to disposal. The Act defines medical waste, establishes acceptable techniques for treatment and disposal, and establishes a department with jurisdiction to enforce the new laws. Several states have implemented the federal guidelines and incorporated additional requirements. The guidelines cover any healthcare-related facility, including blood banks, clinics, research laboratories, hospitals, emergency centers, clinical laboratories, and physicians' offices.

Agencies other than OSHA also have regulations that affect clinical laboratories; these agencies include the EPA, Department of Transportation (DOT), and Nuclear Regulatory Commission (NRC). In addition, local and state laws regulate sewage disposal, fire and building codes, and hazardous waste disposal. Voluntary safety standards, codes, and guidelines have been developed by several government and private agencies such as the National Fire Protection Association (NFPA), the National Committee for Clinical Laboratory Standards (NCCLS), the Centers for Disease Control and Prevention (CDC), the National Institute of Occupational Safety and Health (NIOSH), and the American Conference of Governmental Industrial Hygienists (ACGIH). Voluntary accrediting agencies such as CAP and the Joint Commission for Accreditation of Healthcare Organizations (JCAHO) have adopted standards for inspection and accreditation that include laboratory safety. JCAHO publishes a yearly accreditation manual for hospitals that includes a detailed section on safety requirements.

Safety Practices

According to the NCCLS document on clinical laboratory safety,[4] a laboratory safety officer should be appointed to provide guidance to management officials and supervisors who are responsible for creating a safe workplace for all of their employees. The safety officer may propose safety programs; provide advice on safety issues; propose, provide, or obtain safety orientation and training; serve as a member of the safety committee; and survey worksites for safety deficiencies. Figure 1-1 provides examples of warning symbols commonly used in the laboratory.

The NCCLS recommends establishing a safety audit—an ongoing program to review safe operations and equipment. The NCCLS document GP17-T provides suggested forms that can be used for this purpose.[4] The worksite should be surveyed and inspected at least annually to ensure the proper state of readiness and function of firefighting apparatus and emergency showers, and the proper containment and permissible volumes of flammable and combustible liquids. It is a good idea for the safety committee to be involved in these surveys.

The laboratory should also develop a written chemical hygiene plan that includes a protocol for chemical hazard communication. The plan should define the safety procedures to be followed for handling hazardous chemicals in the laboratory, and should include:

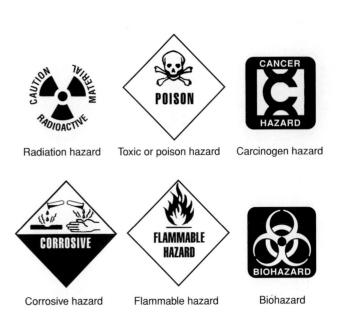

Radiation hazard   Toxic or poison hazard   Carcinogen hazard

Corrosive hazard   Flammable hazard   Biohazard

FIGURE 1-1 Common warning symbols used in the clinical laboratory.

1. Procedures for monitoring inventory for identification of hazardous chemicals, requirements for adequate labeling, and proper storage and disposal
2. Procedures for prudent practices in handling chemicals
3. Method and documentation of employee training
4. Procedures for obtaining, maintaining, and distributing Material Safety Data Sheets (MSDS) for each laboratory chemical used to ensure that employees have 24-hour access to this information

Items reflecting compliance with this plan may be included in laboratory safety inspection checklists. All employees should participate in a safety training program at the time of hire and then annually, unless federal, state, or local laws recommend otherwise. A safety manual should be available in the work area and should be required reading for all new employees. The manual should be specific for the laboratory's needs under the major categories of "Fire Prevention," "Electrical Safety," "Chemical Hazards," "Radiation Hazards," "Microbiologic Hazards," and "Hazardous Waste Disposal."

Proper records and documentation are an integral part of laboratory safety. Management officials need to document employee training. Hazardous waste disposal records and survey and inspection reports should be retained and abatement actions recorded. The laboratory should have a program for reporting laboratory incidents and potential hazards. Reports should be filed for all incidents, and the reports should be reviewed by the safety committee and officer. Appropriate corrective actions should be taken to avoid their recurrence.

General requirements for personal and laboratory safety include the following items:

- Smoking is prohibited in technical work areas because of the risk of igniting flammable solvents. Handling smoking materials (bench to mouth) also poses a risk of exposure to infectious agents and toxins.
- Eating and drinking in technical work areas is prohibited because of the risk of contaminating food and drink with infectious agents. Food should never be stored in technical refrigerators, but only in those reserved exclusively for that purpose in areas designated for eating and drinking.
- Application of cosmetics in technical work areas is not allowed, although employees performing frequent handwashing may apply hand creams.

- Suitable eye and face protection must be used when working with materials that are caustic, toxic, or infectious to guard against splashing.
- The use of gowns, aprons, or laboratory coats is required when it is likely that body fluids may contaminate skin or clothing. Shoes should be made of leather or a synthetic, fluid-impermeable material, and sandals or shoes with open toes or negative heels are not recommended.
- Hair should be tied back and off the shoulders to avoid contact with contaminated materials or surfaces in the work area. Hair should be kept out of moving equipment such as centrifuges.
- Hands should be washed frequently during the day, after removing gloves, before leaving the laboratory, before and after contact with patients, and before eating or smoking. Eye-wash stations and emergency showers should be conveniently located wherever acids, caustics, corrosives, and other hazardous chemicals are in use.
- Appropriate respiratory protection should be provided to employees to prevent them from breathing air contaminated with harmful dust, gases, fumes, and the like. **Mouth pipetting is strictly prohibited**.
- Caution must be exercised when handling sharps such as needles, scalpels, lancets, or broken glass. Used sharps should be immediately placed in proper containers for disposal. **Used needles must not be clipped, bent, broken, recapped, resheathed by hand, or removed from disposable syringes.**

Biohazard Safety

PERSONAL PROTECTION

Blood-borne disease is of increasing concern in the laboratory community, particularly with the epidemic spread of acquired immunodeficiency syndrome (AIDS). Workers in the clinical laboratory are recognized as a high-risk group for job-related infection with HBV (hepatitis B virus) and HIV (human immunodeficiency virus). The CDC (1988) has recommended that to protect healthcare workers and others from acquiring HIV infection, blood and body fluids precautions should be consistently used for all patients and patient specimens. This guideline has become known as "universal precautions." The CDC revision removed certain specimens from the list of body substances requiring universal precautions, but because this caused confusion, many institutions advocate "body substance isolation" (BSI). *The best procedure is to treat ALL body substances as potentially infectious.*

The 1991 OSHA final rule for Occupational Exposure to Blood Borne Pathogens requires that an employer provide personal protective equipment that prevents potentially infectious materials from reaching an employee's clothes, skin, eyes, and mouth under normal conditions of use.[6] Also required are provisions for safe disposal of sharps and other biohazardous waste. In addition, it requires that HBV vaccine and postexposure treatment be made available without charge to all employees who are at risk of exposure. The rule requires annual training for employees to provide information on the risks of exposure and transmission, necessary precautions to avoid exposure, the exposure control plan, interpretation of all signs and warnings, and appropriate actions to take when an emergency arises. Last, the final rule addresses handwashing, specimen transport, use of pipette devices, spill cleanup, waste disposal, and decontamination of equipment.

The universal biohazard symbol is included in Figure 1-1. This symbol is available on gummed labels or tags to be attached to waste containers, equipment, cabinets, rooms, and the like, and it is also printed on plastic bags and other containers used for disposal of biohazard waste.

The NCCLS has provided an excellent summary of the recommendations for protecting laboratory workers from infectious disease transmitted by blood, body fluids, and tissue. These recommendations are summarized in Table 1-1.

DECONTAMINATION OF BIOHAZARDOUS SPILLS

NCCLS Document M29-T2[10] provides guidelines for decontamination of spills of blood, body fluids, or other infectious materials:

- Wear gloves and a gown
- Avoid touching broken glass with the hands
- Absorb the spill (e.g., paper towels, granular absorbent) and discard the used absorbent in the biohazard waste container
- Clean the spill site with aqueous detergent solution
- Disinfect the site using an intermediate or high-level disinfectant
- Absorb the disinfectant solution with disposable material and discard the material in the biohazard waste container

A "biohazard spill kit" containing all the materials and protective equipment needed should be prepared and readily available in all areas where spills are likely to occur. A portable "biohazard spill cart" should also be available for use in areas remote from the laboratory.

WASTE DISPOSAL

NCCLS Document GP5-A[5] divides concerns over medical waste into two categories: health problems and environmental problems. As a health problem, infectious waste is primarily an occupational hazard for healthcare workers and waste haulers.

Infectious waste can be defined as waste capable of producing infectious disease. This involves four necessary factors:

- Presence of pathogens capable of producing disease
- Pathogens of sufficient virulence to produce disease
- Portal of entry
- A susceptible host

Categories of infectious waste include cultures and stocks of infectious agents and associated biologics, pathologic waste, human blood and blood products, contaminated sharps, contaminated animal waste, and isolation wastes.

When handling infectious waste or any other potentially hazardous waste, gloves and protective clothing must be worn. Infectious waste should first be segregated from the general waste stream, then separated into categories to allow for the safest, most efficient, and most economic treatment or disposal options. Once separated, the infectious waste may be further segregated by treatment method. The disposal of sharps requires special attention. These materials should be placed in a prominently labeled, leak-resistant, puncture-resistant container with a molded seam.

All containers used for the collection of infectious waste should be labeled with the "biohazard" symbol. The red (formerly orange) plastic bags used in disposal operations have been generally recognized as containing untreated infectious waste. After collection, the waste must be treated before disposal. The treatment is designed to reduce or eliminate the potential for causing disease. Steam sterilization and incineration (also considered as disposal options) are the most frequently used methods of treatment. Other treatment methods include gas-vapor sterilization, chemical disinfection, sterilization by ionizing radiation, and pulverization combined with chemical disinfection.

After treatment but before disposal, waste should be stored for as brief a time as possible. Temporary storage areas must be properly identified with the biohazard symbol, have restricted access, and be located near the site of generation.

TABLE 1-1
Protection of Laboratory Workers from Infectious Disease Transmitted by Blood, Body Fluids, and Tissue: Summary of Recommendations (NCCLS Document M29-T2)

Universal Precautions
1. Barrier protection at all times.
2. Gloves for blood and body fluids. Gloves in volunteer donor sites optional.
3. Plebotomist wears gloves:
   • With uncooperative patient.
   • With nonintact skin.
   • When performing skin puncture.
   • When in training.
4. Change gloves between patients.
5. Facial protection from splashing.
6. Gown and apron for splashes.
7. Wash hands if contaminated.
8. Wash hands after removing gloves.
9. Avoid accidental injuries.
10. Rigid needle containers.
11. Don't handle needles.
12. Reprocess sharps carefully.
13. No mouth-to-mouth resuscitation contact.
14. Minimize spills and spatters.
15. Decontaminate all surfaces and devices after use.

Protection Techniques
1. Wash hands after contamination, removing gloves, and work.
2. Wear gloves; change after contamination.
3. Full face shield, or goggles and mask for spatter.
4. Occlusive bandages as needed.
5. Wear gown/lab coat always; apron as needed.
6. Use personal respirator if risk of aerosolized M. *tuberculosis* is present.

Decontamination of Spills
1. Tuberculocidal hospital disinfectant.
   • Wear gloves and gown.
   • Absorb spill.
   • Clean with detergent.
   • 1:10 dilution bleach.
   • Wash with water.
   • Biohazard disposal.

Laboratory Procedures
1. Biosafety level 2.
2. No warning labels.
3. Reduce needles/syringes.
4. No mouth pipetting.
5. Leakproof primary and secondary containers.
6. Use centrifuge safety cups.
7. Use biohazard disposal techniques.
   • Infectious waste in "Red Bag."
   • "Red Bag" in rigid container.
   • Sharps in rigid container.
   • Proper storage, transport, and disposal of waste.
8. Service personnel follow universal precautions.
9. "One handed" technique with evacuated tube adapters.

Accidents
HBV— HB vaccine + HBIG if high risk source.
HIV — In clinical setting:
   Voluntary HIV antibody test from source and worker.
   — In laboratory setting:
   Test source specimen and worker.

Consider AZT prophylaxis within 1 hour of exposure. 200 mg every 6 hours. Follow-up 1.5, 3, and 6 mos.

The Autopsy
1. May modify universal precautions.
2. Circulator recommended.
3. Barrier protection:
   • Head-to-toe fluid resistant garb and apron.
   • Double gloves/heavy-duty gloves/ stainless steel mesh gloves.
4. Procedures:
   • Modified Rokitansky or Virchow evisceration.
   • Confine all contaminated materials to autopsy table or photo-stand.
   • One scalpel blade at table.
   • One prosector.
   • Fix all tissues at table.
   • No frozen sections.
   • Decontaminate completely.

Surgical Specimens
1. Follow universal precautions.
2. Use gloves for frozen sections.

Regulatory Compliance
   • Administrative—Develop SOPs.
   • Training and education.
   • Engineering controls.
   • Safe work practices.
   • Personal protective equipment.
   • Medical—HB vaccine.
   • Recordkeeping.

HBV, hepatitis B virus; HBIG, hepatitis B immune globulin; HIV, human immunodeficiency virus; AZT, azidothymidine; SOPs, standard operating procedures.

(*Protection of laboratory workers from infectious disease transmitted by blood, body fluids, and tissues; tentative guideline*—second edition. NCCLS Document M29-T2. National Committee for Clinical Laboratory Standards [NCCLS], Villanova, PA: 1991.) Permission to reproduce this Summary from M29-T2 has been granted by NCCLS. This Summary highlights recommendations described in detail in M29-T2. Users of this summary should have M29-T2 available, and should be familiar with the recommendations it contains. If you do not have this guideline, the current M29 edition may be obtained from NCCLS, 940 West Valley Road, Suite 1400, Wayne, PA 19087, USA.

Chemical Safety

MATERIAL SAFETY DATA SHEETS

OSHA expanded the Federal Hazard Communication Standard (HCS; 29CFR 1919.1200) in August of 1987 to apply to all industries, including healthcare facilities. Also known as the Employees' Right to Know Rule, this regulation states that employees have the "right to know" about all chemical hazards they may work with; it was implemented to reduce the incidence of chemically related work illnesses.[8] The rule mandates that employers identify hazardous chemicals that may be present, provide MSDSs for their employees, ensure that containers are labeled properly, maintain a chemical inventory and hazardous chemical list, provide a program for employee training and information, and develop a written hazard communication program. Under this standard, manufacturers are also required to provide an MSDS for any chemical they manufacture. The MSDSs must be available to employees at all times and must include the following information: identification of the material, hazardous ingredients and identity information, physical and chemical characteristics, fire and explosion hazard data, reactivity data, health hazard data, precautions for safe handling and use, and control measures. It is the responsibility of the employee to read the MSDSs for all products and follow the appropriate precautions in handling and disposal.

CHEMICAL HYGIENE PLAN

Another OSHA regulation (29CFR 1910.1450), which became effective May 1, 1990,[4,6] addresses the occupational exposure to hazardous chemicals in laboratories. It requires laboratories to have a written chemical hygiene plan (CHP) as of January 31, 1991. The rule includes clinical and research laboratories in hospitals as well as private clinical laboratories. The written CHP must include designation of a chemical hygiene officer or committee, criteria for and methods of monitoring chemical exposure, standard operating procedures for handling hazardous chemicals, criteria for implementing engineering controls such as fume hoods, regulations for use of personal protective equipment and other hygiene practices, special precautions for extremely hazardous chemicals, specific measures to ensure that fume hoods and other protective equipment are properly working, provisions for employee information and training, provisions for medical consultation and examination, and designation of a chemical hygiene officer responsible for implementation of the CHP. This regulation basically directs laboratory employers to comply with existing OSHA exposure limits and right-to-know requirements, and to provide medical surveillance programs.

CATEGORIES OF CHEMICALS

The hazard categories of chemicals[6] include corrosives (acids and bases); toxic substances (poisons, irritants, asphyxiants); carcinogens, mutagens and teratogens (causing chromosomal aberrations or congenital malformations); ignitable (flammables and combustibles); and reactive (explosives, oxidizers). Many chemicals are classified as "incompatible" because contact with certain other chemicals may result in a fire or explosion, or in the formation of substances that are toxic, flammable, or explosive.[9] This is especially important to remember when transporting, using, storing, or dispensing such chemicals. Proper storage of chemicals is essential in the prevention as well as the control of laboratory fires and accidents.

HANDLING AND LABELING

Workers should wear personal protective equipment when handling chemicals. Chances of severe injury when handling chemicals can be minimized by using a laboratory coat or rubber apron, eye protection, and gloves. Toxic volatile liquids should be handled using a fume hood or appropriate respirator. Primary and secondary containers of chemicals must be labeled with the name of the chemical and any hazards, as appropriate.

STORAGE

Chemicals should be stored in an area that is properly ventilated and not close to a heat source. Inorganic chemicals generally should be stored separately from organics. Nitric acid should be isolated from the other acids. Flammable liquids should be stored in an appropriate safety cabinet designed to keep fire away from such chemicals. Toxic chemicals should be in clearly marked containers and stored separately from acids and oxidizing agents. A separate, locked cabinet for toxic chemicals can be used to provide greater safety.

DECONTAMINATION OF CHEMICAL SPILLS

The laboratory needs to develop a written plan for containing and cleaning up chemical spills. The MSDSs may be consulted for information on personal protective equipment and spill cleanup procedures. Commercially available spill control kits containing neutralizing and absorbing materials are available. When a chemical is spilled on the skin, the worker should follow recommendations described in the appropriate MSDS. These may include prompt removal of contaminated clothing; flushing the body area with water using a faucet, eye wash, or safety shower; cleansing the affected area with soap and water; and obtaining prompt medical attention.

WASTE DISPOSAL

Disposal of chemicals is closely controlled by state and local laws as well as by specific EPA regulations. In some cases, it is permissible to flush water-soluble substances down the drain with copious quantities of water.[9] However, strong acids or bases should be neutralized before disposal. The possible reaction of chemicals in the drain and potential toxicity must be considered when deciding if a particular chemical can be dissolved or diluted and then flushed into the sanitary sewer. Sodium azide, a common preservative in reagents used in the clinical laboratory, forms explosive salts with metals such as the copper in pipes. Other wastes, including flammable solvents, must be collected in approved containers and segregated into compatible classes for disposal. Many laboratory chemicals need to be disposed of by an EPA-licensed chemical hauler or disposal company.

Fire Safety

CLASSES OF FIRE

Fires can been divided into four classes based on the nature of the combustible material and the substance needed to extinguish the flames:

- Class A: ordinary combustible solid materials such as paper, wood, plastic, and fabric
- Class B: flammable liquids and gases, and combustible petroleum products
- Class C: energized electrical equipment
- Class D: combustible or reactive metals such as magnesium, sodium, and potassium

Extinguishers are also divided into classes corresponding to the type of fire to be extinguished. Using the wrong type of extinguisher may be dangerous. For example, water should not be used for burning liquids or fires involving electrical equipment.

CAUSES AND PREVENTION

Laboratory fires are most commonly caused by carelessness, lack of knowledge about chemicals being used, unattended operations, circuit overload, and open flames. Most institutions have periodic safety in-service education classes to remind employees about safe work practices to prevent fires and other accidents.

Laboratory workers should memorize the location and type of portable fire extinguisher provided in each area of the workplace and should know how to use the equipment before a fire occurs. In the event of a fire, the first thing to do is evacuate all personnel, patients, and visitors who are in immediate danger. Next, the fire alarm should be activated and the fire reported; then an attempt to extinguish the fire safely can be made. If several people are available, they can work as a team to carry out emergency procedures.

Electrical Safety

Electricity can be a direct hazard and cause shock or burns, or it can be an indirect hazard and result in fire or explosion. To minimize these hazards, follow several precautionary procedures when operating or working around electrical equipment:

- Use only explosion-proof equipment in hazardous atmospheres.
- Be particularly careful when operating high-voltage equipment, such as electrophoresis apparatus.
- Use only properly grounded equipment (three-prong plug), and be sure the ground connection on the wall receptacle is really a ground.
- Check for "frayed" electrical cords.
- Promptly report for repair any malfunctioning equipment or equipment producing a "tingle" due to a short circuit.
- Do not work on "live" electrical equipment.
- Never operate electrical equipment with wet hands.
- Know the exact location of the electrical control panel for your work area.
- Use only approved extension cords, and do not overload circuits.
- Have periodic preventive maintenance performed on equipment.

As part of the preventive maintenance program on laboratory instruments, annual electrical safety checks should be conducted and documented.[4] Grounding and polarity checks should be conducted on all electrical outlets at least annually, and the results of these tests should be documented. Portable equipment should be grounded or otherwise arranged with an approved method to protect against shock. The only exceptions to this rule are items strictly encased in plastic so that grounding is impossible. New equipment brought into service should also undergo electrical safety checks. Power cords should be inspected annually for integrity.

In general, no electrical repairs should be attempted on any instrument while it is plugged in.[4] An exception to this is the calibration of instruments that require adjustment in an operational phase. In this case, be sure that hands are dry, remove all jewelry (bracelets, watches, and rings), and proceed with caution. Electrical equipment must be grounded or must be double insulated. Flexible cable, electrical outlets, and plugs must be free from damage. Ground fault circuit interrupters must be installed in wet locations.

Radiation Safety

ENVIRONMENTAL PROTECTION

Environmental and personnel protection should be part of any radiation safety policy. The areas where radioactive materials are used or stored must be posted with caution signs, and traffic in the areas should be restricted to essential personnel only. The standard radiation hazard symbol is shown in Figure 1-1. Regular and systematic monitoring is essential, and decontamination of laboratory equipment, glassware, and work areas must be scheduled as part of routine procedures.

PERSONAL PROTECTION

Only properly trained personnel should work with radioisotopes. Users must be monitored to ensure that the maximally permissible dose of radiation is not exceeded. Good work practices dictate the laboratory maxims of no eating, drinking, smoking, or mouth pipetting when working in the laboratory.

Each person involved in radiation procedures must take the responsibility to minimize his or her own exposure. This is done by keeping as much distance and lead shielding between the radioactive source and operator as possible, and by minimizing the time spent in the vicinity of the radioactive material. General rules to follow when working with radiation are:

- Wear gloves when handling radioactive material, and thoroughly wash hands with soap and water after removing the gloves.
- Work in a contained area lined with absorbent paper to pick up possible spills and to facilitate cleanup.
- Report accidental inhalation, ingestion, or spills immediately.
- Use a sharps container stored in a lead housing to dispose of syringes, needles, and vials contaminated with radioactive materials.

MONITORING RADIATION EXPOSURE

Because radiation cannot be seen and affects none of the senses, film badges are the special means used to record the exposure received by an individual. Each badge contains two pieces of film sensitive to different amounts of radiation. The exposed films document the wearer's exposure to radiation and are examined on a regular basis, and complete records are kept. The estimation of radiation exposure made from the film badge will be correct only if the following rules regarding the wearing of the badge are observed:

- Wear badge on hip or chest at all times while on duty.
- Leave the film badge in a safe place in your work area when not on duty. Do not take it out of the facility.
- Never wear a film badge issued to another person.
- Take care not to send a film badge to the laundry with a uniform or linen.
- The film badge issued to you is your responsibility. Exchange at the proper time for a new one with the same number.
- Report the loss of your badge immediately to your supervisor.
- Report any other incident relative to the wearing of the film badge (such as possible accidental exposure when badge is not worn) to your supervisor.

DECONTAMINATION OF RADIOACTIVE SPILLS

A spill involving radiation must be taken seriously. Even though the amount of radiation present in the clinical laboratory setting is usually minimal, a spill can be dangerous. All people in the vicinity and the supervisor should be notified immediately if a spill occurs. All traffic should be diverted from the spill area and this procedure followed:

- To prevent the spread of the spill, cover it with absorbent paper or gauze.
- Use disposable gloves and tongs to handle contaminated items. Clean with a radioactive decontamination agent from the outer edge to the center of the spill. Carefully fold the absorbent paper and insert into a plastic bag.
- Insert gloves and all other contaminated materials into the plastic bag, seal, label and dispose of properly.
- Wash hands thoroughly with copious amounts of soap and cool water.
- With a radiation survey meter, check the area around the spill, hands, and clothing for contamination.

● If the spill involves skin contact, soap and water should be used for cleansing and care taken to avoid abrading the skin or getting material into open wounds or onto mucous membranes. The area of contact should be monitored for radioactivity after cleansing.

GENERAL INFORMATION

The biologic effect of all types of ionizing radiation is damage to the DNA in the cell nucleus.[6] This damage can lead to mutation, cancer, or cell death. The clinical diagnostic laboratory does not usually use radioisotopes in concentrations high enough to cause immediate cell damage, but exposure should always be controlled because the effects of exposure may be cumulative.

HANDLING

Many institutions have a radiation safety officer and a committee with representation from all the departments that use radioisotopes in the facility (radiology, nuclear medicine, clinical laboratory). Written procedures for receiving shipments and using, storing, and disposing of the material should be available. Written procedures for spill cleanup and monitoring protocols should also be on hand.

Procedures using radioisotopes should be performed in a separate room, with the door labeled "Radioactive Material—Authorized Personnel Only." Waste containers should also be clearly labeled. Areas in which radioisotopes are used should be monitored periodically with a survey meter and a series of wipe tests. A record of all survey results must be kept, as well as a record of corrective actions carried out.

Most clinical *in vitro* radioimmunoassay (RIA) kits use ^{125}I as the tracer. Ingested ^{125}I may be concentrated in the thyroid gland and cause damage to that organ. *When working with radioisotopes, it is therefore particularly important to observe the rule for no eating, drinking, or smoking in the laboratory workplace.*

WASTE DISPOSAL

A clinical laboratory must have a general license issued by the Nuclear Regulatory Commission for the use of RIA kits, even when exempt material is used.[6] Under these guidelines, effluents from RIA *in vitro* tests may be flushed into the sanitary sewer with large amounts of water. However, local and state regulations regarding disposal of radioisotopes must also be fol-

lowed. The sink used for disposal of radioisotopes should be clearly labeled and routinely monitored with a wipe test for residual radioactivity. The laboratory's NRC license should be consulted for guidelines as to disposal of materials such as tubes and pipettes that have been used in radioisotope work.

Other Hazards

COMPRESSED GASES

Compressed gases serve a number of functions in the laboratory and present a unique combination of hazards: fire, explosion, asphyxiation, or mechanical injuries.[9] Safety considerations include:

● Secure cylinders in a vertical position at all times.
● The proper regulator for each type of gas should be used.
● Keep removable protection caps in place until the cylinder is in use.
● Use a hand truck to transport large tanks.
● Make certain that the cylinder is properly labeled to identify the contents.
● Empty cylinders should be marked "empty."

CRYOGENIC MATERIALS

Liquid nitrogen is a widely used cryogenic fluid in the laboratory. Hazards associated with such materials include fire or explosion, asphyxiation, pressure buildup, embrittlement of materials, and tissue damage similar to that of thermal burns.

Special containers designed to withstand ultralow temperatures must be used for cryogenic work. Personal protection includes eye safety glasses and impermeable, loosely fitting gloves that can be quickly removed if the liquid is spilled on them. Specimens to be frozen should be slowly immersed into the coolant to avoid violent boiling, frothing, and splashing. Storage containers should be well insulated to minimize loss of fluid by evaporation, but they should be loosely stoppered to prevent "plugging" and pressure buildup.

MECHANICAL HAZARDS

Centrifuges, autoclaves, and homogenizers are mechanical hazards in the laboratory. Before operating a centrifuge, opposing weights must be balanced so that the loads placed on the rotor are distributed equally. The lid should never be opened while the rotor is moving, nor should a moving rotor be stopped by hand.

REFERENCES

1. Batalden PB, Stoltz PK. A framework for the continual improvement of health care: Building and applying professional and improvement knowledge to test changes in daily work. *Journal on Quality Improvement* 1995;19:424–445.
2. *Clinical laboratory safety; Tentative guideline.* NCCLS Document GP17-T. Villanova, PA: National Committee for Clinical Laboratory Standards (NCCLS), 1994.
3. *Clinical laboratory waste management: Approved guideline.* NCCLS Document GP5-A. Villanova, PA: National Committee for Clinical Laboratory Standards (NCCLS), 1993.
4. Conner SW. Laboratory safety. In: Anderson SC, Cockayne S, eds. *Clinical chemistry: Concepts and applications.* Philadelphia: WB Saunders, 1993.
5. Howanitz PJ, Howanitz JH. *Laboratory quality assurance.* New York: McGraw-Hill, 1987.
6. Luebbert PP. *Laboratory safety and infection control.* Chicago: ASCP Press, 1990.
7. Michael BS, Cavender KD. Laboratory safety. In: Bishop ML, Duben-Engelkirk JL, and Fody EP, eds. *Clinical chemistry.* Philadelphia: JB Lippincott, 1992.
8. *Protection of laboratory workers from infectious disease transmitted by blood, body fluids, and tissue: Tentative guideline—second edition.* NCCLS Document M29-T2. Villanova, PA: National Committee for Clinical Laboratory Standards (NCCLS), 1991.
9. Stewart CE, Koepke JA. *Basic quality assurance practices for clinical laboratories.* Philadelphia: JB Lippincott, 1987.
10. Westgard JO, Klee GG. Quality management. In: Burtis CA, Ashwood ER, eds. *Tietz textbook of clinical chemistry.* 2nd ed. Philadelphia: WB Saunders, 1994.
11. Yablonsky MA. Total quality management in the laboratory. *Laboratory Medicine* 1995;26:253–260.

BIBLIOGRAPHY

Bakes-Martin RC. Quality assurance. In: Anderson SC, Cockayne S, eds. *Clinical chemistry: Concepts and applications.* Philadelphia: WB Saunders, 1993.

Brunzel NA. *Fundamentals of urine and body fluid analysis.* Philadelphia: WB Saunders, 1994.

Ringsrud KM, Linné JJ. *Urinalysis and body fluids: A color text and atlas.* St. Louis: Mosby–Year Book, 1995.

Rose SL. *Clinical laboratory safety.* Philadelphia: JB Lippincott, 1984.

Routine urinalysis and collection, transportation, and preservation of urine specimens: Tentative guideline. NCCLS Document GP16-T. Villanova, PA: National Committee for Clinical Laboratory Standards (NCCLS), 1992.

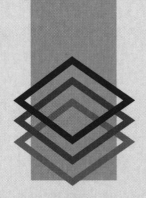

2

Introduction to Urinalysis and Body Fluids

Body Fluids: General Concepts

Body Fluids and Fluid Compartments

Cells are the simplest living entities that still retain all of the functions that characterize life. Even though the body is composed of many different cell types, the basic life processes of these cells are very similar—exchanging materials with their immediate environment, obtaining energy from organic nutrients, synthesizing complex molecules, and reproducing themselves. Most of the cells of a complex multicellular organism are isolated from the surrounding external environment. The life processes of these cells take place in an aqueous, internal environment—the body fluids. Living cells require that the volume and content of these fluids be precisely regulated within a narrow physiologic range.

Body fluids are largely water. This body water contains certain dissolved substances or solutes characteristic for each body fluid.

Body fluids are contained in two major "compartments." The intracellular compartment contains the intracellular fluid found collectively within the body's trillions of cells. The extracellular compartment consists of the extracellular fluid, which includes all the rest of the body fluids: interstitial fluid, the fluid occurring outside body cells and between parts or in the interspaces of tissue; plasma, the fluid portion of the blood; lymph, the fluid derived from interstitial fluid and carried in the lymph vessels; cerebrospinal fluid, the fluid that fills spaces within and around the central nervous system; gastrointestinal tract fluids; synovial fluid, the fluid found in the joint cavities, bursae, and tendon sheaths; the fluids of the eyes and ears; pleural, pericardial, and peritoneal fluids, fluids of the "potential spaces" formed by the pleurae, pericardium, and peritoneum; and the glomerular filtrate, which becomes urine.

Water and solutes are in a constant flux from one body fluid compartment to another. In homeostasis, the volume of fluid in each compartment remains stable. Cell membranes constitute the primary barrier to the movement of substances between the extracellular and intracellular compartments. The ability of a substance to cross cell membranes depends on its solubility in the membrane or its ability to pass through special openings or channels in the cell membrane. Body water moves between the intracellular and extracellular compartments by means of osmosis, which means that the main determinant for fluid balance is the concentration of solutes in the fluids. Because most of the solutes in body fluids are electrolytes, fluid balance is firmly linked with electrolyte balance.

Water

The largest single constituent of the body is water, with a range of from 45% to 75% of the total body weight. The percentage mainly depends on two parameters—an individual's age, and the amount of fatty tissue present in the body. An infant has the highest content of water as percentage of the total body weight (as high as 75%). The proportion of water progressively decreases from birth to old age, with most of the decrease occurring in the first 10 years of life.

Because fat is basically water-free, individuals with a greater amount of lean body mass have a greater proportion of water to total body weight than do those with more fatty tissue (where the percentage of water in the body may be as low as 45%). Women characteristically have more subcutaneous fat than men, so that water averages about 55% of body weight in women in contrast to about 65% in men.

INTAKE AND OUTPUT

The main source of body water is the alimentary canal, from ingested liquids (e.g., 1600 mL) and from water in foods (700 mL), for a total of approximately 2300 mL water daily. Metabolic water is produced by oxidative metabolism of foodstuffs and adds another 200 mL/day to the body. The average total water input is therefore approximately 2500 mL/day.

Water is eliminated from the body in several ways. Water loss through the kidneys averages about 1500 mL/day; from the skin, about 500 mL/day; from the lungs, about 300 mL/day; and from the gastrointestinal tract, about 200 mL/day. Thus, the total average water output from the body is about 2500 mL/day. Normally, the body maintains a constant volume of water because water intake is balanced by water output.

REGULATION OF WATER INTAKE

When water loss exceeds water intake, the resulting dehydration stimulates the sensation of thirst. Locally, dehydration creates dryness of the mouth and pharynx, and the brain interprets this as a sensation of thirst. Dehydration also increases the osmotic pressure of the blood, which stimulates the thirst center of the hypothalamus, again resulting in the sensation of thirst. In response to the thirst stimulus, the individual consumes water (or fluids containing a large proportion of water) and the water loss is balanced.

REGULATION OF WATER OUTPUT

Under the influence of antidiuretic hormone (ADH) and the renin–angiotensin–aldosterone system, the kidneys normally regulate water loss through adjustments in the volume of urine produced. Under abnormal circumstances, other factors may also significantly affect water output. For example, if the body is dehydrated, the blood pressure falls so that the glomerular filtration rate decreases and less filtrate is formed. In the opposite case, excessive body water produces an elevated blood pressure, an increased glomerular filtration rate, and an increased water output. Hypertension leads to increased water loss (increased glomerular filtration rate), and hyperventilation has a similar effect (through increased loss of water vapor through the lungs). Vomiting and diarrhea both may result in a massive loss of water from the gastrointestinal tract.

Solutes

Figure 2-1 shows the principal chemical constituents of the three major fluid compartments (i.e., plasma, interstitial fluid, and intracellular fluid). A comparison of plasma and interstitial fluid shows that plasma contains significantly more protein anions than does inter-

stitial fluid. Because capillary membranes are normally almost impermeable to protein, the protein remains in the plasma and does not leave the circulatory volume or enter the interstitial fluid. The two fluids are similar in most other respects, except that plasma contains more sodium ions but fewer chloride ions compared with the interstitial fluid.

The intracellular fluid and extracellular fluid are quite different. The major extracellular cation is sodium, and the most abundant anion is chloride. Conversely, for intracellular fluid, potassium is the most abundant cation and phosphate the most abundant anion. The concentration of protein anions in the intracellular fluid is much greater than that in the extracellular fluid.

Movement of Body Fluids Between Plasma and Interstitial Compartments

The movement of water back and forth between the plasma and the interstitial fluid occurs across capillary membranes in response to the combined effects of the hydrostatic pressure of the blood, the hydrostatic pressure of the interstitial fluid, the osmotic pressure of the

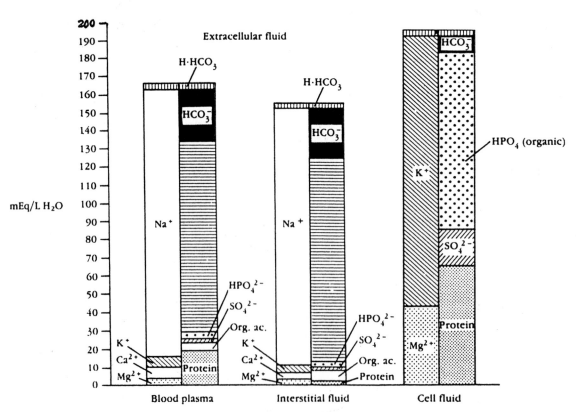

FIGURE 2-1 Electrolyte composition of the body fluid compartments. (From Bullock BL. *Pathophysiology: Adaptations and alterations in function.* 4th ed. Philadelphia: Lippincott–Raven, 1996.)

blood, and the osmotic pressure of the interstitial fluid.

Blood pressure is the hydrostatic pressure within a capillary that tends to force fluid out of the plasma compartment. This hydrostatic pressure in most capillaries is approximately 35 mm Hg at the arterial end and approximately 15 mm Hg at the venous end.

Interstitial fluid hydrostatic pressure tends to push the fluid out of the interstitial compartment into the capillary. It is approximately 2 mm Hg at both the arterial and venous ends of a capillary.

The osmotic pressure of the blood tends to pull water into the plasma (circulatory volume) and averages 25 mm Hg at both ends of a capillary. The protein anions in plasma are mainly responsible for the higher osmotic pressure of blood (also termed colloid osmotic pressure or oncotic pressure).

Interstitial fluid osmotic pressure tends to draw water into the interstitial compartment and is zero at the arterial end of the capillary and approximately 3 mm Hg at the venous end.

The effective filtration pressure (P_{eff}) is the difference between the forces tending to move fluid out of the circulatory volume and those that tend to move fluid in. The P_{eff} determines the direction fluid will move and may be represented as follows:

$$P_{eff} = (\text{blood hydrostatic pressure} + \text{interstitial fluid osmotic pressure}) - (\text{interstitial fluid hydrostatic pressure} + \text{blood osmotic pressure})$$

Using the values given previously, the P_{eff} at the arterial end of a capillary may be calculated:

$$P_{eff} = (35 + 0) - (2 + 25) = 35 - 27 = 8 \text{ mm Hg}$$

This result means that fluid moves into the interstitial fluid from the plasma at the arterial end of a capillary because the sum of the blood hydrostatic pressure and the interstitial fluid osmotic pressure exceeds the sum of the interstitial fluid hydrostatic pressure and the blood osmotic pressure.

The P_{eff} at the venous end of a capillary is:

$$P_{eff} = (15 + 3) - (1 + 25) = 18 - 26 = -8 \text{ mm Hg}$$

In this case, fluid moves from the interstitial compartment back into the plasma because the sum of the interstitial fluid hydrostatic pressure and blood osmotic pressure exceeds the sum of the blood hydrostatic pressure and the interstitial fluid osmotic pressure.

This movement of water between plasma and interstitial fluid across the membranes of capillaries is referred to as Starling's law of the capillaries. Although the calculation indicates that the amount of fluid leaving the plasma at the arterial end of a capillary equals the amount returned to the plasma at the venous end, in actuality, the amount of fluid returned to the plasma is slightly less than the amount leaving the circulatory volume to enter the interstitial space. This slight excess of leftover fluid does return to the plasma but through the lymphatic system by way of the thoracic duct. Thus, under normal conditions, a balance exists between the plasma and the interstitial fluid.

Sometimes the balance between the interstitial fluid and the plasma is upset. One example of fluid imbalance is edema, the abnormal increase in interstitial fluid that results in swelling of the tissues. Another cause of edema is hypertension, which raises the hydrostatic pressure of the blood. Yet another cause of edema is inflammation, in which the capillaries become more permeable and allow proteins to leave the plasma and enter the interstitial fluid. As a result, the osmotic pressure of the blood decreases while the osmotic pressure of the interstitial fluid increases and draws water out of the circulatory volume.

Movement of Body Fluids Between Interstitial and Intracellular Compartments

The movement of water between the interstitial fluid and the intracellular fluid is a result of the same forces that exist between the plasma and the interstitial fluid. Intracellular fluid has a higher osmotic pressure than interstitial fluid; in addition, the principal cation inside the cell is potassium, in contrast to sodium, which is the principal cation outside the cell. In the normal situation, forces that move water out of the cell balance the higher intracellular osmotic pressure so the water balance inside the cell remains normal. Changes in the concentration of sodium or potassium usually are the cause of a fluid imbalance between the two compartments.

Aldosterone and ADH normally control the sodium balance in the body. Aldosterone regulates extracellular fluid volume by adjusting the amount of sodium reabsorbed by the kidney tubules; this, in turn, affects the amount of water retained in the body. ADH contributes to the regulation of the electrolyte concentration of the extracellular fluid by adjusting the amount of water reabsorbed by the kidney tubules—water that makes its way back into the blood through the renal interstitium to the renal venous system.

Under certain conditions, the sodium concentration in the interstitial fluid of the body may decrease. For instance, sodium is excreted by the skin along with water during sweating, and sodium may also be lost through vomiting or diarrhea. If sodium intake is not adequate, a sodium deficit may be produced. A decreased sodium concentration in the interstitial fluid, in turn, lowers the interstitial fluid osmotic pressure. As a result, water moves from the interstitial fluid into the cells. This effect may be quite serious for two reasons.

In the first instance, an increase in intracellular water concentration—termed *overhydration*—is very disruptive to nerve cell function. This "water intoxication" produces neurologic symptoms such as disoriented behavior, convulsions, and coma, and may result in death. The second effect of overhydration is a loss of interstitial fluid volume, leading to a decrease in the interstitial fluid hydrostatic pressure. As this pressure drops, water moves out of the plasma, reducing the blood volume so that an individual may go into shock.

Urinalysis: History and Importance

An examination of the urine, in one way or another, has been used in the diagnosis and treatment of disease for many centuries. Hieroglyphics inscribed by early peoples on the walls of caves and tombs associate certain types of disease with changes in the urine. Sumerian, Babylonian, and Egyptian physicians were highly skilled in the examination of urine (uroscopy) and used the color, odor, taste, and other attributes of urine in diagnosis. "Honey urine" and "black urine" were familiar to these ancient practitioners, whose descriptions of different urine characteristics were well documented in their writings. During mummification of a body, the Egyptians often left the kidneys in situ because they believed that they were sacred.

One of the earliest known records of a urine test may have been the procedure of pouring urine on the ground to observe whether the specimen attracted ants. Honey urine, which attracted the ants, was known to be excreted by individuals who were often suffering from boils. Untreated diabetics still suffer from boils, but thankfully we no longer need to use ants to test for "honey urine."

Urine was often mentioned in the writings of Hippocrates (c. 460–c. 375 BC) and Galen (c. 129–c. 200). These early Greek physicians were concerned with the physical characteristics of urine in various disease states (observing to see if the urine was clear, cloudy, bloody, yellow, milky, and so forth), and were also interested in how the ingestion of water altered the urine. During the Middle Ages and the Renaissance, uroscopy became an important diagnostic tool. Urine became the subject of several treatises, as the ancient Greek and Roman teachings were compiled and revised.

Perhaps the earliest recognition of proteinuria was made by Theophillus (603–641) when he heated urine and noted that it became cloudy in certain disease states. Alchemical methods were applied to the study of urine by Paracelsus (1493–1541), who invented a special flask for use in the distillation of urine that had graduations on its sides and was in the form of a human body. As the specimen was distilled, various metallic salts (such as copper sulfate) were added. A precipitin line might form at a level in the flask corresponding to a part of the body, such as the umbilicus. Because the precipitin band was in the general midabdominal region, the source of the illness was thus concluded to reside in that area of the body.

During this time and beyond, unfortunately, charlatans and quacks often duped the public and collected huge fees for diagnosing illnesses (and forecasting the future) through uroscopy. These "pisse-prophets" used special bladder-shaped vessels to contain the urine specimen, and provided their "diagnosis" while the unfortunate patient watched in fascination. In 1627, Thomas Bryant published a book ridiculing such quackery, urging that uroscopy be carried out only by university-trained professionals. Although Bryant's treatise is considered the inspiration for passage of the first medical licensure laws in England, "urine gazing" continued for some time before gradually dying out on its own.

In 1827, Richard Bright, MD, working in Guy's Hospital in London, described what later came to be known as "Bright's disease" (probably glomerulonephritis). He began using an examination of the urine (e.g., volume, color, pH, protein, but excluding sediment studies) as part of the routine medical examination of his patients. Dr. Bright conducted autopsies and correlated his observations on diseased kidneys with the patient's clinical picture (e.g., edema, proteinuria). In 1846, another physician, Golding Bird, also working at Guy's Hospital, demonstrated the importance of studying the urinary sediment, and described urinary casts in the urine sediment from patients suffering from Bright's disease. Dr. Bird thus combined chemical tests on urine with an examination of the urine sediment, just as we do today in the modern clinical laboratory.

When properly performed, using modern chemical methods and sophisticated microscopic techniques, urinalysis is an accurate science. The examination of urine provides a wide variety of useful medical information regarding diseases of the urinary tract as well as certain systemic diseases that produce quantitative or qualitative alterations of urine constituents or the excretion of abnormal substances. A properly performed urinalysis provides data and interpretations obtained without pain (usually) or danger, and with only minimal inconvenience to the patient.

The evaluation of urine involves several clinical laboratory disciplines, including chemistry, microbiology, urinalysis, and body fluids, as well as cytology and other specialty sections. Urinalysis may be used for screening, diagnosis, monitoring, or prognosis, and urine specimens may be collected with relative ease in a variety of settings, including the home, workplace, physician's office, emergency room, clinic, and hospital.

The National Committee for Clinical Laboratory Standards[1] has defined routine urinalysis as "the testing of urine with procedures commonly performed in an expeditious, reliable, and cost-effective manner in clinical laboratories." Because it offers an inexpensive way to test large numbers of people for a variety of systemic disease syndromes in addition to diseases of the urinary tract, modern urinalysis is definitely in step with the current trends toward preventive medicine and lower medical costs.

REFERENCE

1. National Committee for Clinical Laboratory Standards. *Urinalysis and collection, transportation, and preservation of urine specimens: Approved guideline.* NCCLS Document GP16-A, Vol. 15, No. 15. Wayne, PA: NCCLS, December, 1995:1.

BIBLIOGRAPHY

Bullock BL, Rosendahl PP. *Pathophysiology: Adaptations and alterations in function.* 3rd ed. Philadelphia: JB Lippincott, 1992.

Free HM, ed. *Modern urine chemistry: Application of urine chemistry and microscopic examination in health and disease.* Elkhart, IN: Ames Division, Miles Laboratories, Inc., 1987.

Haber MH. *A primer of microscopic urinalysis.* 2nd ed. Garden Grove, CA: Hycor Biomedical, Inc., 1991.

Kaplan LA, Pesce AJ. *Clinical chemistry: Theory, analysis, and correlation.* 2nd ed. St. Louis: CV Mosby, 1989.

Porth CM. *Pathophysiology: Concepts of altered health states.* 4th ed. Philadelphia: JB Lippincott, 1994.

Ringsrud KM, Linné JJ. *Urinalysis and body fluids: A color text and atlas.* St. Louis: Mosby–Year Book, 1995.

Ross DL, Neely AE. *Textbook of urinalysis and body fluids.* Norwalk, CT: Appleton-Century-Crofts, 1983.

Strasinger SK. *Urinalysis and body fluids.* 3rd ed. Philadelphia: FA Davis, 1994.

Tortora GJ, Anagnostakos NP. *Principles of anatomy and physiology.* 3rd ed. New York: Harper & Row, 1981.

Vander AJ, Sherman JH, Luciano DS. *Human physiology: The mechanisms of body function.* 6th ed. New York: McGraw-Hill, 1994.

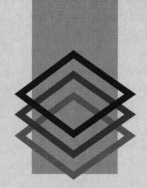

3 Anatomy and Physiology of the Urinary Tract

ABBREVIATIONS USED IN THIS CHAPTER

ADH = antidiuretic hormone	GFR = glomerular filtration rate	PAH = paraaminohippuric acid
DCT = distal convoluted tubule	JGA = juxtaglomerular apparatus	RBF = renal blood flow
ERPF = effective renal plasma flow	MCD = medullary collecting duct	RPF = renal plasma flow
GBM = glomerular basement membrane		

The Urinary System

Two kidneys, two ureters, the urinary bladder, and the urethra make up the urinary system, as illustrated in Figure 3-1. Urine is produced by the kidneys, flows through the ureters to the urinary bladder for storage, and is eliminated through the urethra.

The Kidneys

The two kidneys are protected by the lower ribs, where they lie against the muscles of the back in the upper abdomen in the retroperitoneal space under the dome of the diaphragm. Blood is supplied to each kidney by a renal artery that branches from the abdominal aorta (see Fig. 3-1). In the kidney, the renal artery subdivides into smaller and smaller branches that eventually make contact with the renal corpuscles (Fig. 3-2) Blood leaves the kidney in vessels that finally merge to form the renal vein, which then connects with the inferior vena cava so that blood is returned to the heart.

The Ureters

The ureters are long, slender, muscular tubes extending from the pelvis of the kidney down to the urinary bladder (see Fig. 3-1) and range from 25 to 32 cm in length, depending on the size of the individual. The ureter wall consists of a lining of epithelial cells, a layer of involuntary muscle, and an outer coat of fibrous connective tissue. The lining is continuous with that of the renal pelvis and the bladder. Urine flow through the ureters to the bladder occurs continuously by peristalsis.

The Urinary Bladder

The urinary bladder when empty is located below the parietal peritoneum, behind the pubic joint. When it is full, the bladder pushes the peritoneum upward and may extend into the abdominal cavity. The bladder is a balloon-like chamber with walls of smooth muscle that are capable of extensive stretching. A circular portion of this muscle layer at the neck of the bladder, called the internal sphincter, contracts to keep urine in the bladder. When the bladder is relaxed, the outlet is closed, but when the bladder either actively contracts or is passively distended, the outlet is pulled open by changes in bladder shape. Urine is expelled from the bladder by a process called urination or micturition. Stretch receptors in the bladder send impulses to a center in the lower part of the spinal cord as the bladder fills. Motor impulses are then sent out to the musculature of the bladder, and it is emptied. There is a voluntary external sphincter located below the internal sphincter so that urination can be voluntarily controlled unless the bladder becomes too full.

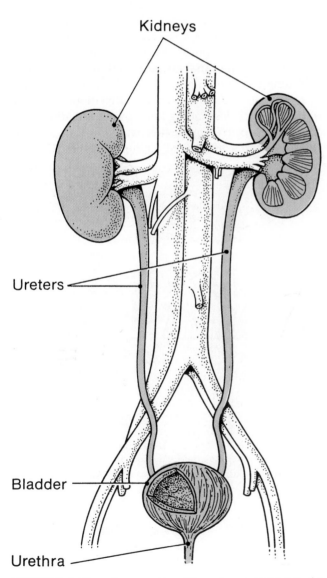

Kidneys

Ureters

Bladder

Urethra

FIGURE 3-1 The urinary system. (From American Society for Clinical Laboratory Science: *Urinalysis, an educational program.* 1979, Bethesda: ASCLS.)

The Urethra

The bladder is emptied by means of the urethra, the tube extending from the bladder to the outside. The male urethra is also part of the reproductive system, and is much longer than the female urethra. The female urethra is a thin-walled tube about 4 cm long located behind the pubic joint and embedded in the muscle of

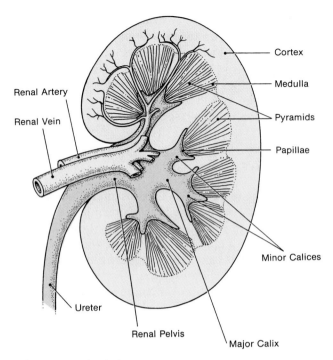

FIGURE 3-2 The kidney in sagittal section. (From American Society for Clinical Laboratory Science. *Urinalysis, an educational program,* 1979. Bethesda: ASCLS.)

the front wall of the vagina. The urethral meatus (the external opening) is located just in front of the vaginal opening between the labia minora. The male urethra, which is about 20 cm long, passes through the prostate gland, where it is joined by the two ducts that carry the sperm, and then proceeds through the penis to the outside.

Renal Anatomy

In the average human adult, the kidney weighs about 150 g, and is a somewhat flattened organ about 12 cm long, 6 cm wide, and 2.5 cm thick.[11] On the concave, inner (medial) border is a notch called the hilum, an area where nerves enter, blood and lymph vessels enter and exit, and the ureter connects with the kidney. As observed in sagittal section (see Fig. 3-2), the kidney is divided into three macroscopic regions: an outer portion, the renal cortex; a darker central portion, the renal medulla; and the renal pelvis, which forms the upper end of the ureter.

As discussed in more detail later, the functional unit of the kidney is the nephron. Each nephron is capable of producing urine. A nephron consists of a dilated portion, the renal corpuscle (glomerulus enclosed in Bowman's capsule); the proximal tubule; the loop of Henle; and the distal convoluted tubule (DCT). The renal corpuscles are all located in the cortex of the kidney along

with the convoluted tubules. The renal medulla is shaped into pyramids consisting mostly of the loops of Henle together with the collecting ducts (or tubules). The apex of each pyramid is formed into a cone-shaped papilla containing a papillary duct that opens into a cavity termed a calyx. The calyces are cuplike extensions of the renal pelvis, and normally there are about 12 minor calyces that unite to form two or three major calyces (see Fig. 3-2). Urine from the papillary ducts enters the calyces and flows onward into the renal pelvis, then into a ureter, and finally into the bladder.

The Nephron

Each kidney contains approximately 1 million nephrons (from the Greek, *nephros*, kidney). A nephron is essentially a renal tubule with its vascular component. As shown in Figure 3-3, several distinct areas can be identified in the nephron, beginning with a dilated or swollen area, the renal corpuscle (Bowman's capsule enclosing a tuft of capillaries—the glomerulus), then proceeding to the proximal convoluted tubule, the loop of Henle (thick descending limb, thin descending limb, the sharp hairpin turn, the thin ascending limb, and the thick ascending limb), and ending with the DCT. The

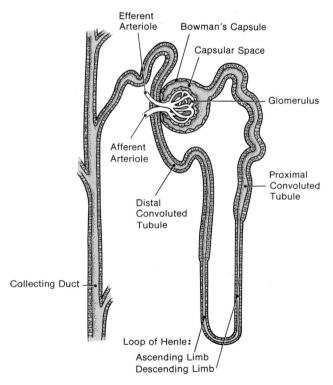

FIGURE 3-3 The nephron. (From American Society for Clinical Laboratory Science. *Urinalysis, an educational program,* 1979. Bethesda: ASCLS.)

individual DCTs connect at some point with a common collecting duct (or tubule), each of which conveys the urine from several nephrons to a papilla.

Although all the renal corpuscles are found in the cortex of the kidney, there are two general types of nephrons, the cortical and the juxtamedullary nephrons. The renal corpuscle of a cortical nephron is found in the outer cortical zone of the kidney; the remainder of the nephron rarely penetrates into the medulla (Fig. 3-4). These outer cortical nephrons have short loops of Henle, and each efferent arteriole branches into a plexus of peritubular capillaries that entirely envelope the tubules (see Fig. 3-4). There are two types of juxtamedullary nephrons—the mid-juxtamedullary and deep juxtamedullary nephrons. These nephrons have long loops of Henle. The efferent arterioles of these nephrons first branch into a peritubular capillary bed that enmeshes the cortical portions of the tubules. They divide then into a series of long, U-shaped vessels, the vasa recta, which descend deep into the renal

medulla alongside the loops of Henle. The ascending vasa recta form the beginnings of the venous renal circulation, emerging from deep in the medulla to form venules that drain into the renal veins. Although all nephrons function in the processes of filtration, absorption, and secretion, these juxtamedullary nephrons are of critical importance in establishing the gradient of hypertonicity in the medullary interstitium, which is the basis for the kidney's ability to produce either a concentrated or a dilute urine, as will be discussed later.

The Renal Corpuscle or Glomerulus

The term "glomerulus" was originally used to designate the tuft of capillaries covered by the visceral layer of Bowman's capsule. The term may also be used in reference to the entire renal corpuscle—that is, Bowman's capsule and the enclosed glomerular tuft of capillar-

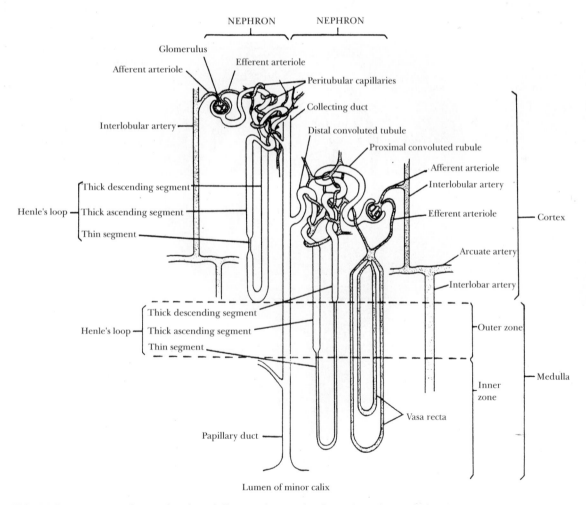

FIGURE 3-4 Structure of cortical and medullary nephrons. Blood supply to the nephron. The vasa recta are shown schematically; this capillary structure normally surrounds Henle's loop. (From Bullock BL, Rosendahl PP. *Pathophysiology*. 3rd ed. Philadelphia: Lippincott–Raven Publishers, 1992.)

ies.[10,19] Functionally, a renal corpuscle is a filtration device, in which a constant fraction of the plasma flowing to the kidney is filtered and delivered to the tubule for processing.

Bowman's capsule, the proximal end of a renal tubule, is a double-walled globe with an inner and an outer layer (see Fig. 3-3). The inner layer (or wall) of the capsule is known as the visceral layer and consists of specialized epithelial cells, called podocytes, which envelop the capillary tuft. The outer or parietal layer of the capsule is separated from the visceral layer by a space called Bowman's space or the urinary space. The parietal layer is composed of simple squamous epithelium supported by a basal lamina and a thin layer of reticular fibers.[8] Each renal corpuscle has a vascular pole, where the afferent and efferent arterioles protrude, and a urinary pole, where the epithelium changes to the simple, columnar epithelium characteristic of the proximal tubule. Inside the renal corpuscle, the afferent arteriole branches into two to five primary

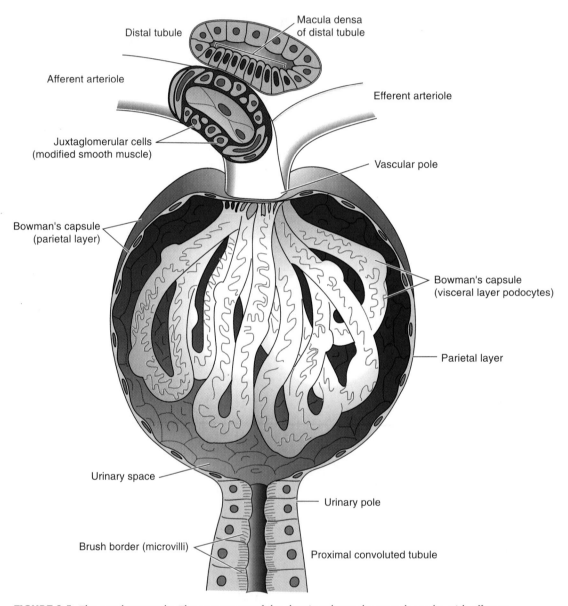

FIGURE 3-5 The renal corpuscle. The upper part of the drawing shows the vascular pole, with afferent and efferent arterioles and the macula densa. Note the juxtaglomerular cells in the wall of the afferent arteriole. Podocyte processes cover the outer surfaces of the glomerular capillaries; the part of the podocyte containing the nucleus protrudes into the urinary space. Note the flattened cells of the parietal layer of Bowman's capsule. The lower part of the drawing shows the urinary pole and the proximal convoluted tubule. (From Junqueira LC, Carneiro J, Kelley RO. *Basic histology*. 7th ed. Norwalk: Appleton & Lange, 1992.)

branches, each subdividing and anastomosing to form the glomerular (or capillary) tuft. These aspects are illustrated in Figure 3-5.

The visceral layer of Bowman's capsule and the endothelium of the capillary tuft form an endothelial–capsular membrane that is the actual glomerular filtration barrier. The three parts of this membrane are the endothelium of the capillary tuft; the epithelium of the visceral layer of Bowman's capsule; and, sandwiched between the two, a distinct trilayer basement membrane, the glomerular basement membrane (GBM).

The first part of the barrier that is crossed by substances filtering from the blood is the capillary endothelium of the glomerular tuft. The cells of this endothelium are fenestrated, that is, they contain large, open pores that are approximately 50 to 100 nm in diameter. Figure 3-6 shows how these pores look when viewed from the lumen of the capillary. On the luminal side, these cells are covered by a negatively charged cell coat that adds to the selectivity of this barrier, as discussed later.

The capillary endothelium rests on the second part of the filtration barrier, the GBM or basal lamina. When studied by transmission electron microscopy with conventional staining, as shown in Figure 3-7, the GBM consists of three layers: the electron-lucent lamina rara interna (facing the capillary endothelium); the central electron-dense lamina densa; and the electron-lucent lamina rara externa. Heparin sulfate, a polyanionic molecule, has been detected in the electron-lucent zones, where it is thought to retard the passage of negatively charged proteins across the GBM. In humans, the GBM is about 200 nm thick and is a gelatinous structure consisting of a cross-linked mesh of polymer chains with hydrated interstices.[10] It contains collagenous and noncollagenous fibrillar proteins together with proteoglycans of the heparin sulfate type.

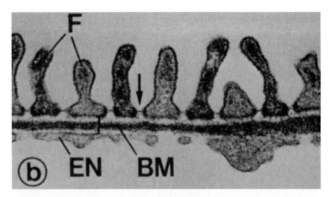

FIGURE 3-7 An electron micrograph of the filtration barrier which is part of the capillary wall. Note the various cell types: endothelium (EN) and epithelium (EP) with foot processes. (F). The glomerular basement membrane (BM) consists of three distinct layers, namely, the lamina rara interna (facing the endothelium), the lamina densa, and the lamina rara externa (facing the epithelium). Note the slit membrane (*arrow*) between the foot processes.

The two lamina rarae contain more of the polar noncollagenous material (the heparin sulfate) and are therefore strongly anionic, whereas the nonpolar collagenous components are concentrated in the lamina densa. The GBM has been referred to as the "dialyzing membrane" of the nephron.[19]

Because it contains no pores, the GBM is a selective macromolecular filter in which the type IV collagen present in the lamina densa acts as a physical filter, and the anionic sites in the laminae rarae act as a charge barrier. Particles greater than 10 nm in diameter do not readily cross the GBM, and negatively charged proteins with molecular weights (MW) greater than that of albumin (MW, 69,000 daltons [da]) pass across only sparingly. In diseases such as diabetes mellitus and glomerulonephritis, the glomerular filter becomes much more permeable to proteins, with the subsequent release of protein into the urine (proteinuria).

The third part of the filtration barrier is the epithelium of the visceral layer of Bowman's capsule. The epithelial cells of this layer are referred to as "podocytes." They have large cell bodies that bulge into the capsular space and many cytoplasmic processes (primary processes) that interdigitate and embrace or clasp the capillaries, thereby covering the entire outer capillary surface. These relationships are illustrated in Figures 3-5 and 3-8. Because of their appearance in cross-section (see Fig. 3-7), the finger-like processes are called "foot processes"—hence the term "podocytes" for the cells.

The foot processes are anchored to the GBM but do not touch each other. They are separated by narrow spaces of a fairly constant width (20–30 nm) that form a zig-zag channel, the so-called "filtration slit" or "slit pore" (see Fig. 3-8). A slit membrane or diaphragm (an extracellular structure about 6 nm thick) forms the

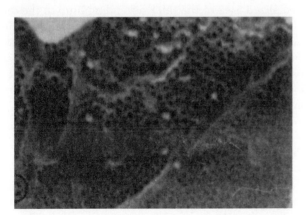

FIGURE 3-6 The surface aspect of the endothelium viewed from the capillary lumen. The fenestrations appear as real pores and are not closed by a diaphragm.

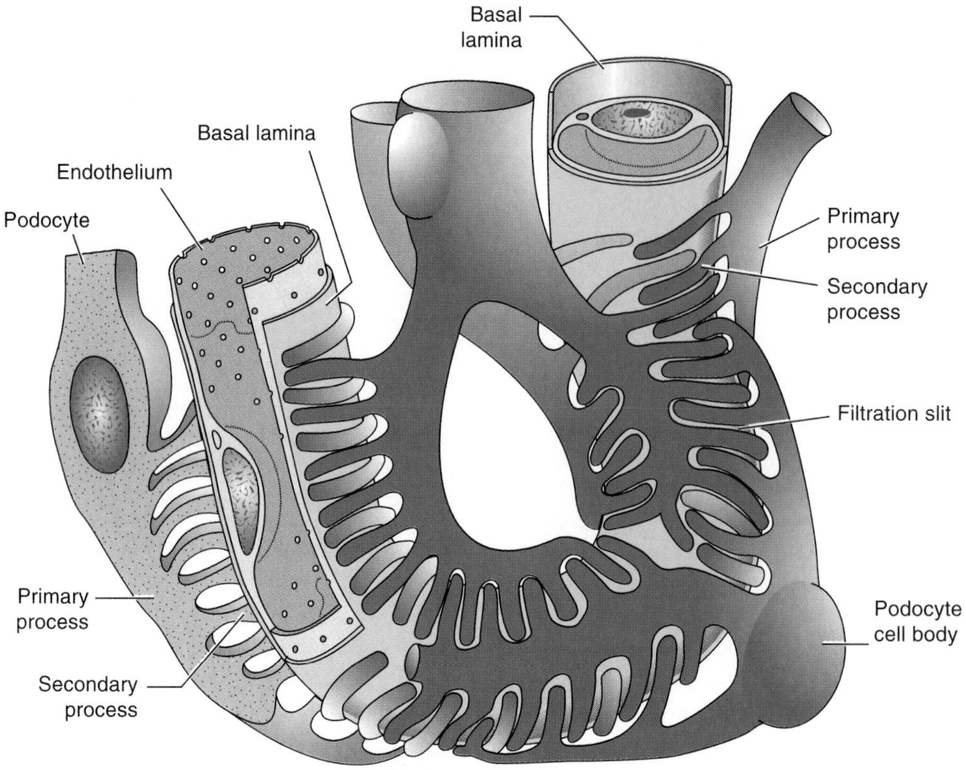

FIGURE 3-8 Schematic representation of a glomerular capillary with the visceral layer of Bowman's capsule (formed by podocytes; shown in color). In this capillary, endothelial cells are fenestrated, but the basal lamina on which they rest is continuous. At left is a podocyte shown in partial section. As viewed from the outside, the part of the podocyte containing the nucleus protrudes into the urinary space. Each podocyte has many primary processes, from which arise an even greater number of secondary processes that are in contact with the basal lamina. (From Ham AW. *Histology*. 6th ed. Philadelphia: Lippincott–Raven Publishers, 1969.)

floor of the filtration slit and rests on the GBM (see Fig. 3-7).

The podocytes are metabolically active cells. They contain numerous organelles and extensive lysosomal elements, features that correlate directly with their phagocytic activities. Macromolecules that are unable to proceed through the slit diaphragm or return to the capillary lumen are rapidly phagocytized by the podocytes to prevent occlusion of the filtration barrier. Like the capillary endothelium, all surfaces of the podocytes, filtration slits, and slit diaphragms that line the urinary space are covered with a thick, negatively charged coating.

The mesangium (Greek, *mesos*, middle, + *angeion*, vessel) is also part of the renal corpuscle and forms a stabilizing core of tissue. The mesangium is located within the anastomosing lobules of the glomerular tuft and is continuous with the extraglomerular mesangium. These features are illustrated in Figure 3-9. The mesangial cells have the capacity for phagocytosis and pinocytosis, so they may also be important in helping to remove entrapped macromolecules from the filtration barrier. As shown in Figure 3-9, there is

no basement membrane between the capillary endothelium and the mesangium.

The juxtaglomerular apparatus (JGA) is located at the vascular pole of Bowman's capsule. It consists of portions of the afferent and efferent arterioles, the extraglomerular mesangium, and the macula densa (a specialized area of the thick ascending limb of the distal tubule). The JGA is the source of the hormone renin, secreted by granular cells (which are differentiated smooth muscle cells) found mainly in the wall of the afferent arteriole (see Fig. 3-9). The renin–angiotensin–aldosterone system is discussed later in the section on renal physiology.

The Tubule

The nephron is said to be the structural and functional unit of the kidney, but depending on one's viewpoint, the term "renal tubule" may or may not include the collecting ducts together with the tubular parts of the nephron.[10] Along the way from Bowman's capsule to the papillary duct, the epithelium lining the renal

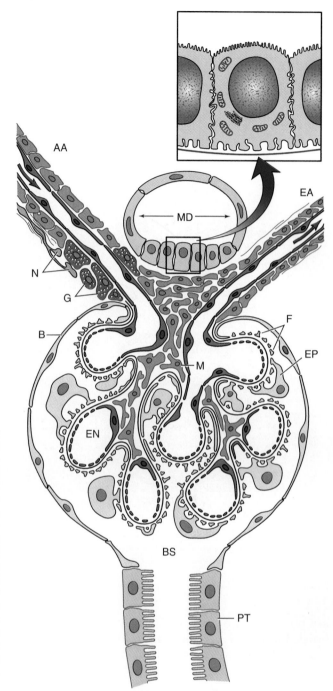

FIGURE 3-9 An overview of a renal corpuscle and JGA. At the vascular pole, an afferent arteriole (AA) enters and an efferent arteriole (EA) leaves the glomerulus. At the urinary pole Bowman's space (BS) becomes the tubular lumen of the proximal tubule. The epithelial cells comprising Bowman's capsule (B) enclose Bowman's space. Smooth muscle cells proper of the arterioles and all cells derived from smooth muscle are shown in black, including the granular cells (G). The afferent arteriole is innervated by sympathetic nerve terminals (N). The extraglomerular mesangial cells are located at the angle between AA and EA, and continue into the mesangial cells (M) of the glomerular tuft. The glomerular capillaries are outlined by fenestrated endothelial cells (EN) and covered from the outside by the epithelial cells (EP) with foot processes (F). The glomerular basement membrane (BM) is continuous throughout the glomerulus. At the vascualr pole, the thick ascending limb touches with the macula densa (MD) the extraglomerular mesangium. The *inset* shown at the top depicts the ultrastructural organization of the macula densa epithelium. (From Koushanpour E, Kriz W. *Renal physiology.* 2nd ed. New York: Springer-Verlag, 1986.)

tubule changes through several distinct areas. One version of this sequence is the proximal convoluted tubule, the loop of Henle, the DCT, and the collecting ducts. These segments are illustrated in Figure 3-10.

PROXIMAL CONVOLUTED TUBULE

As it starts out at the renal pole of Bowman's capsule, the proximal tubule consists of an extensive convoluted portion (the pars convoluta) followed by a straight portion (the pars recta). The tall epithelial cells (see Fig. 3-10) have abundant membrane invaginations and lateral interdigitations with neighboring cells. The Na^+/K^+-adenosine triphosphatase (ATPase) pump responsible for the active transport of sodium ions out of the cells is localized in the basolateral membranes of the cells. Numerous mitochondria are concentrated at the base of the cells arranged in parallel to the cellular long axis, a pattern typical for cells engaged in active transport of solutes. The luminal surfaces of the cells

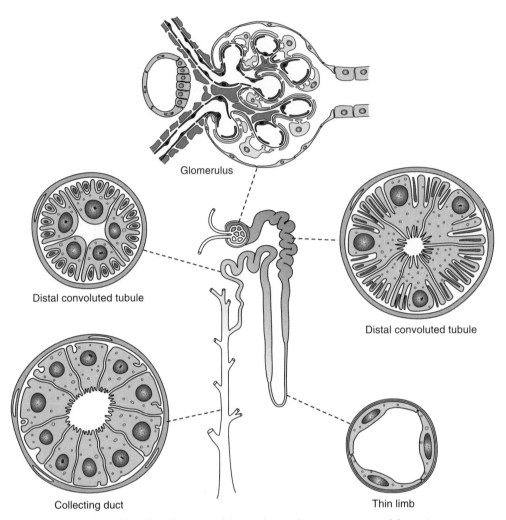

FIGURE 3-10. General histologic features of the nephron. The cross sections of the various segments of the tubule roughly indicate the cellular morphology and the relative size of the cells and tubules at these sites. (From Bennington JL, ed. *Saunders dictionary and encyclopedia of laboratory medicine and technology.* Philadelphia: WB Saunders Company, 1984.)

are provided with microvilli that form an extensive brush border, greatly magnifying the surface area available for filtrate reabsorption.

LOOP OF HENLE

The three types of loops of Henle are cortical, short, and long loops.[8] Cortical loops originate from the most superficially located glomeruli and do not enter the renal medulla. Short loops, reaching down to a position roughly between the inner and outer medulla, originate from superficial and mid-cortical glomeruli. Long loops originate from deep mid-cortical and juxtamedullary glomeruli. In the thin descending limb of the loop of Henle, the epithelium consists of flat, non-interdigitating cells (see Fig. 3-10); then, at the hairpin turn of the loop, the epithelial cells are again interdigi-

tated but remain flat. The cells of the thick ascending limb of the loop of Henle are tall with basolateral membranes extensively enlarged by cellular interdigitation, and large mitochondria are present—features that are characteristic for solute-pumping cells. We touch on this point again later in the discussion of the countercurrent mechanism.

DISTAL CONVOLUTED TUBULE AND COLLECTING DUCTS

The DCT, which begins after the macula densa, is much shorter than the proximal convoluted tubule, and after two or three coils passes over into a short "connecting tubule" and then leads into a collecting duct. The characteristics of the DCT cells and those of the collecting duct are illustrated in Figure 3-10.

Renal Physiology and Formation of Urine

Functions of the Kidney

As the kidneys process blood, some substances are removed from the blood and some substances are added back to the blood.[21] The kidneys regulate the chemical composition of the internal environment of the body by a complex process that involves filtration, active absorption, passive absorption, and active secretion. Table 3-1 summarizes the variety of functions performed by the kidneys. Gluconeogenesis is a relatively new function to be added to the many activities the kidneys carry out. During prolonged fasting, the kidneys synthesize glucose from amino acids and other precursors, releasing it into the blood, just as the liver does at such times.[20]

Nephron Physiology

URINE FORMATION

Figure 3-11 illustrates the three basic renal processes: glomerular filtration, tubular reabsorption, and tubular secretion. Urine formation begins with glomerular filtration, the formation of an ultrafiltrate of blood plasma. The formed elements and most of the proteins are retained in the glomerular capillaries so that the filtrate is essentially protein free and contains all of the crystalloids in the same osmolar concentration as in the aqueous phase of the plasma. Certain low–molecular-weight substances that would other-

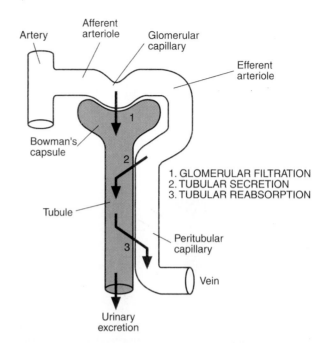

FIGURE 3-11 The three basic renal processes. This figure illustrates only the directions of reabsorption and secretion, not specific sites or order of occurrence. Depending on the specific substance, reabsorption and secretion can occur at various sites along the tubule. (From Vander AJ. *Renal physiology*. New York: McGraw–Hill, Inc., 1995.)

wise be filterable are bound to proteins and therefore are not filtered.

Urine entering the renal pelvis on its way to the ureter is quite different from the glomerular filtrate because as the filtrate flows from Bowman's capsule through the tubule, its composition is altered by tubular reabsorption and secretion. The tubule is closely associated at all points with the peritubular capillary network, permitting the transfer of materials between peritubular fluid and the tubular lumen. When the direction of transfer is from the tubular lumen to the peritubular capillary plasma, the process is termed reabsorption. Transfer of materials from the peritubular capillary plasma to the tubular lumen is called tubular secretion, or simply secretion.

Figure 3-12 shows the renal manipulation of three hypothetical substances: one that is filtered and secreted but not reabsorbed; one that is filtered, and a fraction then reabsorbed; and one that is filtered but is completely reabsorbed. Through the processes of filtration, reabsorption, and secretion, the kidneys play a critical role in the removal of metabolic waste products, the regulation of water and electrolytes, and the maintenance of the acid–base equilibrium in the body. No matter what the body has ingested or produced, the kidneys are the body's "true regulators," controlling which substances are retained and which are excreted.

TABLE 3-1
Functions of the Kidneys

1. Regulation of water and inorganic ion balance
2. Removal of metabolic waste products from the blood and their excretion in the urine
3. Removal of foreign chemicals from the blood and their excretion in the urine
4. Secretion of hormones:
   a. Erythropoietin, which controls erythrocyte production
   b. Renin, which controls formation of angiotensin, which influences blood pressure and sodium balance (this chapter)
   c. 1,25-Dihydroxyvitamin D$_3$, which influences calcium balance
5. Gluconeogenesis

(From Vander AJ, Sherman JH, Luciano DS. *Human physiology*. 6th ed. New York: McGraw–Hill, 1994.)

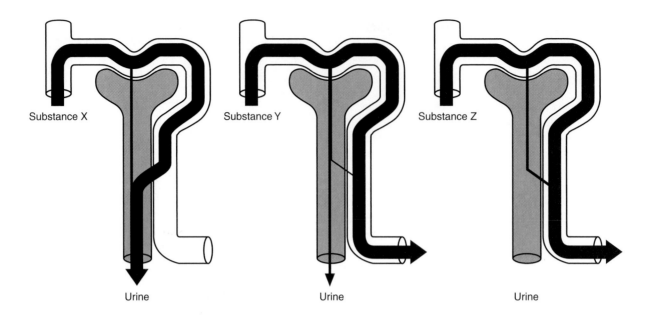

FIGURE 3-12 Renal manipulation of three hypothetical substances, X, Y, and Z. X is filtered and secreted but not reabsorbed. Y is filtered, and a fraction is then reabsorbed. Z is filtered but is completely reabsorbed. (From Vander AJ. *Renal physiology.* New York: McGraw–Hill, Inc., 1995.)

An average daily volume of 180 L of glomerular filtrate is converted by the kidneys to a final urine volume of from 600 to 1800 mL of urine. Urea, chloride, sodium, and potassium are the principal solutes, with lesser amounts of phosphates, sulfates, creatinine, and uric acid. Other substances that were initially present in the ultrafiltrate, such as glucose and amino acids, are almost completely reabsorbed by the tubules and do not normally appear in the urine. If we assume an average normal urine output of 1200 mL/day, which is approximately 1% of the ultrafiltrate volume, then 99% of the initial ultrafiltrate volume is actually reabsorbed.

GLOMERULAR FILTRATION

As discussed earlier in the section on the nephron, the glomerular filtration barrier is composed of the endothelium of the capillary tuft, the GBM, and the filtration slits (with their slit diaphragms) between the foot processes of the podocytes. In addition, the negatively charged coating on the cells on both sides of the ultrafilter is essential for barrier function as well as the strongly anionic character of both lamina rarae of the GBM. The glomerular barrier, compared with the barrier formed by most capillaries, has a unique combination of functional characteristics.[10] It has an extremely high permeability for water and ions but a very low permeability for plasma proteins. The slit diaphragm, which comprises only about 3% of the entire GBM area, appears to be the major hydraulic barrier.

For macromolecules, the barrier function is selective with respect to charge and with respect to size—including configuration.[10] Size selectivity resides in the dense network of the GBM. Compounds that are uncharged or neutral with an "effective radius" of 1.8 nm freely pass through the filter. Effective radius is an empirical value that compares the configuration of molecules and also attributes a "radius" to nonspherical molecules. Larger molecules are increasingly restricted up to an effective radius of 4 nm, where absolute restriction begins. Because plasma albumin has an effective radius of 3.6 nm, it would pass through the filter in considerable amounts were it not for the repulsion due to the negative charge on the cell coats on both sides of the barrier as well as within the GBM itself. Plasma proteins usually carry a net negative charge at the normal pH of arterial blood.

The slit membrane is apparently the final trap for macromolecules that have escaped the rest of the barrier.[10] Trapped molecules are phagocytized by the podocytes, and those trapped proximally to the slit membranes are believed to be taken up by the mesangial cells.

Blood flow to the kidneys is normally about 1200 mL/minute, which corresponds to a plasma flow of about 660 mL/minute, assuming a hematocrit of 0.45. During this same time, a volume of 125 mL of glomerular filtrate is formed. The ratio of the glomerular filtration rate (GFR) to the renal plasma flow (RPF) is the filtration fraction. This is 125/660 = 0.19, which means that 19% of the entering plasma volume is removed as filtrate.

Forces Involved in Filtration

As with filtration across any capillary, glomerular filtration is a process of bulk flow (i.e., all constituents move together).[21] This filtration is determined by opposing forces: the hydrostatic pressure difference across the capillary, which favors filtration, and an opposing osmotic force (oncotic pressure), the protein concentration difference across the wall. This is illustrated in Figure 3-13.

The hydrostatic force favoring filtration is the glomerular capillary blood pressure of 60 mm Hg. Because of the larger diameter of the afferent arteriole of the nephron, this pressure is higher than in other capillaries of the body. The fluid in Bowman's capsule opposes filtration with a hydrostatic pressure of 15 mm Hg, and a second force opposing filtration is the oncotic pressure in the plasma of the glomerular capillary. The net glomerular filtration pressure is approximately 18 mm Hg, which initiates urine formation by forcing an essentially protein-free filtrate of plasma through the ultrafilter into Bowman's space. Once the

ultrafiltrate has reached Bowman's space, hydrostatic pressure alone moves it through the remaining tubular portions of the nephron.[4]

The volume of fluid filtered from the glomerular capillaries into Bowman's capsule per unit time is the GFR. The average volume filtered into Bowman's capsule, for a 70-kg person, is 180 L/day. Forming such a huge volume of filtrate means that the kidneys receive from 20% to 25% of the total cardiac output. If the total plasma volume in the cardiovascular system is assumed to be about 3 L, this means that the entire plasma volume is filtered by the kidneys about 60 times a day.

For any nonprotein substance (and one not bound to protein), the total amount that is filtered into Bowman's capsule can be determined by multiplying the GFR by the plasma concentration of the substance. By comparing the filtered load of the substance to the amount of the substance excreted, it is possible to determine if the substance undergoes net tubular reabsorption or net secretion. Tubular reabsorption is indicated if the quantity of a substance excreted in the urine is less than the filtered load. On the other hand, if the amount excreted in the urine is greater than the filtered load, tubular secretion has occurred.

THE TUBULES AND TUBULAR FUNCTION

Tubular reabsorption and secretion are accomplished by tubular transport mechanisms that are either active or passive. Active transport requires the direct expenditure of energy and moves a substance across cell membranes against a concentration gradient. Passive transport requires no direct expenditure of energy and involves movement along an osmotic gradient (from an area of higher concentration to one of lower concentration), such as for the reabsorption of urea.

Proximal Convoluted Tubule

The processes of reabsorption and excretion begin as the glomerular filtrate formed in the renal corpuscle passes into the proximal convoluted tubule. Although tubular reabsorption takes place throughout the nephron, the proximal convoluted tubule segment actively reabsorbs essentially 100% of the glucose, amino acids, and proteins, along with about 85% of the sodium contained in the filtrate. The glucose, amino acids, and sodium are reabsorbed by an active cotransport mechanism involving the Na^+/K^+-ATPase pump located in the basolateral cell membranes. Other solutes such as bicarbonate, phosphate, sulfate, magnesium, calcium, and uric acid are actively reabsorbed as well. Water diffuses passively, following the osmotic

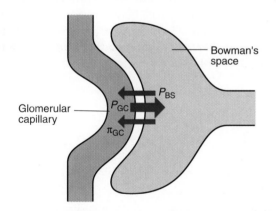

Forces	mmHg
Favoring filtration:	
Glomerular capillary blood pressure (P_{GC})	60
Opposing filtration:	
Fluid pressure in Bowman's space (P_{BS})	15
Osmotic force (due to protein in plasma) (π_{GC})	27
Net glomerular filtration pressure	18

FIGURE 3-13 Forces involved in glomerular filtration. The symbol π denotes an osmotic force due to differences in solute and hence water concentration. The difference in solute concentration is due solely to the presence of protein in plasma but not in Bowman's space, since the filtrate is essentially protein-free plasma. The rate at which fluid is filtered–the glomerular filtration rate–averages 180 L/day. (From Vander AJ, Sherman JH, Luciano DS. *Human physiology*. 6th ed. New York: McGraw-Hill, 1994.)

gradient, and chloride passively follows the electro-chemical gradient. The reabsorption of the small amount of protein that may appear in the filtrate takes place by pinocytosis, followed by lysosomal digestion to release amino acids that can be reused. Even though the fluid volume and the concentrations of specific solutes have been significantly reduced, the osmolality of the proximal tubular filtrate remains the same as that of the original ultrafiltrate.

Tubular secretion, an active process, takes place in the proximal convoluted tubule as well as throughout the nephron, just as does tubular reabsorption. As discussed later in the section on tubular reabsorption and secretion, the renal tubule is able to secrete substances from the interstitial plasma into the tubular filtrate. Substances secreted by the proximal convoluted tubule include those incompletely metabolized by the body (thiamine), as well as foreign substances such as radiopaque contrast media, mannitol, penicillin, and salicylate. In addition, the proximal tubule participates along with the rest of the renal tubule in maintaining a proper acid–base equilibrium in the body, as is discussed later.

Loop of Henle

The loop of Henle is involved in water retention and participates with the vasa recta, by means of an "active" countercurrent multiplier mechanism, to create a gradient of hypertonicity in the medullary interstitium that influences the concentration of the urine as it flows through the collecting ducts. This function is discussed in more detail later, in the section on the countercurrent multiplier system.

Distal Convoluted Tubule

Under the control of aldosterone, sodium is absorbed and potassium is secreted in the DCT. As part of the maintenance of acid–base balance in the body, the distal tubule also secretes hydrogen and ammonium ions into the glomerular filtrate. At the vascular pole of the renal corpuscle of its parent nephron, the DCT is modified to form the macula densa—a component of the juxtaglomerular apparatus. The cells of the macula densa are part of the network regulating the secretion of renin, discussed later under the heading Renin–Angiotensin–Aldosterone System.

The Collecting Ducts

Traversing both the renal cortex and medulla, the collecting ducts are the final site for concentrating the urine or diluting it. The cells of the collecting duct epithelium have intercellular junctions or spaces between them that extend from their luminal surfaces to their bases. Under the influence of antidiuretic hormone (ADH), secreted by the posterior pituitary if water intake is limited, the spaces between the cells dilate so that the epithelium becomes very permeable to water. In contrast, when ADH is absent, the spaces are tightly joined. This is illustrated in Figure 3-14.

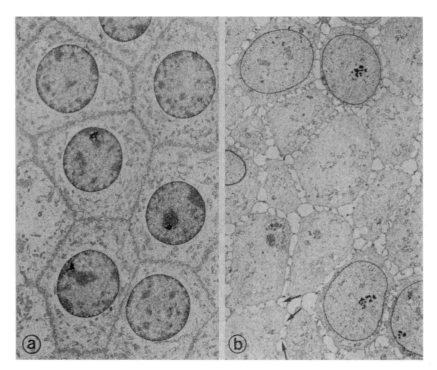

FIGURE 3-14 Electron micrographs of cross-sections through the inner MCD epithelium. In A, the intercellular spaces are narrow, and in B, they are dilated. The dilated intercellular spaces are probably the result of an ADH-induced water flow through the epithelium. Note that the extent of intercellular space dilation is limited by the lateral microfolds that are connected by desmosomes (*arrows*). (From Koushanpour E, Kriz W. *Renal physiology.* 2nd ed. New York: Springer-Verlag, 1986.)

REGULATION OF ACID–BASE EQUILIBRIUM

The two physiologic acid–base regulators, the pulmonary and renal systems, share one regulatory component in common: the blood buffer system. There are three renal secretory mechanisms that aid in maintaining the blood pH at the normal range. Each system relies directly or indirectly on the tubular secretion of hydrogen ions.[10]

In the first mechanism, as shown in Figure 3-15, 80% to 90% of the bicarbonate in the ultrafiltrate is reabsorbed along the proximal tubule. In this obligatory bicarbonate reabsorption, the electroneutral exchange of hydrogen ions for sodium ions across the luminal border of the proximal cell membrane is a key factor. Once in the tubular lumen, the H^+ combines with the filtered bicarbonate to form carbonic acid, which is then converted to carbon dioxide and water by the carbonic anhydrase present in the brush border of the luminal membrane. This carbon dioxide diffuses into the cell, where it is converted to bicarbonate and hydrogen ions, again by the enzyme carbonic anhydrase. This "reabsorbed" bicarbonate resupplies the blood buffer system by diffusing back into the peritubular capillary blood.

The second secretory mechanism is illustrated in Figure 3-16. This mechanism involves the formation and excretion of titratable acid in which the kidney conserves Na^+ and replenishes the body bicarbonate pool, thus acidifying the urine. In this case, the exchange of hydrogen ions for sodium ions converts disodium phosphate to monosodium phosphate and, as a consequence of this exchange, sodium and bicarbonate

are returned to the peritubular capillary blood. In this way, the body's stores of bicarbonate are replenished. The "titratable acids" (monobasic phosphates) in the urine can be titrated to pH 7.4 using standardized NaOH and a pH meter.

The third mechanism for acid removal, shown in Figure 3-17, depends on the secretion of ammonia followed by the exchange of sodium ions for ammonium ions. The tubular cells produce ammonia by the partial deamination of glutamine (the amide of glutamic acid) to yield glutamic acid and ammonia, and the ammonia diffuses into the tubular lumen, where it combines with hydrogen ions (which have been secreted by the tubular cell) to form ammonium ions, which then may combine with chloride or sulfate ions to form neutral salts. Again, bicarbonate and sodium are available for return to the peritubular capillary blood. The proximal tubule and collecting duct cells are both able to produce ammonia for these reactions, but final urine acidification occurs mainly in the collecting ducts.[4] The rate of ammonia synthesis responds directly to the systemic acid–base status, so that an increased extracellular hydrogen ion concentration lasting for more than 1 to 2 days stimulates the rate of tubular cell ammonia production.[21]

FORMATION OF HYPERTONIC OR HYPOTONIC URINE

The collecting ducts passing through the medulla toward the renal pelvis are responsible for adjusting the final solute concentration of the urine. This process

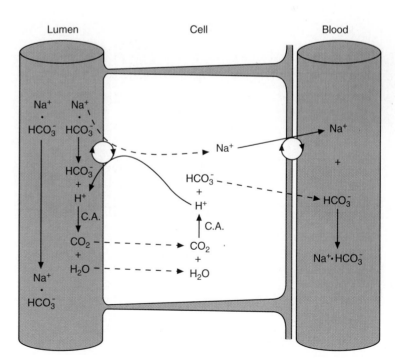

FIGURE 3-15 Mechanism of obligatory bicarbonate reabsorption in the proximal tubule.

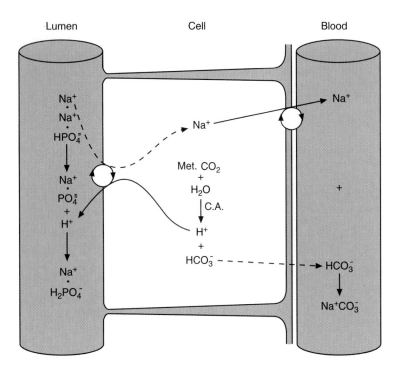

FIGURE 3-16 Mechanism of controlled excretion of titratable acid in the collecting duct.

depends on the maintenance of a gradient of increasing osmolality along the medullary pyramids toward the papillae. The interstitial fluid surrounding the ducts is very hyperosmotic. If ADH is present, the ducts become more permeable to water, which is then drawn out of the ducts into the hyperosmotic interstitial fluid so that a hypertonic urine is produced. Without ADH the ducts are not permeable, water does not pass out of the fil-

trate into the interstitium, and a hypotonic (or dilute) urine is produced.

The maintenance of this gradient of increasing osmolality along the medullary pyramids toward the papillae depends on the loops of Henle operating as countercurrent multipliers (an "active" process) and the vasa recta acting as countercurrent exchangers (a "passive" process). The nephrons involved in renal con-

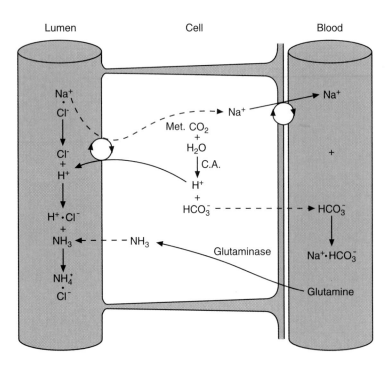

FIGURE 3-17 Mechanism of controlled excretion of ammonium ions in the collecting duct.

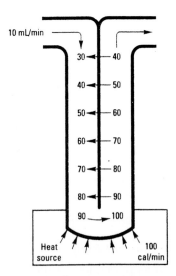

FIGURE 3-18 Operation of a countercurrent system. The heater raises the temperature of the water 10 degrees Celsius or C, but the heated water flowing away from the heater warms the inflow. A gradient of temperature is thus set up along the pipe, so that at the bend the temperature is raised not from 30 to 40 degrees but from 90 to 100 degrees. (From Ganong WF. *Review of medical physiology*. 15th ed. Norwalk: Appleton & Lange, 1991.)

The Countercurrent Multiplier System

In a countercurrent system, the inflow runs parallel to, counter to, and in close proximity to the outflow for some distance. Such an arrangement is shown in Figure 3-18, which uses temperature changes to illustrate the countercurrent multiplier concept. In this model, the countercurrent system results in a temperature at the apex of the loop of the pipe far in excess of that caused by the heater. Some of the heat in the outgoing fluid is transferred to the incoming fluid, setting up a gradient, so that by the time the incoming fluid reaches the heater, its temperature is 90°C instead of 30°C, and the heater therefore raises the fluid temperature from 90° to 100°C rather than from 30° to 40°C.

Although it is analogous to this model, the operation of the countercurrent multiplier system in the kidney depends on fundamental differences between the descending and the ascending loop of Henle. The thin descending limb is highly permeable to water but relatively impermeable to solute. On the other hand, the thin ascending limb is relatively impermeable to water and relatively permeable to solutes. The thick ascending limb is relatively impermeable to both water and solute, and it is adapted for actively cotransporting sodium and chloride into the interstitium. The hyperosmolality produced draws water out of the collecting ducts into the interstitium to produce a concentrated urine in the ducts.

As shown in Figure 3-19, the osmolality of the filtrate entering the loop of Henle is 300 mOsm/L, the

centration are the juxtamedullary nephrons, with their loops of Henle extending into the medulla of the kidney. These loops are surrounded by vessels of the vasa recta. Both the loops of Henle and the juxtamedullary capillary system (vasa recta) work together to concentrate urine.

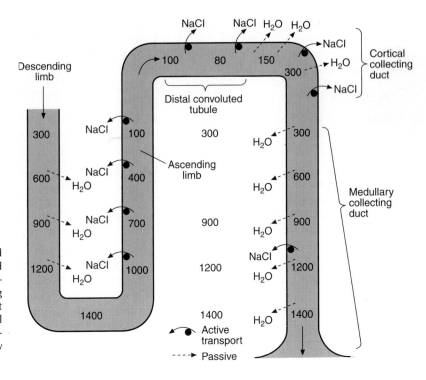

FIGURE 3-19 Interactions of Henle's loop and collecting duct in formation of a concentrated urine. ADH, acting on the principal cells, increases water permeability of the collecting ducts, both cortical and medullary. Note that interstitial osmolarity at every level is identical to descending limb and collecting duct osmolarity. (From Vander AJ. *Renal physiology*. New York: McGraw-Hill, Inc., 1995.)

same as plasma. The thick ascending limb actively co-transports (reabsorbs) sodium and chloride from the filtrate out into the interstitium. Because the thick ascending limb is relatively impermeable to water, little water follows the solute. In contrast, there is a net diffusion of water out of the descending limb into the more concentrated interstitial fluid that was created by the pumping action in the thick ascending limb. Although a gradient of only 200 mOsm/L is maintained across the ascending limb at any given horizontal level in the medulla, there is a much larger osmotic gradient from the top of the medulla to the bottom (~300 vs. ~1400 mOsm/L). The intratubular fluid is progressively concentrated as it flows down the descending limb, and the medullary interstitial fluid is progressively concentrated to the same degree.

The active ion transport mechanism in the ascending limb is the essential component of the entire system. The countercurrent flow itself would have no effect without the active pumping mechanism. The osmolality of the fluid in the descending limb approaches that in the interstitium but is diluted by the NaCl cotransporter as the filtrate passes through the thick ascending limb. This fluid now enters the collecting ducts, which become highly permeable to water under the influence of ADH. Water diffuses out into the interstitial fluid as a result of the high osmolality set up there by the loop countercurrent multiplier system. This water enters the medullary capillaries and is carried out of the kidneys in the venous blood.

Because water is reabsorbed all along the lengths of the collecting ducts, the fluid at the end of the collecting ducts has essentially the same osmolality as the interstitial fluid surrounding the bend in the loops (i.e., at the bottom of the medulla). This is the mechanism for producing a hyperosmotic urine, allowing the kidneys to compensate for a water deficit in the body.

The Role of Urea

In addition to the sodium and chloride in the interstitium, approximately 50% of the medullary osmolality consists of urea. As water is reabsorbed, the urea concentration in the filtrate rises progressively along the cortical collecting ducts (as well as along the outer medullary collecting ducts [MCDs]). However, urea is not reabsorbed because these tubular segments are impermeable to urea. The high urea concentration in the tubular fluid drives the reabsorption out of the inner MCDs (which contain a facilitated diffusion transporter for urea), and ADH activates this urea transporter.[20] Even though urea is being lost from these ducts, the simultaneous movement of water out of the inner MCDs maintains a high urea concentration in the tubular fluid. In this way, the urea concentration of the inner medullary interstitial fluid comes to approximate the urea concentration of the luminal fluid within adjacent, inner MCDs. The net result is that urea within the tubule is balanced by urea within the interstitium so that the sodium and chloride within the interstitium need balance only the solutes other than urea in the tubular fluid. Without urea in the interstitial fluid, more sodium chloride would have to be transported by the ascending limb of Henle's loop. It is possible for a maximally concentrated urine (1400 mOsm/L), under conditions of extensive sodium chloride reabsorption, to contain almost no sodium chloride, so that urea, creatinine, uric acid, and potassium make up much of the solute.

The Countercurrent Exchange System

The hairpin-loop anatomy of the medullary blood vessels (the vasa recta) that run parallel to the loops of Henle (and the MCDs) is essential for the maintenance of the osmolality gradient in the interstitium. With ordinary capillaries, the interstitial gradient would be lost because there would be massive, net diffusion of sodium chloride into and water out of the capillaries. In a hairpin loop of the vasa recta, blood enters the loop at an osmolality of 300 mOsm/L, and as it flows down the capillary into the medulla, sodium chloride diffuses into and water diffuses out of the vessel. After the bend in the loop is reached, the blood then flows up the ascending vessel loop and the process is almost completely reversed—sodium chloride diffusing out of and water diffusing into the vessel. In this way, the vessel loop acts as a so-called countercurrent exchanger (an exchanger because the process is passive), and this process prevents the solute gradient from being dissipated (Fig. 3-20).

THE RENIN–ANGIOTENSIN–ALDOSTERONE SYSTEM

Juxtaglomerular Apparatus

Earlier in this chapter, in connection with the renal corpuscle, mention was made of the JGA and the production of renin. Referring again to Figure 3-9, note the granular cells (differentiated smooth muscle cells in the wall of the afferent arteriole), the extraglomerular mesangial cells, and the macula densa cells that are part of the late, thick, ascending limb of the corpuscle's loop of Henle. This entire area of the renal corpuscle is known as the JGA. Renal sympathetic noradrenergic neurons are distributed to the afferent and the efferent arterioles, the JGA, and many portions of the tubule. Secretory vesicles in the granular cells of the JGA are the source of the hormone renin, which is the starting point for the effects of the renin–angiotensin–aldosterone system.

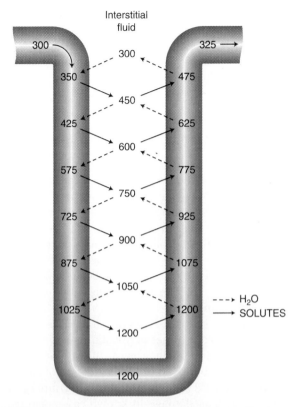

FIGURE 3-20 Vasa recta as countercurrent exchangers. All movements of water and solutes shown are by diffusion. Not shown is the simultaneously occurring uptake of interstitial fluid by bulk flow. (Vander AJ. *Renal physiology.* New York: McGraw-Hill, Inc., 1995.)

The Renin–Angiotensin–Aldosterone Pathway

The substrate for renin (which is an enzyme) is angiotensinogen, a large α_2-globulin containing more than 400 amino acid residues. Angiotensinogen is produced by the liver and is normally present at all times in the circulation. Once renin has been released by the juxtaglomerular (granular) cells, it splits off a small, inactive decapeptide, angiotensin I, from the angiotensinogen. Next, angiotensin-converting enzyme removes two carboxy-terminal amino acid residues from the angiotensin I to form angiotensin II, which is the active molecule in this system. Angiotensin-converting enzyme is found in very high concentration on the luminal surface of capillary endothelial cells, particularly in the lungs. Therefore, most of the conversion of angiotensin I to angiotensin II occurs as blood flows through the lungs.

Factors that bring about the release of renin into the bloodstream include decreased blood volume, decreased arterial pressure, sodium depletion, vascular hemorrhage, or increased potassium.[4] The end-product of this system, angiotensin II, is a potent vasoconstrictor that also stimulates the adrenal glands to se-

crete aldosterone. Both of these effects counteract the conditions that bring about the release of renin.

As a vasoconstrictor, angiotensin II not only constricts renal arterioles but also arterioles in most organs and tissues of the body, so that an increased plasma angiotensin II concentration increases total peripheral resistance and raises arterial blood pressure. By stimulating the adrenal glands to secrete aldosterone, angiotensin II indirectly brings about increased reabsorption of sodium and chloride, mostly in the late distal tubules and collecting ducts. This, in turn, expands the fluid volume because of water retention, leading to an increase in blood pressure. In addition, the exchange of potassium for sodium during the reabsorption of sodium restores the balance of potassium to normal if increased potassium was the factor causing the release of renin.

Composition of Urine

Urine is a complex, yellowish fluid consisting of approximately 95% water and 5% dissolved solids. The actual composition varies according to such factors as an individual's diet, physical activity and health, nutritional status and metabolic rate, the general state of the body, and the state of the kidneys. As it reaches the bladder, urine represents an ultrafiltrate of the plasma with selected solutes reabsorbed, other solutes secreted, and the final water volume adjusted according the body's state of hydration. The major nitrogenous waste products include urea (which accounts for about 50% of the dissolved solids in the urine), uric acid, and creatinine. The major electrolytes found are sodium chloride, potassium chloride, calcium, magnesium, phosphates, and sulfates. Table 3-2 illustrates the composition of urine from healthy individuals. In addition to solutes, normal urine may also contain a few cells from the blood and the lining of the urinary tract, together with a few hyaline casts and certain kinds of crystals, topics discussed in Chapter 9.

Volume of Urine

Urine volume is discussed as part of the section on Physical Examination of Urine in Chapter 6. Because water is a major body constituent, the amount excreted is usually determined by the body's state of hydration. Many factors influence the volume of urine produced, including fluid intake, loss of fluid from nonrenal sources, level of ADH, and increased amounts of solutes that must be excreted in the urine. Although the average daily volume of urine for a normal adult is

TABLE 3-2
Composition of Urine From Healthy Subjects

Constituent	Value
Albumin	<15–30 mg/L
Calcium	100–240 mg/24 hr
Creatinine	1.2–1.8 g/24 hr
Glucose	<300 mg/L
Ketones	<50 mg/L
Osmolality	>600 mOsm/L
Phosphorus	0.9–1.3 g/24 hr
Potassium	30–100 mEq/24 hr
pH	4.7–7.8
Sodium	85–250 mEq/24 hr
Specific gravity	1.005–1.030
Total bilirubin	(Not detected)
Total protein	<150 mg/24 hr
Urea nitrogen	7–16 g/24 hr
Uric acid	300–800 mg/24 hr
Urobilinogen	<1 mg/L

(Kaplan LA, Pesce AJ. *Clinical chemistry*. 3rd ed. St. Louis: The CV Mosby Company, 1996.)

1200 to 1500 mL, the normal range is about 600 to 2000 mL/day. Polyuria (>2000 mL/24 hours), oliguria (<500 mL/24 hours), and anuria (virtual absence of urine) are discussed in Chapter 6, together with a brief review of clinical correlations.

Renal Function Tests

Renal function testing and liver function testing share many of the same problems. In both the kidney and the liver a multiplicity of enzyme and transport systems co-exist—some related, others both spatially and physiologically quite separate. Like the liver, the kidney has not one but a great many functions that may or may not be affected in a given pathologic process. By measuring the capacity to perform these individual functions, one hopes to extract anatomical and physiologic information. Unfortunately, the tests available to the clinical laboratory are few and gross compared with the delicate network of systems at work. One can measure only what passes into and out of the kidney. What goes on inside is all-important but must be speculated on by indirect means.[14]

Ravel thus expresses the tremendous handicap that results from this situation: the inability of function tests to reveal the etiology of the dysfunction. All we learn is whether a certain degree of dysfunction is present and a rough estimate of its severity.

The three basic renal processes are glomerular filtration, tubular reabsorption, and tubular secretion. These were illustrated in Figures 3-11 and 3-12.

Glomerular Filtration

Glomerular filtration, the first event in the formation of urine, is the bulk flow of fluid from the glomerular capillaries into Bowman's capsule. Bulk flow means that all constituents move together. This glomerular filtrate normally contains no cells and is an ultrafiltrate of plasma, essentially protein free, containing most of the inorganic ions and low–molecular-weight organic solutes (e.g., glucose) in nearly the same concentrations as in the plasma. The GFR is the volume of filtrate formed per unit time.

In disease states, a reduction in GFR is most often due to a decrease in net permeability resulting from a loss of filtration surface area due to some form of glomerular injury. Rather than detection of early renal disease, the GFR is most useful in determining the extent of nephron damage in known cases of renal disease; in monitoring the effectiveness of treatment designed to prevent further nephron damage; and in determining the feasibility of administering medications, which can build up to toxic levels in the blood if the GFR is markedly reduced.

Some type of clearance test is used to estimate the GFR. Clearance may be defined as the volume of plasma from which a measured amount of substance can be completely eliminated (cleared) into the urine per unit of time. Renal clearance is estimated by UV/P, where U is the urine concentration of the substance (in mg/dL), V is the rate of urine flow (in milliliters per minute), and P is the plasma (or serum) concentration of the substance (in milligrams per deciliter). To be useful, the substance measured must have certain characteristics: It is freely filtered by the glomerulus, it is not reabsorbed or secreted, and it is neither synthesized nor broken down by the tubules.[20]

INULIN CLEARANCE

The reference method for measuring the GFR is the inulin clearance test. Inulin, an exogenous, nontoxic, fructopolysaccharide (MW, 5200 da) meets all of the theoretic criteria of the ideal substance for a clearance test. However, there are certain drawbacks to its routine use. Inulin must be continuously infused into the patient throughout the duration of the test to maintain a constant plasma level. Also, available analytical methods for inulin are difficult and time consuming.

UREA CLEARANCE

The earliest of the clearance tests for routine determination of the GFR was the urea clearance test. Urea, an endogenous, nitrogen-containing waste product of protein metabolism, is synthesized in the liver from ammonia and is freely filtered by the glomerulus. Because approximately 40% of the filtered urea is reabsorbed, normal values had to be adjusted to reflect this, and patients needed to be well hydrated to produce a urine flow of 2 mL/minute to make sure that no more than 40% of the filtered urea was reabsorbed. Another drawback to the use of urea for a clearance test is that its clearance depends on the rate of urine flow. At low levels of flow (<2 mL/minute), the values are very inaccurate. In addition, the levels of urea in the blood change to some extent during the day and can also change a great deal with variations in diet.

CREATININE CLEARANCE

The endogenous creatinine clearance test is a significant improvement on the use of urea clearance to measure GFR. Creatinine, the anhydride of creatine, is a byproduct of the metabolism of creatine (and phosphocreatine) in muscle. Because creatinine is produced at a relatively constant rate, the plasma concentration and urinary excretion rate are also relatively constant. Because the creatine in the body is related to muscle mass, creatinine formation is related to a patient's sex, physical activity, and age. To take into account this dependence on individual muscle mass, creatinine clearance values are often normalized to the external body surface area of an "average" individual: 1.73 m^2.

Creatinine is freely filtered by the glomerulus, is secreted by the tubules, but is also reabsorbed to an equal extent. The *net* effect is that the amount filtered is the amount excreted.[12–14] The GFR has been shown to decrease with increasing age, one study indicating a 4 mL/minute decrease for each decade after age 20 years. Values for creatinine clearance as low as 50 mL/minute in clinically healthy, elderly people have been found in several studies, and one study found values between 40% to 70% of normal.[14] Because creatinine formation is related to muscle mass, decreased muscle mass as seen in the elderly exaggerates any apparent decrease in clearance due to a diminished GFR. On the other hand, if meat is consumed in sufficiently large quantity, the level of serum creatinine may increase and therefore the creatinine clearance will decrease.

Usually creatinine clearance is determined on a 24-hour timed collection of urine because of the diurnal variation in the GFR. A standard version of the calculation including a correction for the body surface area of the patient is:

$$C \text{ (mL/min)} = \frac{U \times V}{P} \times \frac{1.73 \text{ m}^2}{SA}$$

where C = creatinine clearance, U = urine creatinine concentration in mg/dL, V = urine volume in mL/minute, P = plasma or serum creatinine concentration in mg/dL, 1.73 m^2 = the body service area of the "average person," and SA = the body surface area of the patient determined from a nomogram (see Appendix B) or calculation. No matter what units are used for the urine and plasma/serum creatinine concentrations, they must be the same so they will cancel each other out in the renal clearance calculation.

The body surface area as related to body weight and height may be calculated as follows:

$$\text{Log SA} = (0.425 \times \log \text{weight}) + (0.725 \times \log \text{height}) - 2.144$$

where SA = body surface area in m^2, weight is in kg, and height is in cm.

Formulas have been developed to estimate the creatinine clearance from the serum creatinine when it is necessary to prescribe medications rather than waiting for the collection of a 24-hour urine specimen, the analysis, and the traditional calculation. The most frequently used formula[14] was developed by Cockcroft and Gault:

$$C_{cr} = f([140 - \text{age}][\text{weight in kg}] \div 72 \times \text{serum creatinine in mg/dL})$$

where C_{cr} = creatinine clearance.

Because the weight of an average man is about 72 kg, the formula can be simplified to:

$$C_{cr} = \frac{140 - \text{age}}{\text{serum creatinine}}$$

The results are multiplied by 0.9 for women.[14]

Tubular Reabsorption

Included here are determinations of specific gravity and osmolality, fluid deprivation tests, osmolar clearance, and solute-free water clearance.

As discussed in Chapter 6, specific gravity and

osmolality both reflect the concentration of urinary solute. Specific gravity is the ratio of the mass of a solution compared with the mass of an equal volume of pure water. Osmolality reflects the number of dissolved particles in solution. Although plasma specific gravity remains fairly constant, ranging from 1.010 to 1.012, the urine specific gravity varies from 1.003 to 1.035 as the urine is either diluted or concentrated by the tubules. The normal osmolality of serum ranges from 285 to 319 mOsm/kg water. Urine osmolality varies between 50 to 1400 mOsm/kg water.[13] In nondisease states, urine osmolality corresponds closely with urine specific gravity, but with renal disease, solutes such as protein contribute much more to the specific gravity than to the osmolality.[13]

According to Pincus and colleagues, the best method to determine maximal concentration and dilution of urine is by urine osmolality studies, and withholding fluids is judged to be the simplest test to evaluate concentrating ability.[13] Normally, urine specific gravity should exceed 1.025 after 16 hours of fluid deprivation. A normal response is for the urine osmolality to exceed 800 mOsm/kg water, or for the ratio of urine osmolality to serum osmolality (U/S) to exceed

---

TABLE 3-3
A Method to Evaluate Concentrating Ability

1. Patient consumes evening meal.
2. After 6:00 P.M., patient is deprived of all fluid intake but is allowed to consume solid food. The patient voids at 8:00 A.M. next day.
3. At 10:00 A.M., serum (S) osmolality and urine (U) osmolality are determined. If U/S is greater than 3.0 (or urine osmolality exceeds 850 mOsm), the test response is considered normal and no vasopressin (Pitressin) is needed. Test is terminated.
4. If U/S is less than 3.0 (or urine osmolality is below 850 mOsm). 5 units of Pitressin tannate in oil are given subcutaneously.
5. Urine and serum osmolality are then determined at 2:00 P.M. (20 hours) and, if necessary, at 6:00 P.M. (24 hours).
6. If U/S osmolality ratio reaches or exceeds 3.0 (or urine osmolality exceeds 850 mOsm) at any time, test is immediately terminated and patient is allowed fluids.
7. If patient does not attain an osmolality of 850 mOsm/kg or a U/S of 3.0 by 6:00 P.M., test is terminated regardless.
8. Urine osmolality is determined on A.M. specimen the next day.

(From Pincus MR, Preuss HG, Henry JB: Evaluation of renal function, water, electrolytes, acid–base balance, and blood gases. In Henry JB: ed, *Clinical diagnosis and management.* 19th ed. Philadelphia: WB Saunders Co, 1996.)

3.0. A common method that may be used to assess concentrating ability is described in Table 3-3.

The ability to form a dilute urine can be evaluated by giving the patient a water load and observing the change in urine osmolality. For a patient who is already normally hydrated, the accepted response after drinking 500 mL of water is a reduction in the urine osmolality to the range of 40 to 80 mOsm/kg water.[13] A more precise challenge is to give an oral water load of 20 mL/kg body weight and then to replace the subsequent urine volume with an equal volume of water. With maximal water diuresis, urine osmolality decreases to the range of 50 to 100 mOsm/kg.

With some chronic renal diseases (e.g., chronic glomerulonephritis, chronic pyelonephritis), the ability of the tubules to form a concentrated urine is often affected rather early and slowly declines until the specific gravity and the osmolality of the excreted urine remain fixed at 1.010 and 290 mOsm/kg, respectively, which are the values for the ultrafiltrate.

A different approach in evaluating the concentrating and diluting capacities of the kidneys is to calculate the osmolar clearance and the free water (solute-free water) clearance. The U/S (or U/P) osmolality ratio is converted to a clearance value when it is multiplied by the volume of urine (V):

$$C_{osmol} = \frac{U_{osmol} \times V}{S_{osmol}}$$

where C_{osmol} is the osmolar clearance, U_{osmol} is the osmolality of the urine, V is the volume of urine, and S_{osmol} is the osmolarity of the serum. The osmolar clearance represents the amount of water cleared from the plasma that results in a urine having the same osmolarity as the plasma. The free water (solute-free water) clearance, C_{H2O}, is the difference between the total urine volume and the osmolar clearance:

$$C_{H2O} = V - C_{osmol}.$$

A positive value for C_{H2O} indicates that the urine is dilute compared with serum; conversely, a negative value for C_{H2O} indicates that the urine is more concentrated than serum. The highest possible free water clearance is 10 to 15 mL/minute. With acute tubular necrosis or with chronic renal failure, free water clearance values are usually near zero or are positive.

Tubular Secretion and Renal Blood Flow

The major pathway for substances to reach the ultrafiltrate is by glomerular filtration. A second pathway into the tubular lumen is by secretory processes across the tubular epithelium. Substances must first diffuse out of the peritubular capillaries into the interstitial fluid. A transcellular route of elimination involves entering the tubular cells though the basolateral membranes by an active process, resulting in a high intracellular concentration that drives "downhill" movement across the luminal membrane into the filtrate. If there is a favorable electrochemical gradient between the interstitial fluid and the tubular lumen for a given substance (and the plasma membranes or tight junctions are permeable to the substance), then passive secretion can occur by diffusion by either paracellular or transcellular means.[20]

Even substances that are mainly bound to plasma proteins and are not filtered by the glomerulus may be secreted by the tubules. An equilibrium exists between molecules of a substance bound to plasma proteins and those not bound. Free molecules are able to diffuse out of the peritubular capillaries into the interstitium and from there reach the tubules. As free molecules diffuse out of the capillaries, others are released from the proteins (by mass action) and diffuse out into the interstitium, and so on. Release from the carrier protein and diffusion into the interstitium occurs rapidly enough so that in those cases in which an active secretory system exists for a substance, nearly all of the substance originally bound to the protein undergoes secretion, often during only a single passage of blood through the renal system.[20] A large number of different organic anions, those endogenously produced (urate, oxalate, fatty acids) and those that are exogenous (hippurate, salicylates, sulfonamides, penicillin), are secreted by the proximal tubular cells.

One organic anion that has been intensively studied and that is secreted by this pathway via the proximal tubules is para-aminohippuric acid (PAH). The rate of PAH secretion increases as the plasma concentration increases until the transport maximum (T_m) is reached. PAH is also filtered at the glomerulus, and when its plasma concentration is fairly low, almost all of the

PAH that is not filtered is secreted. PAH is not reabsorbed, so that the net effect is that PAH is completely cleared from all the plasma supplying the nephron. This pattern is like substance X in Figure 3-12. Because PAH is completely removed from the plasma in its first pass through the glomerulus and the peritubular capillaries, the actual plasma flow in milliliters per minute can be estimated using the traditional clearance equation:

$$C_{PAH} = \frac{U \times V}{P}$$

where U is the PAH concentration in the urine (mg/dL), V is the volume of urine (ml/min), and P is the PAH concentration in the plasma/serum (mg/dL). In theory, one could measure the total RPF if PAH were completely cleared from all of the plasma flowing through the entire kidney. However, approximately 10% to 15% of the total RPF supplies renal tissue that is nonfiltering and nonsecreting, so that PAH is not removed from that fraction. Therefore, the PAH clearance in reality measures about 85% to 90% of the total RPF, which is termed the effective RPF (ERPF).

For normal renal function, there must be an adequate renal blood flow (RBF). The RBF is related to the RPF according to the following expression:

$$RBF = \frac{RPF}{1 - Hct}$$

where Hct is the hematocrit. The normal range for RPF as determined by the PAH clearance test is from 600 to 700 mL/minute.[4] If we assume an average normal Hct of 42%, then normal values for the RBF would range from about 1000 to 1200 mL/minute. Even though the PAH clearance test is the reference method for determining RPF and RBF, PAH is an exogenous substance and must be infused, and current methods for PAH analysis in both urine and plasma are not suited to routine laboratory testing.

REFERENCES

1. Brunzel NA. *Fundamentals of urine and body fluid analysis*. Philadelphia: WB Saunders, 1994.
2. Burtis CA, Ashwood ER, eds. *Tietz' fundamentals of clinical chemistry*. 4th ed. Philadelphia: WB Saunders, 1996.
3. Junqueira LC, Carneiro J, Kelley RO. *Basic histology*. 7th ed. Norwalk, CT: Appleton & Lange, 1992.
4. Koushanpour E, Kriz W. *Renal physiology*. 2nd ed. New York: Springer-Verlag, 1986.
5. Memmler RL, Cohen BJ, Wood DL. *The human body in health and disease*. 7th ed. Philadelphia: JB Lippincott, 1992.
6. Pincus MR. Interpreting laboratory results: Reference values and decision making. In: Henry JB, ed. *Clinical diagnosis and management*. 19th ed. Philadelphia: WB Saunders, 1996: 74–91.
7. Pincus MR, Preuss HG, Henry JB. Evaluation of renal function, water, electrolytes, acid–base balance, and blood gases. In: Henry JB, ed. *Clinical diagnosis and management*. 19th ed. Philadelphia: WB Saunders, 1996:139–161.
8. Ravel R. *Clinical laboratory medicine*. 6th ed. St. Louis: Mosby, 1995.
9. Tortora GJ, Anagnostakos NP. *Principles of anatomy and physiology*. 3rd ed. New York: Harper & Row, 1981.
10. Vander AJ. *Renal physiology*. New York: McGraw-Hill, 1995.
11. Vander AJ, Sherman JH, Luciano DS. *Human physiology*. 5th ed. New York: McGraw-Hill, 1990.
12. Vander AJ, Sherman JH, Luciano DS. *Human physiology*. 6th ed. New York: McGraw-Hill, 1994.

BIBLIOGRAPHY

Anderson SC, Cockayne S. *Clinical chemistry*. Philadelphia: WB Saunders, 1993.

Bennington JL, ed. *Saunders' dictionary and encyclopedia of laboratory medicine and technology*. Philadelphia: WB Saunders, 1984.

Berkow R, ed. *The Merck manual of diagnosis and therapy*. Rahway, NJ: Merck & Co., Inc., Publications Department, 1982.

Bullock BL, Rosendahl PP. *Pathophysiology*. 3rd ed. Philadelphia: JB Lippincott, 1992.

Ganong WF. *Review of medical physiology*. 15th ed. Norwalk, CT: Appleton & Lange, 1991.

Kaplan LA, Pesce AJ. *Clinical chemistry*. 3rd ed. St. Louis: CV Mosby, 1996.

Ringsrud KM, Linné JJ. *Urinalysis and body fluids: A color text and atlas*. St. Louis: Mosby–Year Book, 1995.

Rose BD, Rennke HG. *Renal pathophysiology*. Baltimore: Williams & Wilkins, 1994.

Sampaio FJB, Uflacker R. *Renal anatomy applied to urology, endourology, and interventional radiology*. New York: Thieme Medical Publishers, 1993.

Strasinger SK. *Urinalysis and body fluids*. 3rd ed. Philadelphia: FA Davis, 1994.

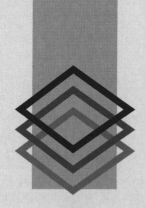

4

Urine Specimens

Types of Specimens

The National Committee for Clinical Laboratory Standards (NCCLS) denotes three types of urine specimens: patient collection, supervised collection, and assisted collection.[2]

Patient Collection

Specimens collected by cooperative patients after instruction and without direct supervision include random specimens; first-morning or 8-hour specimens; and timed specimens, including 24-hour collections. Random specimens may be collected at unspecified times and are the most convenient for the patients. They are usually satisfactory for routine screening even though they may not accurately reflect the patient's status because antecedent conditions such as hydration can directly affect urine composition. For the first-morning specimen (also known as an overnight specimen), the patient voids at bedtime and discards this urine. Immediately on arising from sleep, the patient collects the "first-morning" specimen. Because this urine was retained in the bladder for approximately 8 hours, it is the most concentrated of the day's urine and is also the most acid, so that formed elements such as cells and casts are more stable than in dilute, less acid urines.

A timed short-term specimen may be collected with respect to another activity, such as a specimen collected 2 hours after a meal (postprandial). A timed long-term specimen would be one collected over a predetermined length of time, such as 12 or 24 hours. The 24-hour specimen is especially useful for quantitative analyses because the extended collection period averages out fluctuations in analyte concentration caused by diurnal variations in the excretion of hormones, proteins, metabolites, and the like. Accurate timing of the collection as well as accurate measurement of the total volume are essential. In general, the patient should empty the bladder and discard the urine at the beginning of the timed period, collect all urine voided during the designated period, and at the end of the period empty the bladder and add this urine to the timed collection. Proper preservation of timed specimens is discussed later in the section dealing with preservatives.

Supervised Collection

Trained personnel from the clinical laboratory staff may be required to supervise or participate in the collection of midstream, clean-catch specimens and specimens for microbiologic culture. A midstream specimen is obtained by having the patient start voiding into a receptacle (e.g., bedpan) or toilet, then having the patient fill the collection container by inserting it into the urine stream, and voiding any remaining urine into the receptacle or toilet. This procedure ensures that the urine collected is more representative of what was stored in the bladder because materials in the urethra are first flushed out.

For a clean-catch specimen, the patient first cleanses the urethral meatus (female) or glans penis (male) and surrounding area according to instruction, then voids while preventing tissues surrounding the urethral orifice from coming in contact with the urine. The clean catch specimen avoids contamination from areas surrounding the urethral orifice and provides an excellent specimen for both routine urinalysis and microbiologic testing. For microbiologic testing, the container must of course be sterile and the patient should be instructed not to contaminate it with fingers, toilet paper, and so forth.

Assisted Collection

The following types of specimens require the active participation of trained personnel: catheter specimens and suprapubic aspiration specimens. For catheter specimens, a sterile catheter is inserted into the bladder through the urethra. Urine flows directly through the indwelling catheter from the bladder and is collected in a plastic reservoir bag. A single urine specimen may be collected from the urine outflow, or a specimen may be collected at any time from the bag.

A suprapubic specimen is one collected by aspirating urine from the distended bladder through the abdominal wall by means of needle and syringe, using aseptic technique. This procedure is most often used for bacteriologic examination (especially for anaerobes) and for infants, in whom specimen contamination may otherwise be unavoidable.

Containers: Specimen Handling and Preservation

Specimen containers should be clean and dry, and must be sterile for microbiologic testing. Some laboratories prefer to use sterile containers for all urine collections. Disposable plastic containers are the type most commonly used; they have capacities ranging from 50 to 100 mL. The base of the container should be wide enough to avoid accidental spillage and the opening should be at least 4 cm in diameter.[2]

For transportation to the laboratory, the container needs to have a lid that is easily fitted to and removed from the container but does not leak. As needed, a secondary container (e.g., plastic bag) may be used to ensure containment of possible spills.[2] Containers for 12- and 24-hour collections usually have a capacity of at least 3 L and have a wide mouth and a leakproof closure. They often are made of opaque, brown plastic to protect the specimen from light, and should be resistant to chemical preservatives.

Because newborns and pediatric patients at certain ages cannot urinate voluntarily, commercially available plastic urine collection bags with a hypoallergenic skin adhesive may be used. The perineal area is cleaned and dried before placement of the bag onto the skin. The bag is placed over the penis for boys and around the vagina (excluding the rectum) for girls. The adhesive is firmly attached to the perineum and checked frequently to see if an adequate specimen has been collected. The bag should be removed as soon as possible, labeled, and the specimen transported to the laboratory. When the patient has been appropriately prepared, bag specimens are usually satisfactory for routine screening and quantitative assays. For microbiologic testing, a catheterized specimen or one collected by suprapubic aspiration may be necessary.

The container should be designed to accept a label that resists moisture and adheres during refrigeration.[2] Space on the label should accommodate the patient's full name, identification number, date and time the specimen was collected, and the name of the preservative used, if applicable. Some laboratories may require other information or a bar code. Many laboratories use computer-generated labels. To ensure proper specimen identification, a label should be placed on the container itself rather than on the lid. The container should be labeled immediately before or after collection of the urine. If a special preservative is required, it should be added to the collection container before urine collection.

Because the physical, chemical, and microscopic characteristics of a urine specimen begin to change as soon as the urine is voided, urine specimens (except for long-term collections) should ideally be delivered to the laboratory for analysis immediately after collection. Because this is not always possible, steps should be taken to minimize the deterioration of the specimen until it can be transported to the laboratory. Refrigeration at 4°C is adequate for most specimens, and is especially important if the specimen is for microbiologic studies. Refrigeration retards bacterial growth, and the specimen remains suitable for microbiologic studies for up to 24 hours.

Once the specimen arrives in the laboratory, it should be analyzed promptly, although how this is defined depends on the laboratory in question. A common rule is that the specimen should be analyzed within 1 or 2 hours of the time of voiding. If this is not possible, the specimen should be refrigerated or a preservative added. Refrigeration at 4°C is the most commonly used means to preserve urine specimens for delayed analysis, although certain complications result: It induces precipitation of amorphous or crystalline deposits, which often seriously interfere with the urine microscopic examination. The specimen must be allowed to come to room temperature before dipstick testing is performed because low temperatures alter the time required for reactions to come to completion. Although freezing destroys the formed elements in urine specimens, it can be used to preserve bilirubin, urobilinogen, and porphobilinogen for analysis. Chemical preservatives usually act as antimicrobial agents, and their use depends on the analyte and the analytical procedure.[4]

Nonrefrigerated specimens for long-term collections (12 or 24 hours) may be kept in a specified area or in the patient's bathroom. If storage in the cold is necessary, the collection bottle may be kept in an iced container or stored in a refrigerator. When a preservative is added to the collection container (e.g., hydrochloric acid), the patient must be instructed to take precautions against spilling the contents. Preservatives used are determined by the urine substance for which the test is designed. The NCCLS provides an extensive listing of preferred 24-hour urine preservatives as recommended by some of the major reference laboratories in the United States.[2]

The results of a routine urinalysis can be seriously affected if the specimen is improperly handled or not properly preserved.

Several changes[5] may occur in a specimen if it is allowed to remain unpreserved at room temperature for longer than 1 hour:

1. The pH may increase because of the breakdown of urea to ammonia by urease-producing bacteria.
2. Glucose may decrease because of metabolic breakdown by body cells and microorganisms.
3. Ketones may decrease because of volatilization.
4. Bilirubin may decrease because of photooxidation.
5. Urobilinogen may decrease because of oxidation to urobilin.
6. Nitrite may increase because of bacterial reduction of nitrate.
7. Bacteria may multiply.
8. Turbidity may increase because of bacterial growth and possible precipitation of amorphous material.

9. Body cells and casts may disintegrate, especially in a dilute, alkaline urine.
10. Color may change because of oxidation or reduction of metabolites.

Quality Control

To ensure suitability for analysis, the NCCLS recommends[2] inspecting a urine specimen for the following:

- Information on the requisition and container must agree.
- The time elapsed from collection of the specimen to receipt in the laboratory must be acceptable.
- If transport to the laboratory was delayed, proper preservation procedures must have been used.
- Container must be suitable and sealed.
- Volume must be adequate and specimen free of contaminating materials.

- Depending on analyses requested, a proper chemical preservative must have been used.

The NCCLS also recommends[2] that if the specimen does not meet the criteria for acceptability, the attending physician or the nursing station should be contacted immediately for a decision on further action. The "unacceptable" specimen should be retained until clinical personnel have been consulted and a mutually agreeable decision has been reached. The NCCLS also suggests[2] that the laboratory establish a quality assurance program for urine specimens to ensure that the following information is documented:

- Consistency in correct specimen type, adequate volume, suitable containers, and proper labeling
- Timely transportation to the laboratory
- Prompt inspection and proper handling of specimens after arrival in the laboratory

REFERENCES

1. National Committee for Clinical Laboratory Standards. *Urinalysis and collection, transportation, and preservation of urine specimens: Approved guideline.* NCCLS Document GP16-A, Vol. 15, No. 15. Wayne, PA: NCCLS, December, 1995.

2. Schumann GB, Schweitzer SC. Examination of urine. In: Henry JB, ed. *Clinical diagnosis and management by laboratory methods.* 18th ed. Philadelphia: WB Saunders, 1991:387–444.
3. Strasinger SK. *Urinalysis and body fluids.* 3rd ed. Philadelphia: FA Davis, 1994.

BIBLIOGRAPHY

Brunzel NA. *Fundamentals of urine and body fluid analysis.* Philadelphia: WB Saunders, 1994.

Ringsrud KM, Linné JJ. *Urinalysis and body fluids: A color text and atlas.* St. Louis: Mosby–Year Book, 1995.

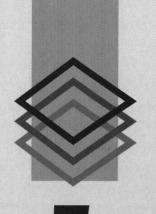

Instrumentation in the Urinalysis and Body Fluids Laboratory

5

ABBREVIATIONS USED IN THIS CHAPTER

ADH = antidiuretic hormone
CSF = cerebrospinal fluid
CUA = CHEMSTRIP Urine Analyzer
ID = identification

IRIS = International Remote Imaging Systems, Inc.
LCD = liquid crystal display
LED = light-emitting diode

LIS = laboratory information system
SG = specific gravity
SI = Système International
STAT = statim, immediately

Osmometers and the Measurement of Osmolality

The inability to produce a concentrated urine is often the first sign of renal disease, and it may also be a sign of hormone deficiency (e.g., ADH [antidiuretic hormone]). The solute concentration of urine can be quantitated by measuring either the specific gravity (SG) or the osmolality. Osmolality depends on the number of dissolved particles in solution and reflects the concentrating ability of the kidney more than does SG.

Dissolved solutes change the colligative properties of solutions: osmotic pressure, vapor pressure, boiling point, and freezing point. The extent of these changes at a constant temperature is determined only by the number and *not* by the nature or mass of the particles in solution. Methods to measure osmolality could be developed based on any one of the colligative properties, but in practice, freezing point depression and vapor pressure (or dew point) depression have been the favored approaches. The time-honored approach has been to use the freezing point osmometer.

One gram molecular weight (6.023×10^{23} particles) of a nonelectrolyte such as glucose dissolved in 1 kg of distilled water (i.e., a 1-molal solution) will increase the boiling point 0.52°C, increase the osmotic pressure 17,000 mm Hg, lower the vapor pressure 0.3 mm Hg, and lower the freezing point 1.858°C. This solution contains 1 Osm/kg H_2O or is said to have an osmolality of 1. A related expression is osmolarity, defined as 1 osmol of nonelectrolyte dissolved in 1 L of distilled water. Osmolality is the preferred unit of measurement because it is a constant weight-to-weight relationship rather than weight-to-volume. Osmolarity is affected by the volume-expanding effect of dissolved solute as well as the direct effect of temperature on fluid volume.

The osmolality of a 1-molal solution of an electrolyte (e.g., NaCl) is greater than 1 owing to the disso-ciation of the electrolyte into component atoms when in solution. The osmolality of an electrolyte solution is determined by the formula: osmolality = fnC, where n is the number of atoms that dissociate in solution, C is the concentration of the electrolyte in moles per kilogram of water, and f is the osmotic coefficient. For example, n for NaCl = 2 (Na^+ and Cl^-).

Freezing Point Osmometer

Freezing point osmometry is the indirect determination of the osmolality of a sample by measuring its freezing point depression. For each molal weight of particles added to the solution, the freezing point is lowered 1.858°C. In this technique, the freezing point depression is determined by monitoring the sample temperature with a thermistor as the sample is first subjected to supercooling and then allowed to freeze. The difference between the measured freezing point temperature of the solution and standard freezing point temperature of the solvent is the freezing point depression.

This process is illustrated in Figure 5-1, which shows the effect of the heat of fusion released during the formation of the ice as the heat of fusion temporarily raises the temperature of the solution to its freezing point. Contemporary instruments measure the freezing point depression, compute the osmolality, and display the results as milliosmoles per kilogram. A typical freezing point osmometer is illustrated in Figure 5-2. Normal urine values range from 50 to 1400 mOsm/kg.

Vapor Pressure Osmometer

The vapor pressure of a solution is lowered 0.3 mm Hg for every molal weight of particles added to the solution. Related to the vapor pressure is the dew point, the

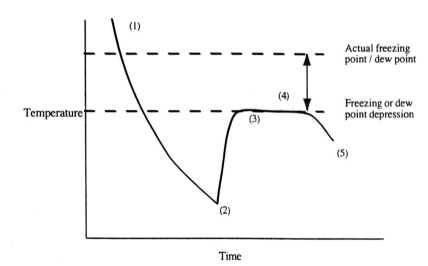

FIGURE 5-1 Freezing point depression curve. (1) Forced cooling begins. (2) Point of supercooling agitation is initiated. (2,3) Heat of fusion released into sample. Temperture increases. (4) Freezing point equilibrium is maintained for a short time. (5) Forced cooling begins again. (From Karselis TC. *The pocket guide to clinical laboratory instrumentation.* Philadelphia: FA Davis Company, 1994.)

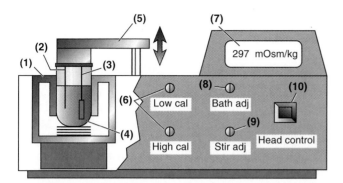

FIGURE 5-2 A typical freezing point osmometer. The sample is placed into the sample cup, and the agitator head (5) is lowered by the operator depressing the head control button (10). The temperature of the sample chamber (1) is slowly lowered by the temperature control module (4), until it is below freezing (called supercooling), at which time the stirring rod/agitator (2) is activated to promote crystal formation. The heat of fusion released by the formation of ice crystals is measured by the thermistor probe (3). When the temperature stabilizes, the temperature is read and recorded as the freezing point depression. The osmolality is displayed as a function of the difference between the sample temperature reading and the temperature readings previously obtained from a high and low standard solution. The instrument is calibrated (6) by the use of known (low and high) standards (6). The temperature of the bath can be adjusted (8) by the operator, as can the vibrational or stirring rate of the agitator (9) head. (From Karselis TC. *The pocket guide to clinical laboratory instrumentation*. Philadelphia: FA Davis Company, 1994.)

temperature at which a condensate (re-formation of liquid) begins to form on a cold surface at a given humidity. There is a linear function between depression of the vapor pressure and the dew point temperature depression.[11] With fewer water molecules in the vapor phase above a solution, the drop in temperature necessary for these water molecules to recondense into a liquid (i.e., reach the dew point) is greater.

In one fairly representative version of a vapor pressure osmometer, the dew point temperature depression of a sample is monitored by means of a fine-wire thermocouple.[11] After the sample is placed into a sealed chamber and allowed to reach equilibrium, the ambient temperature is read and used as a reference. A current is then passed through the junction of the thermocouple, cooling one arm (by means of the Peltier effect) to a temperature well below that at which water from the vapor phase condenses into liquid droplets on the surface of the metal junction. The current is stopped, and the heat of condensation produced when water molecules from the vapor phase condense to form a liquid causes the temperature of the junction to rise to the dew point. The difference between this dew point temperature and the ambient temperature of the chamber (recorded earlier) is the dew point depression, which is used to calculate the osmolality of the specimen (displayed in milliosmoles per kilogram). This temperature curve is illustrated in Figure 5-3.

Other vapor pressure osmometers use thermistors or mirrors with optical sensors to detect the dew point.

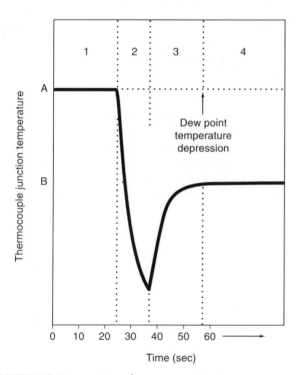

FIGURE 5-3 Temperature changes occurring in vapor-pressure depression (dew point) osmometry. A, Reference-point (starting) temperature. B, Dew point temperature. 1. Sample equilibration time. 2. Maximum thermocouple cooling. 3. Increase to dew point (heat of condensation). 4. Dew point equilibrium. (Modified from 550 Vapor Pressure Osmometer, Wescor, Inc., Logan, UT: 1998)

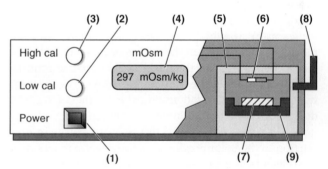

FIGURE 5-4 A typical vapor pressure osmometer. The microcolume sample is placed on a small filter paper disk (7) mounted on a sliding tray (9) and then placed into a chamber (5), which is then sealed by the operator with a spring-loaded locking arm (8). The water from the sample evaporates, forming a vapor, and at equilibrium an initial temperture reading is taken by the thermocouple (6). The thermocouple is electronically cooled (the Peltier effect) until vapor begins to condense onto the thermocouple, at which point the dew point temperature is recorded. This temperature is proportional to osmolality since the instrument response has been previously aligned with the low and high calibration controls (2,3) and appropriate calibration standards. The osmolality is displayed directly in milliosmoles on the digital readout (5). (From Karselis TC. *The pocket guide to clinical laboratory instrumentation*. Philadelphia: FA Davis Company, 1994.)

A vapor pressure osmometer is illustrated in Figure 5-4. The osmolality is displayed directly in milliosmoles per kilogram on the digital readout.

Instruments to Read Reagent Strips

The subjectivity associated with visual evaluation of urine dipsticks has been alleviated by the development of automated reagent strip readers using reflectance spectrophotometry.[16] Automated urine dipstick analyzers currently available include several CLINITEK models and the Atlas (Bayer Corporation, Diagnostics Division [formerly Miles, Inc.], Elkhart, IN); a series of CHEMSTRIP Urine Analyzers (Boehringer-Mannheim Corporation, Indianapolis, IN); and the Rapimat II (Behring Diagnostics, Inc., Westwood, MA).

Reflectance Spectrophotometers

All of the instruments developed for "reading" the reactions on urine reagent strips (dipsticks) use some form of reflectance spectrophotometry, which allows quantitative measurement of reactions on surfaces such as the reagent pads on a dipstick. In this technique, light from a source is directed at 90° relative to the sample surface and the diffuse, reflected light is measured rather than absorbed light. A fraction of the diffuse reflectance that is radiated at 45° relative to the incident beam is collimated by a lens and focused on a detector. An optical filter or monochromatic device, to select a wavelength at which the analyte absorbs, may be placed either in front of the source or in front of the detector, depending on the design of the instrument. In some instruments the source and filter arrangement may be replaced by a light-emitting diode (LED). The detector may be a phototube or a photodiode.

Light reflected from the test pads decreases in proportion to the color produced as the analyte reacts with the reagents in the pads. To establish the instrument response when no absorbing substance is in the optical path, a reagent strip pad consisting of a reflectance standard is used. This may be a highly purified powder of magnesium carbonate or barium sulfate, or a white ceramic material. The intensity of the reflected light from the test pads is compared with the intensity of the light reflected from the reflectance standard. Because the light intensities measured in reflectance spectrophotometry do not follow Beer's law, the instrument uses mathematical algorithms to linearize the relationship between the intensity of reflected light and analyte concentration.

Bayer Corporation—Diagnostics Division

CLINITEK 50 URINE CHEMISTRY ANALYZER

The CLINITEK 50 is a compact, portable unit designed for running urinalysis outside the hospital core laboratory. All tests are performed using Bayer Multistix 10 SG reagent strips, which are automatically analyzed by the CLINITEK 50. The instrument determines urine color and distinguishes between intact red blood cells and hemolyzed occult blood. A battery pack provides a test capacity of approximately 200 analyses, or the unit can be operated on line power. Reporting options include a 2-line, 24-character liquid crystal display (LCD); a hard-copy output from an integral 24-column printer; or direct-to-computer reporting. Results may be reported with semiquantitative values (milligrams per deciliter and millimolar), or with a "plus" system which reports levels of test positivity. Positive results are marked with an asterisk (*) for quick review.

The operator dips the reagent strip in the urine specimen and presses the START button. After blotting the side of the reagent strip, the operator places it on the instrument feed table, which draws the strip into the instrument. From the time the reagent strip is dipped in the sample and drawn into the instrument, it takes 1 minute for the CLINITEK 50 to analyze the specimen, display, and print the results.

CLINITEK 100 URINE CHEMISTRY ANALYZER

The CLINITEK 100 is a semiautomated, benchtop, microprocessor-controlled instrument designed to read Bayer Multistix 10 SG reagent strips. It is intended for laboratories analyzing moderate numbers of urine specimens per day, as in physicians' offices, clinics, and small hospitals. In the CLINITEK 100 optical system, light from three pairs of LEDs is reflected from the surface of the reagent test area and detected by a photodiode. The instrument operates by means of a removable program card that contains information on wavelength, error messages, operating sequence, and algorithms needed to process the reflectance data. With the appropriate program card, the instrument will read Multistix 10 SG, Multistix 9, or Uristix 4 reagent strips.

The operator dips the reagent test strip in urine and places the strip in the strip-loading station of the analyzer. The strip is drawn into the instrument, where the reactions are read. The specimen identification (ID) number, color, and clarity all can be entered on the keypad. There are eight descriptions for color and five for clarity. The approximate time for reading and printing of results from one strip is 77 seconds. Online data processing is available through external interface connectors to a standardized urinalysis form, an 80-column printer, or a computer.

CLINITEK 200+ URINE CHEMISTRY ANALYZER

The CLINITEK 200+ is a semiautomated, benchtop instrument for moderate- to large-volume urine testing. The analyzer reads Bayer Multistix SG reagent strips by reflectance spectrophotometry at a rate of one strip every 10 seconds. An optional bar code reader is available for the CLINITEK 200+, which eliminates operator keystroke entry of the patient ID. The operator dips a reagent strip in urine and places it on the strip-loading station of the analyzer. Once loaded, the strip automatically advances to the readheads. Measurements are taken, a sequential ID number is automatically assigned, and results are printed out and stored in memory. After measurements are taken, the strip is automatically advanced to the waste container.

Reflectance spectrophotometry is accomplished with a halogen lamp light source and photodiodes for sensing reflected light of various wavelengths. For each reagent pad, reflected light is measured at two wavelengths to compensate for any urine pigmentation that could otherwise cause erroneous results. Results are calculated from the ratio of each pair of measurements. Color and clarity can be entered for each patient by choosing from a series of options. Abnormal results can be flagged on the printed report.

CLINITEK ATLAS AUTOMATED URINE CHEMISTRY ANALYZER

The CLINITEK Atlas is an automated urine analyzer for measuring nine urine chemistries (by reagent test strip) and three physical characteristics. The CLINITEK Atlas Reagent Pak contains special reagent strips packaged in continuous rolls of 490 strips. The reagent strips have pads for 10 tests: glucose, protein, pH, occult blood, nitrite, leukocytes, ketones, urobilinogen, bilirubin, and urine color. The chemistries are read by reflectance spectrophotometry, and the urine color is measured by variable wavelength reflectance spectrophotometry. Specific gravity is determined by refractometry and clarity by light scatter (nephelometry).

Samples, calibrators, controls, and STATs are placed in bar coded tubes that are held in a 50-position tray. The automatic pipette senses sample volume, aspirates 700 μL of specimen, and precisely dispenses the volume required onto each reagent pad on the reagent strip, as well as adding the proper volume to the SG cuvet for the determination of SG and clarity. After the

pipetting of urine, the reagent strip is automatically advanced to the dual readheads of the reflectance spectrophotometer. The pipette is automatically washed between specimens. Results can be displayed, printed, or sent to a central computer. On-board memory stores 500 sets of patient results and 200 control/calibration results.

Behring Diagnostics

RAPIMAT II

The Rapimat II is a complete urinalysis analyzer and data management system. The detached terminal can be placed near a microscope for one-touch entry of sediment results and includes a printer for preparation of complete patient reports. The operator can arrange the analyzer position for convenient strip placement for right- or left-handed people.

The analyzer is a 12-channel reflectance spectrophotometer. Each channel includes an LED (which operates at one of four possible wavelengths) and a photodiode detector, both aligned on a single sensor head. Ten of the reflectometers are used to evaluate the reagent strip chemistry tests. Another reflectometer evaluates the urine color compensation pad, and one confirms the appropriate alignment of the reagent strip.

The user dips the reagent strip in the urine and places it on a "conveyor belt," which draws the strip into the instrument for reading. The leukocyte esterase test pad is thermostatically warmed to enhance this particular reaction. At the appropriate timed interval, the reflectance reading for each chemistry reaction is taken and the results are adjusted for urine color, if necessary. The microprocessor can store the results or they can be printed out. Both the physical and microscopic examination results can be entered and included on the printed report. The biohazardous and disagreeable chore of disposing of test strips is eliminated because the strips are individually rolled onto absorbent paper and the operator simply discards the roll. An ascorbic acid pad alerts the operator to false-negative glucose readings caused by the presence of ascorbic acid.

Boehringer-Mannheim Corporation

CHEMSTRIP MINI UA

The readheads of the CHEMSTRIP Mini UA reflectance spectrophotometer operate at three different wavelengths. On the front of the instrument is a door that is hinged to open downward, with a channel to accept the urine test strip. The operator dips the CHEMSTRIP urine test strip in the specimen, places the strip in the channel in the door with test pads facing upward, flips the door shut, and pushes the analyze button. Ninety seconds later, the on-board printer records the results in one of three formats: conventional, SI, or arbitrary units. LEDs visible on the top of the instrument correspond to each of the 10 tests and provide a display for positive or negative results. The instrument is portable.

CHEMSTRIP CRITERION

The CHEMSTRIP Criterion is a more complex analyzer than the Mini UA and provides interfacing capabilities and bar code patient identification. It features custom flagging parameters, 2-week calibration stability, and CHEMSTRIP color compensation.

CHEMSTRIP URINE ANALYZER

The CHEMSTRIP Urine Analyzer (CUA) is a benchtop, semiautomated reflectance spectrophotometer for reading the reactions on CHEMSTRIP 10UA reagent strips. The CUA light source consists of LEDs at three specific wavelengths (555, 620, and 660 nm) in each of the two readheads. A reference calibration strip with specific reflectance values is used to calibrate the system once every 2 weeks. Actual calibration values are automatically printed, a feature that provides the documentation needed to meet regulatory requirements.

To perform an individual analysis, a reagent strip is dipped into a urine sample and then placed on the transport tray at the strip insertion area of the instrument. The strip is automatically drawn into the analyzer, and results are recorded by the thermal printer within 2 minutes. Microscopic results may be entered, if desired, through the sediment terminal (an optional component) or the main unit of the CUA. Sample ID can be entered through a bar code reader, the bidirectional interface with the laboratory computer, or by manual keyboard entry. A disposable transport tray collects used strips and reduces exposure to biohazardous waste. The only maintenance necessary involves the strip transport plate, which slides out for cleaning.

CHEMSTRIP SUPER UA

The CHEMSTRIP Super UA automated urine analyzer is a walk-away instrument that can analyze 55 samples in 11 minutes. Samples are stirred and volume adjusted, reagent strips are robotically dipped, reactions on reagent pads are measured and results are reported—all automatically.

The sample tray (carousel) has a 60-sample capacity (55 sample positions plus 5 STAT positions). The reflectance spectrophotometer has two readheads with three LEDs for each wavelength used (555, 620, 660 nm). The instrument has an integrated bar code reader for sample ID. The humidity-controlled storage compartment keeps CHEMSTRIP reagent strips stable for up to 8 hours.

The strips are stored and automatically "pulled for processing" directly from the 200-strip capacity compartment. The desiccant lids from the strip containers are placed inside the compartment to help provide optimum storage conditions. A displacement rod is automatically inserted into each specimen tube as needed to adjust sample volume to the proper level so volume measuring is not required. Each sample is automatically mixed, then a test strip is robotically dipped into the urine and conveyed to the reflectance spectrophotometer for measurement. The CHEMSTRIP reagent strip has a color-blanking pad to compensate for background color.

Automation of selecting, dipping, and discarding test strips prevents contact with potentially infectious samples. Trays for gathering and discarding used test strips are disposable and collect 200 or more used test strips.

Instruments to Read Reagent Strips and Analyze Sediment

International Remote Imaging Systems

International Remote Imaging Systems, Inc. (IRIS) markets three instruments that perform all elements of routine urinalysis: urine chemistries by CHEMSTRIP reagent test strips (Boehringer Mannheim), SG by harmonic oscillation, and automated sediment microscopic examination.

Test strips are measured using either an integrated or connected reader by the familiar technique of reflectance photometry. Specific gravity is determined using a unique procedure, termed "harmonic oscillation," which is based on the frequency attenuation of sound moving through solutions of varying densities. A known volume of urine is placed in a U-shaped tube, and a resonator at one end sends a sonic wave through the tube at a fixed frequency. As the wave exits the other end, a detector senses the change in frequency, which is inversely and directly related to the density or SG of the urine.

Formed elements such as blood cells and casts are analyzed in uncentrifuged urine without wet mounts or manual microscopic scans. After a specimen is introduced, it is automatically stained to enhance contrast, then injected into a patented, specially designed flow chamber in which sediment particles are hydrodynamically oriented in the correct focal plane. As the urine moves through the flow cell, a high-intensity strobe light flashing at 60 Hz illuminates the chamber interior and "freezes" particle motion, while a synchronized video camera captures images of the particles in the chamber through an objective lens. Each video "frame" is digitized in real time by the system computer, all particles in the frame are detected using edge tracing, and the particle images are computer-sorted by size and other parameters for visual presentation to the operator on a video monitor.

For clear specimens, only a low-power (×100) scan is performed; if particle concentrations exceed user-defined thresholds, an additional high-power scan (×400) is completed to allow full characterization of all analytes. The number of fields examined is fully programmable and can be adjusted for various specimen types. All particles of all types that can be detected microscopically are found and reported, and the instruments produce quantitative counts (per field or per microliter) based on the number of images of each particle type actually identified.

As noted later, the instruments can also perform cell counts on other body fluids, including cerebrospinal fluid (CSF), pleural fluid, peritoneal fluid, peritoneal lavage, peritoneal dialysate, pericardial fluid, seminal fluid, and synovial fluid.

MODEL 300 URINALYSIS WORKSTATION

With the Model 300, the operator begins urinalysis by identifying the specimen using the touch command screen, then wetting the CHEMSTRIP with specimen and placing it on the transport tray of the integrated strip reader. The strip is drawn into the reader and measured by a specially designed photometer, using photodiode detectors. Front-panel color LEDs are used to indicate any abnormal chemistry results.

Uncentrifuged urine (6 mL) is then poured into the entry port, and the specimen is conducted into the automated microscopic and SG subsystems for analysis, as described previously. When the sediment examination is finished, digitally reconstructed images of all particles detected are presorted into "most likely" type categories and displayed in a series of "pages" on the integrated video monitor. Each page contains a "montage" of images of like size; the operator can make any necessary corrections to the computer preclassifica-

tions of each image using simple touch commands. When all image screens have been reviewed and confirmed, the operator touches a final command to accept the results and send the report automatically to the laboratory information system (LIS) or the local printer. Analytical run time for a typical clear urine is less than 1 minute. Abnormals are usually completed in less than 2 minutes.

MODEL 500 URINE/FLUIDS WORKSTATION

The Model 500 operates in the same general manner as the Model 300, using the same CHEMSTRIP reader. Unlike the 300, it features full-color video imaging, which greatly enhances contrast for improved discrimination of casts, crystals, cells, and organisms. The Model 500 also uses a new high-speed image-processing computer, operating over 30% faster than that of the 300, and provides on-board capability to archive specimen image data on removable disk cartridges.

Body fluids analysis is standard on the Model 500 (optional on Model 300). To perform a body fluid examination, the operator selects Body Fluids mode with the touch screen, enters the specimen type, identifies the specimen, and pours 6 mL of fluid (diluted if necessary) into the entry port. The microscopic scan in low and high power and automatic particle enumeration are performed in the same manner as for urine. Chemistries and SG are not determined. For low-volume or highly concentrated specimens, a special diluent and dilution vial system are provided. Fluid counts on the Model 500 typically require no more than 3 minutes, compared with 10 to 15 minutes using manual hemacytometry.

900D_X URINE PATHOLOGY SYSTEM

This fully automated, high-capacity analyzer consists of three modular components: the Boehringer Mannheim Hitachi CHEMSTRIP Super UA Urine Analyzer (described previously in the section on Boehringer Mannheim), the IRIS FlowMicroscope, and an Intel Pentium microcomputer ViewStation running Microsoft Windows NT, which captures, consolidates, and manages the results from the two analytical units. Unlike the Model 300 or 500, the 900UD_x is a batch analyzer capable of processing up to 55 urine samples in an unattended manner.

The workflow sequence begins by loading barcoded tubes containing urine into a disk carousel transfer unit that fits on both the Super UA and the FlowMicroscope. First, the loaded carousel is mounted on the Super UA and the chemistry analyses are started. The Super UA reads each tube bar code, mixes the sample, wets a CHEMSTRIP test strip robotically, and transfers the strip to a photometer unit, where color change in each pad is measured and corrected for background color. Each result is transmitted to the ViewStation computer, where it is logged into an online database according to sample ID. Analysis of a full carousel is completed in 12 minutes with as little as 3 mL urine per tube. STAT samples can be inserted into the carousel for priority processing at any time during the batch.

After the chemistry analyses are completed, the entire carousel is then moved from the Super UA to the autosampler unit of the FlowMicroscope, and a one-touch command is given to start the batch of microscopic analyses. All tubes in the carousel are prescanned for bar code IDs, and the FlowMicroscope queries the ViewStation database in real time for analytical instructions for each individual tube. If so programmed by the user, only urine samples with a positive chemistry profile, or with a certain identification code or work order, will be examined, or the type or intensity of the examination can be automatically adjusted by specimen criteria in the database.

For urine samples that are to receive a sediment examination, SG determination by harmonic oscillation, or automated photometric color and clarity, the autosampler then aspirates sample into the instruments, directs urine to all the appropriate subsystems, and completes the sediment analysis in essentially the same manner as with Models 300 and 500. When each analysis is finished, all microscopic, SG, color, and clarity data are sent serially to the ViewStation, where they are matched with chemistries in the database and saved on the hard disk. Using routine programming, about 55 urine samples per hour can be examined with a full profile of microscopic, SG, and color/clarity, and throughput can increase dramatically if automatic "sieving of abnormals only" is programmed.

At the ViewStation, which can be located remotely from the Super UA and FlowMicroscope, review of the results can be completed at the operator's convenience. The software prioritizes specimens on a STAT and first-in, first-out basis. On beginning a review session, the software displays each specimen record as a single "page" containing all information (sediment particle images, chemistry/SG/color/clarity data, and any specimen-related data) to provide a comprehensive snapshot of the specimen on a high-resolution, 20″, color touch-screen monitor. Normals or urines with no unusual formed elements can be recognized and confirmed at a glance. Touching the "Accept" command ends the review and sends the report to the LIS.

If further visual confirmation of any particle images or corrections in classification are necessary, any group of images can be enlarged with a single touch command. The presence of abnormal chemistry results or unusual particles can be automatically highlighted on screen to draw operator attention. The ViewStation software also automatically tracks and monitors performance of all quality-control samples; permits user customization of screen displays; permits archiving of specimen records and retransmission of reports; and supports networking through the Windows NT operating system.

REFERENCES

1. Karselis TC. *The pocket guide to clinical laboratory instrumentation*. Philadelphia: FA Davis, 1994.

2. Strasinger SK. *Urinalysis and body fluids*. 3rd ed. Philadelphia: FA Davis, 1994.

BIBLIOGRAPHY

Anderson SC, Cockayne S. *Clinical chemistry*. Philadelphia: WB Saunders, 1993.
Bayer Corporation, Diagnostics Division (formerly AMES Division of Miles, Inc.). *Product information*. Elkhart, IN: Bayer Corporation, 1996.
Behring Diagnostics, Inc. *Product information*. Westwood, MA: Behring Diagnostics, Inc., 1996.
Bender GT. *Principles of chemical instrumentation*. Philadelphia: WB Saunders, 1987.
Boehringer-Mannheim Corporation. *Product information*. Indianapolis, IN: Boehringer-Mannheim Corporation, 1996.
Brunzel NA. *Fundamentals of urine and body fluid analysis*. Philadelphia: WB Saunders, 1994.
Burtis CA, Ashwood ER, eds. *Tietz' fundamentals of clinical chemistry*. 4th ed. Philadelphia: WB Saunders, 1996.
Hicks MR, Haven MC, Schenken JR, McWhorter CA, eds. *Laboratory instrumentation*. 3rd ed. Philadelphia: JB Lippincott, 1987.
International Remote Imaging Systems (IRIS). *Product information*. Chatsworth, CA: IRIS, 1996.
Kaplan LA, Pesce AJ. *Clinical chemistry*. 2nd ed. St. Louis: CV Mosby, 1989.
Narayanan S. *Principles and applications of laboratory instrumentation*. Chicago: ASCP Press, 1989.
Pincus MR, Preuss HG, Henry JB. Evaluation of renal function, water, electrolytes, acid–base balance, and blood gases. In: Henry JB, ed. *Clinical diagnosis and management*. 19th ed. Philadelphia: WB Saunders, 1996:139–161.
Ringsrud KM, Linné JJ. *Urinalysis and body fluids: A color text and atlas*. St. Louis: Mosby–Year Book, 1995.
Schoeff LE, Williams RH. *Principles of laboratory instruments*. St. Louis: Mosby–Year Book, 1993.
Ward KM, Lehmann CA, Leiken AM. *Clinical laboratory instrumentation and automation*. Philadelphia: WB Saunders, 1994.

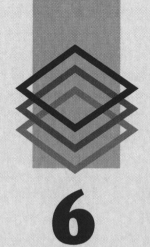

6

Physical Examination of Urine

Appearance

Although there are few occasions when the color, clarity, and odor of urine are of clinical significance, any unusual color, clarity, or odor should be noted on the report form.[2]

Color

Most urines are some shade of yellow; this coloration is largely due to the pigment urochrome and small amounts of urobilins and uroerythrin.[5] The color indicates roughly the degree of hydration and urine con-

---

TABLE 6-1
Appearance and Color of Urine

Appearance	Cause	Remarks
Colorless	Very dilute urine	Polyuria, diabetes insipidus
Cloudy	Phosphates, carbonates	Soluble in dilute acetic acid
	Urates, uric acid	Dissolve at 60°C and in alkali
	Leukocytes	Insoluble i dilute acetic acid
	Red cells ("smoky")	Lyse in dilute acetic acid
	Bacteria, yeasts	Insoluble in dilute acetic acid
	Spermatozoa	Insoluble in dilute acetic acid
	Prostatic fluid	
	Mucin, mucous threads	May be flocculent
	Calculi, "gravel"	Phosphates, oxalates
	Clumps, pus, tissue	
	Fecal contamination	Rectovesical fistula
	Radiographic dye	In acid urine
Milky	Many neutrophils (pyuria)	Insoluble in dilute acetic acid
	Fat	
	Lipiduria, opalescent	Nephrosis, crush injury—soluble in ether
	Chyluria, milky	Lymphatic obstruction—soluble in ether
	Emulsified paraffin	Vaginal creams
Yellow	Acriflavine	Green fluorescence
Yellow-orange	Concentrated urine	Dehydration, fever
	Urobilin in excess	No yellow foam
	Bilirubin	Yellow foam if sufficient bilirubin
Yellow-green	Bilirubin–biliverdin	Yellow foam
Yellow-brown	Bilirubin–biliverdin	"Beer" brown, yellow foam
Red	Hemoglobin	Positive ⎤
	Erythrocytes	Positive ⎬ reagent strip for blood
	Myoglobin	Positive ⎦
	Porphyrin	May be colorless
	Fuscin, aniline dye	Foods, candy
	Beets	Yellow alkaline, genetic
	Menstrual contamination	Clots, mucus
Red-purple	Porphyrins	May be colorless
Red-brown	Erythrocytes	
	Hemoglobin on standing	
	Methemoglobin	Acid pH
	Myoglobin	Muscle injury
	Bilifuscin (dipyrrole)	Result of unstable hemoglobin
Brown-black	Methemoglobin	Blood, acid pH
	Homogentisic acid	On standing, alkaline; alcaptonuria
	Melanin	On standing, rare
Blue-green	Indicans	Small intestine infections
	Pseudomonas infections	
	Chlorophyll	Mouth deodorants

(From Schumann GB, Schweitzer SC. Examination of urine. In Henry JB, ed. *Clinical diagnosis and management by laboratory methods.* 18th ed. Philadelphia: WB Saunders Company, 1991.)

centration; a dilute urine is pale, and a more concentrated urine is darker in color. However, a pale urine with high specific gravity may occur with diabetes mellitus (glucosuria), and after the administration of radiographic contrast dyes. Certain foods and drugs used for investigation and therapy may also impart colors to the urine. Table 6-1 summarizes the various colors that may be observed in urine.

Turbidity

Although a cloudy urine is not necessarily pathologic, turbidity in an uncentrifuged urine needs to be microscopically examined. Turbidity can be due to amorphous or crystalline solids, blood cells, epithelial cells, microorganisms, and spermatozoa. Turbidity may also be caused by blood clots, menstrual discharge, pieces of tissue, small calculi, clumps of pus, and fecal material (sometimes from a fistula between the colon or rectum and bladder).

Chyluria (lymph in the urine) is seldom observed. The appearance of the urine varies with the amount of lymph present, either normal, opalescent, or milky. Chyluria occurs with obstruction to the flow of lymph and rupture of the lymphatic vessels into the renal pelvis, ureters, bladder, or urethra. Chyluria has been associated with filariasis (late in the disease), abdominal lymph node enlargement, and tumors.

Odor

Normal urine has a "faintly aromatic" odor. Unsuitable specimens that have not been properly handled and have developed bacterial growth often produce a fetid or ammoniac odor. Certain foods (e.g., asparagus) impart odors to urine. Some of the aminoacidurias also produce characteristic odors such as the mousy or musty odor associated with phenylketonuria or the "burnt-sugar" odor observed with maple syrup urine disease.

Volume

As an aid in clinical diagnosis, determining the urine volume during timed intervals may be valuable. For a normal adult, the average daily volume of urine is 1200 to 1500 mL, with a normal range of 600 to 2000 mL.[5]

Polyuria refers to a urine volume of more than 2000 mL in 24 hours. An increase in urine volume is called diuresis. It may be associated with increased consumption of water, diabetes insipidus, diabetes mellitus, certain drugs (e.g., diuretics, caffeine, alcohol), and therapy with intravenous saline or glucose solutions. Continuous polyuria is associated classically with diabetes insipidus and diabetes mellitus.

Oliguria refers to the daily excretion of less than 500 mL of urine; anuria means the virtual absence of urine formation. Oliguric levels of urine formation may be associated with prolonged vomiting, diarrhea, or excessive sweating when inadequate replacement of water results in dehydration and hemoconcentration. Oliguria and anuria occur with renal ischemia, in which blood supply to the kidneys is inadequate due to heart failure or hypotension, and may also be observed after a major hemolytic transfusion reaction.

Renal disease and obstruction may also result in oliguria or anuria.

Concentration of Dissolved Solutes

To maintain homeostasis of body fluids and electrolytes, the kidneys vary the volume of excreted urine and the concentration of solute in the urine. This is accomplished by producing a urine that is much more concentrated than the plasma from which it was formed. The inability to produce a concentrated urine is often the first sign of renal disease and may also be a sign of hormone deficiency (e.g., antidiuretic hormone).

The solute concentration of urine can be quantitated by measuring either the specific gravity or the osmolality. The specific gravity is the ratio of the mass of a solution compared with the mass of an equal volume of water. This is actually a comparison of weights; it does not measure the exact number of solute particles. Osmolality is a measure of the number of dissolved particles in solution and reflects the concentrating ability of the kidney more than does specific gravity.

Normal adults with normal diets and normal fluid intake produce urine having a specific gravity of 1.016 to 1.022 during a 24-hour period. If a random specimen of urine has a specific gravity of 1.023 or more, concentrating ability can be considered normal.[5]

Hyposthenuria is a term that refers to urines of low specific gravity, less than 1.007. Isosthenuria means the specific gravity of multiple specimens from a patient remains fixed at about 1.010 and may indicate end-stage renal failure. Hypersthenuria refers to urine specimens with a specific gravity greater than 1.010. Methods that have been used in the routine measurement of specific gravity include the hydrometer, refractometer, dipstick reagent pad, and harmonic oscillation.

The hydrometer, a weighted glass float, uses displacement to estimate specific gravity. When it is calibrated for urine, it is called a urinometer. The device has several disadvantages, including the need for rather large volumes of urine, a correction if the temperature of the specimen is not at 20°C, and a correction for high amounts of glucose and protein. According to the National Committee for Clinical Laboratory Standards, a urinometer is not the method of choice for determining urine specific gravity.[2] This device is illustrated in Figure 6-1.

The refractometer method depends on the fact that light is refracted in proportion to the amount of total solids dissolved in a liquid. The refractometer is temperature-compensated for use between 15° and 38°C. Results should be corrected for large amounts of glucose or protein because they have no relationship to renal concentrating ability but nevertheless increase specimen density. Refractometer determinations of specific gravity are elevated by 0.003 for each gram per deciliter of protein and by 0.004 for each gram per deciliter of glucose. A refractometer is illustrated in Figure 6-2.

The dipstick reagent pad methodology is described in Chapter 7. The special device using harmonic oscillation to measure specific gravity, which is part of a urinalysis instrument produced by the International

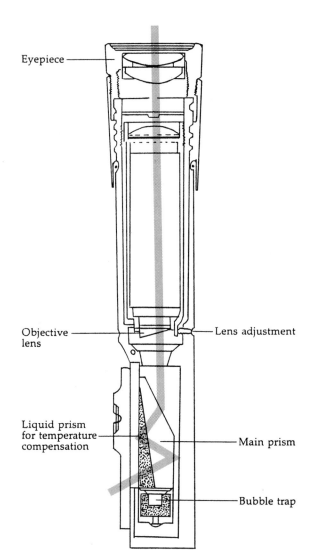

FIGURE 6-2 Schematic diagram of the total solids refractometer. (From Graff Sister L. A *handbook of routine urinalysis*. Philadelphia: Lippincott–Raven Publishers, 1981.)

Remote Imaging Systems corporation, is described in Chapter 5.

The colligative properties of solutions (osmotic pressure, vapor pressure, boiling point, and freezing point) are changed by varying the amounts of dissolved solutes. Note that at constant temperature, the extent of these changes is determined only by the number and *not* by the nature or mass of the particles in solution. A 1-molal solution of a nonelectrolyte such as glucose, which contains 1 g molecular weight (mole) dissolved in 1 kg of water, is defined as having an osmolality of 1 (or 1 Osm/kg water). This solution by definition contains Avogadro's number of particles (6.023×10^{23}). The osmolality of a 1-molal solution of an electrolyte is greater than 1 owing to the dissociation of electrolyte into component atoms in solution.

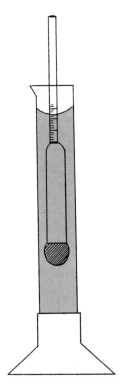

FIGURE 6-1 Urinometer for measuring specific gravity. (From Graff Sister L. A *handbook of routine urinalysis*, Philadelphia: Lippincott–Raven Publishers, 1981.)

The osmolality of an electrolyte solution is determined by the formula: osmolality = fnC, where f is the osmotic coefficient (a physical constant), n is the number of atoms that dissociate in solution, and C is the concentration of the electrolyte in moles per kilogram of water. Coefficients vary for each electrolyte because the dissociation into individual atoms is not complete and the individual particles may form secondary chemical bonds with solvent molecules.

Methods to measure osmolality could be developed based on any one of the four colligative properties. As a practical matter, however, instruments using freezing point depression or vapor pressure (dew point) have been favored. The time-honored approach has been the freezing point osmometer. These methods are discussed in Chapter 5.

Osmolality varies with the state of hydration. Maximally diluted or concentrated urine shows osmolalities between 50 and 1400 mOsm/kg water, respectively.

Urine osmolality corresponds well to urinary specific gravity in nondisease states, but the correlation is less reliable in renal disease states because of the greater contribution of high–molecular-weight substances (e.g., protein) to specific gravity than to osmolality.[3]

A normal adult on a normal diet with a normal fluid intake produces a urine of about 500 to 850 mOsm/kg water. The normal kidney is able to produce urine of osmolality in the range of 800 to 1400 mOsm/kg water in dehydration, and a minimal osmolality of 40 to 80 mOsm/kg water during water diuresis.

Renal function as related to osmolality and specific gravity is discussed in Chapter 3.

Quality Control

Commercial quality-control materials are available for the measurement of dissolved solutes in urine.

REFERENCES

1. Brunzel NA. *Fundamentals of urine and body fluid analysis.* Philadelphia: WB Saunders, 1994.
2. National Committee for Clinical Laboratory Standards. *Urinalysis and collection, transportation, and preservation of urine specimens: Approved guideline.* NCCLS Document GP16-A, Vol. 15, No. 15. Wayne, PA: NCCLS, December, 1995.
3. Preuss HG, Podlasek SJ, Henry JB. Evaluation of renal function and water, electrolyte, and acid–base balance. In: Henry JB, ed. *Clinical diagnosis and management by laboratory methods.* 18th ed. Philadelphia: WB Saunders, 1991:119–139.
4. Ringsrud KM, Linné JJ. *Urinalysis and body fluids: A color text and atlas.* St. Louis: Mosby–Year Book, 1995.
5. Schumann GB, Schweitzer SC. Examination of urine. In: Henry JB, ed. *Clinical diagnosis and management by laboratory methods.* 18th ed. Philadelphia: WB Saunders, 1991:387–444.
6. Strasinger SK. *Urinalysis and body fluids.* 3rd ed. Philadelphia: FA Davis, 1994.

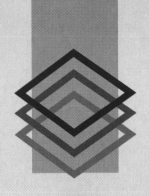

7 Chemical Examination of Urine

ABBREVIATIONS USED IN THIS CHAPTER

ABG = arterial blood gas

ADA = American Diabetic Association

AER = albumin excretion rate

ALA = delta-aminolevulinic acid

ALP = alkaline phosphatase

ALT = alanine aminotransferase

AST = aspartate aminotransferase

BUN = blood urea nitrogen

C&S = culture and sensitivity

CHD = coronary heart disease

CHF = congestive heart failure

CK = creatine kinase

CKMB = CK_3, a CK isoenzyme

CLIA = Clinical Laboratory Improvement Act

CPR = cardiopulmonary resuscitation

DKA = diabetic ketoacidosis

DM = diabetes mellitus

EGTA = ethyleneglycol-bis (aminoethylether) tetra-acetic acid

ER = emergency room

ESRD = end-stage renal disease

FDA = Food and Drug Administration

HPF = high-power field

HTN = hypertension

IDDM = insulin-dependent diabetes mellitus

LD = lactate dehydrogenase

LE = leukocyte esterase

LPF = low-power field

MI = myocardial infarction

NAD = nicotinamide adenine dinucleotide

NIDDM = non–insulin-dependent diabetes mellitus

(continued)

ABBREVIATIONS USED IN THIS CHAPTER		

PBG = porphobilinogen
PCP = phencyclidine
PMN = polymorphonuclear
  neutrophil
PT = prothrombin time
PTT = partial thromboplastin
  time
	QC = quality control
	RBC = red blood cell
	SOB = shortness of breath
	SSA = sulfosalicylic acid
	TCA = trichloroacetic acid
	TNTC = too numerous to
	  count
		U/L = international units per
		  liter
		UAE = urinary albumin
		  excretion
		UTI = urinary tract infection
		WBC = white blood cell

Introductory Case Study

The patient, a 42-year-old woman, was known to have a history of cirrhotic liver disease due to alcohol abuse. At 9:30 A.M. on the day of admission to the hospital, as she was lying in bed, her husband noticed that she was experiencing SOB and then stopped breathing altogether. He called 911, and the paramedics gave her CPR on the way to the hospital. In the hospital she was intubated and placed on a ventilator. Her admission diagnosis was respiratory arrest, hepatic encephalopathy/coma, and alcoholic liver disease.

The admission urinalysis was significant for: bilirubin moderate; blood moderate; pH 5.0; leukocyte esterase moderate; color amber; appearance cloudy; WBCs/HPF 20–50; RBCs 10–20/HPF; bacteria 4+; and Ictotest positive. A drug abuse panel on her urine was positive for PCP (phencyclidine, "angel dust") and for amphetamines. After these analyses, UTI and amphetamines/PCP abuse were added to the admission diagnosis. The urine C&S was positive for *Escherichia coli*.

Admission blood work (reference values in parentheses) was significant for: total bilirubin 4.2 mg/dL (0–1.5); conjugated bilirubin 3.4 mg/dL (0–0.4); ALP 272 U/L (37–107); AST 53 U/L (8–42); ALT 9 U/L (3–36); total protein 5.0 g/dL (6.4–8.2); albumin 1.4 g/dL (3.4–5.0); LD 475 U/L (100–190); uric acid 7.4 mg/dL (2.4–5.1); BUN 37 mg/dL (5–25); creatinine 2.1 mg/dL (0.6–1.0); CO_2 11 mEq/L (24–35); anion gap 27 (1–11); blood ammonia 221 μmol/L (11–35); lactic acid 16 mmol/L (0.3–2.4); PT 16.4 seconds (<13); and PTT 91.9 seconds (25–40). Arterial blood gases (ABG) on admission were significant for: pH 7.03 (7.38–7.46); CO_2 32 mm Hg (32–46); and HCO_3 8 mEq/L (21–29).

The Multistix results on the urine that correlate with the diagnosis of alcoholic liver disease in this case are increased bilirubin and a positive Ictotest. The blood chemistries that correlate with this diagnosis are the increased bilirubin (total and conjugated); the elevated ALP, ALT, and ammonia; the decreased total protein and albumin; and the prolonged PT and PTT. Uric acid, BUN, and creatinine were elevated, suggesting some degree of renal ischemia due to the respiratory and cardiac arrest. The increased anion gap correlates with the elevated lactic acid, which, in turn, is probably correlated with the respiratory arrest and anaerobic metabolism. The impaired liver function probably contributed to the lactate remaining elevated.

The patient was given supportive therapy for her liver disease and drug abuse as well as antibiotics for her urinary tract infection. She was eventually discharged in stable condition.

Reagent Strips

Despite their ease of use, reagent test strips for urine encompass complex, multiple, state-of-the-art chemical reactions. This complexity should not be overlooked or taken for granted. The chemical examination of urine rests on the reagent strip methodology, although confirmatory tests and other procedures may be required for certain patient populations and under special circumstances.[12]

A reagent test-strip (or dipstick) is a narrow band of plastic 4 to 6 mm wide and 11 to 12 cm long with a linear series of small absorbent pads attached to it. Each pad contains reagents for a separate reaction, so several tests can be carried out simultaneously. It is very important that the reactions are read at the prescribed time after the strip is dipped in urine and compared closely with the color chart provided by the manufacturer.

There are three major manufacturers of chemical reagent strips: Bayer Corporation—Diagnostics Division (Elkhart, IN; formerly Ames division of Miles, Inc.), which produces Multistix; Boehringer-Mannheim Corporation (Indianapolis, IN), which manufactures Chemstrip; and Behring Diagnostics, Inc. (Somerville, NJ), which produces Rapignost. With the exception of the test pad for urobilinogen, the chemical methodologies used on all the reagent strips are variations on a theme, as discussed later. Suggestions for the proper storage and use of reagent test strips are provided in Table 7-1.

The colors produced on the various reagent pads can be interpreted visually by means of the color charts provided with the reagent strips, or they can be read

---

TABLE 7-1
Recommendations for Reagent Strips

Storage

Protect from moisture and excessive heat.

Store in cool, dry area but not in a refrigerator.

Check for discoloration with each use; discoloration may indicate loss of reactivity. Do not use discolored strips or tablets.

Keep container tightly stoppered.

Check manufacturer's directions with each new lot number for changes in procedure.

Testing

Test urine as soon as possible after receipt.

Remove only enough strips for immediate use; recap tightly.

Test a well mixed, unspun urine sample.

Urine samples must be at room temperature before testing.

Do not touch the test area with fingers.

Do not use reagent strips in the presence of volatile acids or alkaline fumes.

Dip reagent strip into urine briefly—no longer than 1 second.

Drain excess urine off—run edge of strip along rim of tube, or blot edge on absorbent paper.

Do not allow reagents to run together.

Do not lay reagent strip directly on work bench surface.

Follow exact timing recommendations for each chemical test.

Hold reagent strip close to the color chart and read under good lighting.

Know sources of error, sensitivity, and specificity of each test on the reagent strip.

Think! Make correlations between patient history and individual test, then follow through.

(From Schumann GB, Schweitzer SC: Examination of urine. In Henry JB: [ed]. *Clinical diagnosis and management by laboratory methods*. 18th ed. Philadelphia: WB Saunders Company, 1991.)

---

photometrically using instruments developed by each reagent strip manufacturer. A dipstick reader helps avoid some of the variability in testing related to the differences in color perception from person to person. These instruments, along with the specialized Yellow IRIS workstation developed by International Remote Imaging Systems, are discussed in Chapter 5.

Tablet and Chemical Tests

Tablet and chemical tests are used to confirm results obtained by dipstick methods when there are differences in sensitivity (e.g., bilirubin) and specificity (e.g., sulfosalicylic acid [SSA] for protein, Clinitest for galactose), or to avoid interferences when pigments in the specimens mask the colors obtained on the reagent pads. Tablet tests such as Ictotest (for bilirubin), Clinitest (for reducing sugars), and Acetest (for ketone bodies) are available to confirm results obtained on the reagent test strips, and are discussed later in relation to the applicable reagent strip test. As is true for reagent test strips, reagents in tablet form should be properly stored and used according to manufacturer's instructions, and they should also be included in the QC program.

An entirely new approach, avoiding the need for dipsticks and dipstick readers, has been taken by CRC (Chimera Research and Chemical, Inc., Tampa, Florida) in the development of their UA Perfect 10 Automatic Urinalysis System for human urine. CRC has received U.S. Food and Drug Administration (FDA) clearance for this system using liquid reagents for quantitative urinalysis on automated spectrophotometric analyzers. Application sheets are available for use of the system on the Hitachi 717. The system currently measures pH, specific gravity, ketones (acetoacetic acid), blood (hemoglobin), leukocyte esterase (LE), nitrite, protein, glucose, bilirubin, and urobilinogen. The CRC system also has FDA clearance for creatinine (CR Perfect), and also for glutaraldehyde (AD Perfect), a common adulterant used to interfere with drugs of abuse testing.

pH

As discussed in Chapter 3, the kidneys, along with the lungs and blood buffers, are part of the essential mechanism for the regulation and maintenance of a normal hydrogen ion concentration in the plasma and extracellular fluid. So-called "fixed acids" such as sulfuric, phosphoric, and hydrochloric are produced as byproducts of metabolism along with small amounts of organic acids (pyruvic, lactic, and citric acids and ketone bodies). Unlike carbonic acid, which can be converted to carbon dioxide and eliminated by the lungs, these fixed acids are excreted by the kidneys along with cations such as sodium. The tubular cells reabsorb sodium ions in exchange for hydrogen ions and the urine becomes acid.

The pH of normal urine[12] ranges from about 5 to 8. Because endogenous acid production predominates, the average person excretes a urine that is slightly acid, pH 5.0 to 6.0. After a meal, however, the urine becomes less acid (the so-called "alkaline tide") as the parietal cells of the stomach secrete hydrochloric acid for digestion, leaving behind bicarbonate ion that enters the interstitial fluid and the blood to be finally filtered by the kidneys.

Causes of an acid urine include dietary effects (e.g., large amounts of meat, some fruits such as cranberries), metabolic acidosis, respiratory acidosis, and medications designed to maintain an acid urine in treatment for the formation of some calculi (e.g., calcium carbonate). Causes of an alkaline urine include dietary effects (e.g., a vegetarian diet or high amounts of citrus fruits), metabolic alkalosis, respiratory alkalosis, certain renal diseases (e.g., renal tubular acidosis), and medications designed to maintain an alkaline urine in treatment for the formation of some calculi (e.g., calcium oxalate).

The pH pad on all the different brands of reagent strips functions by means of acid–base indicators in various combinations. The Rapignost system uses bromothymol blue, cresol red, and methyl red; the Multistixpad contains bromothymol blue and methyl red; and the Chemstrip pad contains bromothymol blue, methyl red, and phenolphthalein. With these systems, as the pH shifts from acid to alkaline, the colors range from orange through yellow and green to blue. The range extends from pH 5.0 to 9.0 in either 0.5 or 1.0 pH unit increments, depending on the manufacturer.

Although two manufacturers state that there are no known interferences that affect the results, regardless of the reagent strip used, erroneous results can occur if the specimen is improperly stored or preserved so that bacteria proliferate and convert urea to ammonia, resulting in a strongly alkaline urine.

The UA Perfect Automated Urinalysis System uses the indicator principle; no specific information on the dyes used is available.[14] This system is a spectrophotometric measurement and the reagents give a broad range of color intensity, covering the entire urinary pH range.

Protein

Urinary proteins are normally present in only trace amounts, up to about 150 mg/24 hours or 10 mg/dL, and originate in the plasma and urinary tract.[12] Albumin is about a third of the total; the remaining plasma proteins are small globulins.

Small plasma proteins (molecular weight < 50,000–60,000 daltons) pass through the glomerulus, are normally reabsorbed by the tubular cells, and do not appear in the urine. Albumin, with a molecular weight of approximately 70,000 daltons, is apparently filtered, but only in tiny amounts, and is also reabsorbed. Tamm-Horsfall glycoprotein is secreted by the tubular cells and makes up about one third or more of the total protein normally lost.

Proteinuria is often the first finding in cases of renal disease. The dipstick result should be confirmed by an independent method such as SSA precipitation. Acid precipitation methods detect all proteins, although not with equal sensitivity.[6] Proteinuria may be observed in healthy individuals after strenuous exercise or with dehydration; in patients with hemorrhage or salt depletion; and in febrile illnesses possibly due to dehydration and relative renal ischemia.[12]

Because protein has a very low maximal tubular rate of reabsorption (T_m), increased filtration or production soon saturates the reabsorptive mechanism. Thus, detection of an abnormal amount of protein in the urine is one of the most reliable indicators of renal disease. The degree of protein excretion is determined by analyzing a urine specimen collected over a 24-hour period. Although they are modified by the patient's history and examination, confirmatory tests for protein are usually accompanied by tests of renal function, examination of the urine sediment, and urine culture.[12] Proteinuria can be separated into a glomerular pattern, a tubular pattern, and an overflow pattern.

The glomerular pattern is characterized by proteins that would usually be retained in the plasma, such as albumin, transferrin, prealbumin, and other proteins of similar size or charge. Very small plasma proteins are mostly reabsorbed because tubular functions may still be normal. The nephrotic syndrome is associated with glomerular disease states and is diagnosed when the protein excretion is greater than 3.0 to 3.5 g/dL or 2 g/m²/24 hours. In addition to heavy proteinuria, the nephrotic syndrome is characterized by low serum albumin, generalized edema, and increased serum lipids. Many granular casts, fatty casts, and fat-filled renal tubular epithelial cells (oval fat bodies) as well as cholesterol droplets are found when lipid is lost in the urine. Common causes of the nephrotic syndrome are mentioned later in the discussion of heavy proteinuria.

The tubular pattern is associated with loss of urinary protein that would otherwise be largely reabsorbed and involves proteins of low molecular weight (e.g., alpha$_1$-microglobulin, beta$_2$-microglobulin, and immunoglobulin light chains). The tubular pattern occurs with renal tubular disease such as Fanconi's syndrome, Wilson's disease, and pyelonephritis. With glomerular diseases, the level of proteinuria is lower, approximately 1 to 2 g/day.[12] Because reagent strips are designed primarily to detect albumin, tubular proteinuria may not be detected, although acid precipitation tests are positive.

Increased amounts of proteins appearing in the circulation (e.g., hemoglobin, myoglobin, or immunoglobulins) are filtered by the glomeruli and produce overflow proteinuria. Reabsorption of large amounts of such proteins is damaging to the tubular cells. Myoglobin causes acute tubular necrosis.

Bence Jones proteins are immunoglobulin light chains and are excreted by up to 80% of multiple myeloma patients. Bence Jones proteinuria can be demonstrated in several ways, although electrophoresis and immunoelectrophoresis techniques are best. Bence Jones proteinuria shows up with the SSA precipitation method, although it may not be detected by the reagent strip methodologies because they are most sensitive to albumin. Large amounts of Bence Jones proteins cause the tubular cells to degenerate because of the high levels of protein reabsorbed. Inclusions may form in the cells, and casts containing the desquamated cells are observed in the sediment. The damaged kidney is sometimes called a myeloma kidney.

So-called "functional proteinuria" is associated with conditions that cause a type of mild glomerular or mixed pattern of proteinuria without the presence of renal disease. These include strenuous exercise, fever, hypothermia, emotional distress, congestive heart failure, and dehydration. Mechanisms appear to involve changes in glomerular blood flow or increased glomerular permeability. The conditions are transitory and are resolved with time and supportive treatment. The amount of protein excreted is usually less than 1 g/day.

Postural or orthostatic proteinuria is considered to be a functional proteinuria. In this condition, proteinuria occurs only when the individual is in an orthostatic or upright position. Postural proteinuria is usually less than 1.5 g/dL and is usually considered to be a benign condition, although renal biopsy has revealed glomerular abnormalities in a few patients. The loss of protein in the urine is apparently related to lordosis, producing renal congestion or ischemia.[12]

To test for this condition, an individual collects two urine specimens: a first-morning specimen and a second specimen collected after the patient has been standing and walking about for 2 hours or more. The two urine specimens are tested for protein. If the first specimen is negative while the second is positive for protein, the patient may have postural proteinuria.

The reagent strip methodologies are based on the "protein error of pH indicators." At a constant pH, proteins act as hydrogen ion acceptors and cause certain acid–base indicator dyes to release hydrogen ions and change color. The reagent pad for protein contains various dyes, depending on the manufacturer, and a buffer to keep the pH at 3.0. Rapignost has tetrabromophenol blue, Multistix has tetrabromophenol blue, and Chemstrip has 3', 3″, 5', 5″-tetrachlorophenol-3,4,5,6-tetrabromosulfophthalein. The sensitivity of the reagent test strip methods ranges from 6 to 30 mg/dL protein, depending on the manufacturer.

A major source of error for the reagent pad method occurs with a highly alkaline urine, which neutralizes the buffer system and produces an alkaline reaction that causes a color change unrelated to protein concentration. Allowing the reagent strip to "soak" in the urine leaches the buffer out of the pad and permits a color change also unrelated to protein concentration. Rarely observed with the use of clean, disposable urine containers, contamination of the container with alkaline cleaning agents may cause false-positive results. High salt concentrations decrease the sensitivity of the reagent pad.

The UA Perfect Automated Urinalysis System measures protein spectrophotometrically by means of the dye-binding method. Coomassie blue is dissolved in an acid medium and reacts with protein to form a colored protein–dye complex. The amount of color produced is proportional to the protein concentration. The test is specific for protein, although not all proteins react equally. Elevated hemoglobin (>250 $\mu g/dL$), a highly buffered (1.0 mol/L) urine, or an abnormal urine pH (pH < 4.0 or > 9.0) may alter protein results. Strongly basic urine (pH 9.0+) may result in false-positive results, as may the presence of ascorbic acid (50 mg/dL), certain medications, or quaternary ammonia compounds/detergents contaminating the urine container.

Precipitation tests for protein involve an organic acid like SSA, TCA (trichloroacetic acid), or acetic acid. The most commonly used reagent is SSA. The amount of centrifuged urine, as well as the volume and concentration of acid used, varies greatly among laboratories, although, in general, the final concentration of SSA in the urine is very much the same.

The SSA reagent and urine supernatant are added together, mixed by inversion, and allowed to stand for 10 minutes at room temperature before being evaluated. After 10 minutes, the specimen is mixed again by inversion and observed in ordinary room light. In many laboratories the precipitation reaction is graded as negative, trace, 1+, 2+, 3+, and 4+ according to various protocols involving factors such as turbidity without discrete granulation, ability to read newsprint through the mixture, visibility of a ring or circle in the bottom of the test tube when viewed from above, and so forth. In other laboratories the precipitation reaction is graded with concentration values of milligrams per deciliter (rather than 1+, etc.) corresponding to a series of protein standards. The sensitivity of the method is approximately 5 to 20 mg/dL of protein, depending on the reference consulted.

False-positive results for the SSA procedure include nonprotein substances precipitated by the acid (e.g., radiographic dyes and certain drugs). Such precipitates are seen to be crystalline when viewed microscopically, whereas protein precipitates are amorphous. False-negative results can occur with highly alkaline urine, which neutralizes the SSA.

A considerable body of literature has developed relating minimal proteinuria or "microproteinuria" (Albustix negative) to the subsequent development of clinical proteinuria (Albustix positive) and diabetic nephropathy. This literature also emphasizes the desirability of identifying proteinuric patients early enough to take corrective action by encouraging tighter glycemic control.[1,2]

Most studies have focused on albuminuria and its measurement. As summarized by Hawthorne,[4] later occurrence of major disease events in diabetics is correlated with early and persistent increases in "microalbuminuria." For approximately 80% of patients with insulin-dependent diabetes mellitus (IDDM), persistently increased urinary albumin excretion (UAE) is associated with diabetic nephropathy, end-stage renal disease (ESRD), and proliferative retinopathy. For patients with non–insulin-dependent diabetes mellitus (NIDDM), persistently increased UAE is also associated with diabetic nephropathy (25% of cases), together with increased risk of coronary heart disease (CHD) and mortality.

For patients with IDDM and increased UAE, studies have shown[4] that treatment of hypertension, improved glycemic control, and restriction of dietary protein may reduce, arrest, or reverse the rate of increase of UAE and slow the rate of renal function decline. Further, for obese NIDDM patients with increased UAE, it has been shown[4] that a hypocaloric low-protein diet with concomitant weight loss, reduction in blood pressure, and improved glycemic control can reduce UAE and presumably also decrease the risk for nephropathy and CHD, and reduce patient mortality.

Minimal proteinuria or microproteinuria has been defined in several ways. Perhaps the most accepted definition was formulated in 1985 at a meeting in Europe of researchers from three major diabetes centers. In this formulation, microalbuminuria is defined as an albumin excretion rate (AER) of more than 20 μg/minute but less than or equal ($\leq$) to 200 μg/minute in at least two of three timed urine collections.[7] For random specimens, assuming an average urine flow of 1500 mL/24 hours, these numbers become more than 2 mg/dL but less than or equal to 20 mg/dL.

On the other hand, Hindmarsh[5] pointed out that, in a 24-hour urine collection from a "normal" person, albumin excretion is less than 20 μg/minute (or <2 mg/dL, assuming a urine volume of 1500 mL/day). On this basis, he suggested that the preferred detection limit for microalbuminuria in random specimens should be 0.5 mg/dL, with a range of 0.5 to 20 mg/dL.

Several recently developed methods for measuring trace amounts of proteins include radioimmunoassay, enzyme-linked immunosorbent assay, and immunonephelometric and immunoturbidimetric procedures; however, these methods do not necessarily lend themselves to simple screening for minimal proteinuria. Two screening methods are available, the Micro-Bumintest (Bayer), and the Chemstrip Micral Urine Test Strip (Boehringer-Mannheim).

The Micro-Bumintest is designed to detect minute amounts of albumin in urine (microalbuminuria) to monitor patients for impending diabetic nephropathy. Early detection of microalbuminuria and aggressive control of the diabetes is a means to forestall further damage to the kidney.

The Micro-Bumintest is based on the principle of the protein error of indicators. The test tablet contains salicylic acid and bromophenol blue indicator. A drop of urine containing albumin is placed on the tablet and two drops of water are added to wash the urine through the tablet. The albumin remains on the surface of the tablet, where it reacts with the indicator to produce a bluish-green spot or ring. Any bluish-green spot or ring that is seen on the tablet surface after the water has been absorbed should be considered as a presumptive positive reaction.

Positive reactions are usually found at albumin concentrations between 4 to 8 mg/dL. In some cases, a positive reaction may be found at lower albumin concentrations. Note that the sensitivity of Multistix is stated to be 15 to 30 mg/dL albumin; for Rapignost, the sensitivity is 12 mg/dL; and for Chemstrip it is 6 mg/dL . False-positive results occur with strongly alkaline urines and with contamination of the urine specimen with quaternary ammonium compounds or with skin cleansers containing chlorhexidine. With very low concentrations of albumin and urines with high specific gravity, a background color caused by the salts left behind on the tablet surface may hinder the visibility of the faint bluish-green spot developed with the albumin.

The second method for detecting microalbuminuria is the Chemstrip Micral Urine Test Strip.[3] In this method, a soluble antibody–enzyme complex present on a zone of the test strip specifically binds with the albumin in the urine. In a separation zone containing immobilized human albumin, excess conjugate is retained, allowing only the conjugate–albumin immunocomplex from the sample to reach the reaction zone. In the reaction zone, a red dye is produced from the reaction between beta-galactosidase and a substrate. The color is allowed to develop for 5 minutes, and the intensity is proportional to the amount of albumin in the urine.[3] Levels of the color blocks are 0, 10, 20, 50, and 100 mg/L, and a sensitivity in the range of 1 mg/dL albumin is suggested. The test is specific for human albumin and appears to be free from drug interferences, but specimens should not be collected in containers that have been cleaned with strong oxidizing agents.

Glucose

Glucosuria (or glycosuria) is the presence of glucose in the urine. Glucosuria can be associated with prerenal conditions causing hyperglycemia (elevated blood glucose) or to the renal condition of defective tubular absorption of glucose.

Glucose in the blood is freely filtered by the glomeruli but actively reabsorbed by the renal tubules, so that urine normally contains only trace amounts of glucose. With hyperglycemia, glucose increases to the point that it exceeds the renal threshold (approximately 160–180 mg/dL) and spills over into the urine because the tubules are no longer able to reabsorb all of it. Hyperglycemia may occur with diabetes mellitus (DM), various hormonal disorders, liver and pancreatic disease, and with certain drugs. Defective tubular reabsorption of glucose can be associated with such conditions as Fanconi's syndrome, heavy metal poisoning, and pregnancy.[12]

The reagent strip methodologies for glucose all use a similar double-sequential enzyme system but differ in the type of chromogen used. The first reaction is with glucose and the enzyme glucose oxidase, which results in the production of gluconic acid and hydrogen peroxide. The second reaction is with a peroxidase enzyme that uses the peroxide from the first reaction to oxidize a chromogen on the reagent pad. For the Multistix reagent strip, the chromogen is potassium iodide; for Chemstrip and Rapignost, it is tetramethylbenzidine.

The Chemstrip color chart reports glucose as negative (normal), or from 1/20 to 1 g/dL. The Multistix color chart reports glucose as negative, or from 100 mg/dL to greater than or equal to ($\geq$) 2000 mg/dL (from 0.1% to 2%). The Rapignost color chart reports glucose as negative, 50 mg/dL, 150 mg/dL, but not greater than 500 mg/dL. In dilute urine containing less than 5 mg/dL ascorbic acid, Multistix are sensitive down to 40 mg/dL glucose, and the generally detectable levels are given as 75 to 125 mg/dL.[8] The maximum sensitivity of the Rapignost reagent strip for glucose is stated to be to 20 mg/dL,[10] and for Chemstrip 40 mg/dL[2].

As stated in the product inserts,[2,8,10] the reagent strip test is specific for glucose. No substance excreted in urine other than glucose is known to give a positive result, although reactivity may be influenced by urine specific gravity and temperature. False-positive results occur when strong oxidizing agents (bleach) or peroxides (microbial) are present in the urine. False-negative results occur with reducing agents (ascorbic acid), which prevent oxidation of the chromogen. False-negative results occur by allowing specimens to remain unpreserved at room temperature for extended periods of time so that living cells that may be present in the urine consume the glucose before it can be detected.

The UA Perfect Automated Urinalysis System uses the enzyme glucose dehydrogenase to convert glucose to gluconic acid, with the simultaneous reduction of the coenzyme nicotinamide adenine dinucleotide (NAD). The reduced coenzyme is measured spectrophotometrically. Results may be altered by the presence of hemoglobin (>250 μg/dL), a highly buffered (1.0 mol/L) urine, or an abnormal urine pH (pH < 4.0 or > 9.0). False-positive results may occur as a result of a container contaminated by strong oxidizing agents. Ascorbic acid does not interfere unless the concentration exceeds 100 mg/dL.

Clinitest

One of the earliest chemical tests performed on urine was the measurement of glucose (a reducing sugar) by copper reduction methods. In hot alkaline solution, glucose converts cupric sulfate to cuprous oxide. Other reducing sugars (e.g., galactose) as well as other reducing agents (e.g., ascorbic acid, uric acid) react in the same way. For many years, this methodology has been available in tablet form as the Clinitest for the semiquantitative determination of glucose and other reducing substances in the urine.

The Clinitest tablet contains copper sulfate, sodium carbonate, sodium citrate, and sodium hydroxide. When it is placed in a mixture of water and urine, the tablet is rapidly dissolved by the action of sodium carbonate and citric acid, which act as effervescents. The sodium carbonate releases carbon dioxide which forms a layer over the reaction mixture to prevent room air from interfering with the reduction reaction. The sodium hydroxide provides the alkaline medium necessary for the reaction, and the heat required is provided by the reaction of sodium hydroxide with water and citric acid.

At the conclusion of the effervescent reaction, colors ranging from blue to orange can be compared with the manufacturer's color chart to determine the approximate amount of glucose present. The package insert gives important precautions to be followed in the test, including alertness to excessively high amounts of glucose, which leads to a phenomenon known as the "pass through."

In the presence of high amounts of reducing substances, the reaction mixture "passes through" all possible colors to orange—the highest concentration—and then reverts back to a color (greenish brown) characteristic of a low concentration. What occurs is the re-oxidation of the cuprous oxide back to the original cupric oxide together with other cupric complexes. Thus, falsely low results for glucose would be indicated. This error is avoided if the laboratorian adheres to the manufacturer's procedural directions.

Note that the Clinitest method is nonspecific for glucose and is subject to interference from other reducing sugars and other reducing agents such as ascorbic acid, certain drug metabolites, and antibiotics such as the cephalosporins.

Because the reagent strip methodologies have improved so much in sensitivity and specificity, many laboratories no longer confirm a positive dipstick for glucose by carrying out a copper reduction test. However, various circumstances may result in the appearance of other sugars in the urine. The most important of these is the reducing sugar galactose. Galactose is excreted in the urine of individuals affected by an inherited enzyme deficiency that results in galactosemia. This metabolic defect has several forms; all involve the absence or low activity of one of the enzymes necessary for the conversion of galactose to glucose. Lactose, or milk sugar, is a disaccharide formed from the two monosaccharides glucose and galactose, and is the main dietary source of galactose.

It is important to recognize infants born with this enzyme deficiency as early as possible, in order to remove milk from their diet and thus avoid cataract formation, hepatic dysfunction, and severe mental retardation. These effects are due to the accumulation of toxic intermediates resulting from the impaired metabolism of galactose. At first, the symptoms are vomiting, diarrhea, and failure to thrive, but the more serious effects of the disease develop within a few weeks. Normal growth and development are possible if the condition is recognized early enough and galactose is eliminated from the diet.

Many states now require newborns to be screened for galactosemia. Because galactosuria results from galactosemia, many institutions use the Clinitest initially to screen pediatric urines for this reducing sugar. If the urine test is positive, more definitive studies can then be carried out

Ketones

With incomplete fat metabolism, which is most commonly observed with uncontrolled DM, three compounds ("ketone bodies") are formed, appear in the blood (ketonemia), and are excreted in the urine (ketonuria): acetoacetic acid, acetone, and beta-hydroxy-

butyric acid. The acetoacetic acid is formed from excess acetyl-coenzyme A, which accumulates because of decreased activity of the Krebs cycle associated with low levels of intermediates, which, in turn, associated with decreased utilization of glucose. Acetoacetic acid gives rise irreversibly to acetone by decarboxylation and to beta-hydroxybutyric acid by reduction (which is reversible). In addition to diabetic ketoacidosis (DKA), ketonuria is also observed with acute febrile illnesses, starvation, low–carbo-cal diets, and toxic states accompanied by vomiting and diarrhea.

The basis for all reagent strip testing for ketones is the nitroprusside (sodium nitroferricyanide) reaction. The ketone reagent pad for both the Chemstrip and the Rapignost reagent strips contains sodium nitroferricyanide and glycine, which react with acetoacetic acid as well as with acetone in an alkaline medium to form a violet-colored product. The Multistix ketone reagent pad contains buffers and sodium nitroferricyanide, which react only with acetoacetic acid (but not acetone), producing a pink-maroon color. False-positive results occur in the presence of certain dyes (phthaleins) or large amounts of phenylketones, the preservative 8-hydroxyquinoline, or L-dopa metabolites. The antihypertensive drugs methyldopa and captopril give positive results. False-negative results occur due to decreased reagent reactivity or loss of labile ketones from the specimen.

The UA Perfect Automated Urinalysis System test for ketone bodies is based on the development of color due to the reaction of acetoacetic acid with nitroprusside. The assay detects acetoacetic acid in urine and does not react with acetone or beta-hydroxybutyric acid. The presence of elevated bilirubin (>3.0 mg/dL) or hemoglobin (>250 μg/dL) may increase ketone values.

Acetest

Just as for the reagent strips, the Acetest tablet contains sodium nitroprusside and a strongly alkaline buffer, but it also contains glycine; therefore, it detects both acetoacetic acid and acetone. Whole blood, plasma, serum, or urine can be analyzed. Although a few laboratories may still use the Acetest tablet to confirm a positive reagent strip reaction, the tablet test may be more useful if the urine has an interfering color. The tablet detects 5 to 10 mg acetoacetic acid/dL of urine and 20 to 25 mg acetone/dL of urine. False-positive and false-negative reactions occur for the same reasons as described for the reagent strips.

Blood

As discussed in more detail later, the basis of the method for detecting red blood cells, free hemoglobin, and free myoglobin in the urine depends on the presence of the heme ring (or nucleus). Red blood cells can enter the urinary tract anywhere from the glomeruli to the urethra. Red blood cells also may be present as a contaminant in an improperly collected specimen. The presence of intact RBCs in the urine is termed hematuria, and can be related to several possible causes: renal and urinary tract diseases such as glomerulonephritis, pyelonephritis, cystitis, calculi, and tumors; extrarenal disease; trauma and strenuous exercise; and certain drugs (e.g., cyclophosphamide).

Hemoglobin may enter the urine directly through the glomeruli from the blood. Causes for this situation include intravascular hemolysis, as with transfusion reactions and hemolytic anemias; extensive burns; strenuous exercise (march hemoglobinuria); and certain infections. More commonly, hemoglobinuria occurs when intact RBCs enter the urine through the glomerulus and undergo lysis in the urinary tract, liberating their hemoglobin.

Myoglobin is small enough to pass the glomerular filtration barrier and is increased with muscle trauma (e.g., crushing injury, surgery, ischemia); muscle-wasting diseases and polymyositis; seizures; and severe exercise.

With both hemoglobinuria and myoglobinuria, the urine is dark red or brown, and some erythrocytes are observed in the sediment.[12] Thus, it is difficult to distinguish between hemoglobinuria and myoglobinuria by a simple examination of the urine. Hemoglobin and some myoglobin are bound to proteins in the urine, which contributes to the difficulty of separating them by salt precipitation or cellulose acetate electrophoresis. Immunochemical tests are available and are preferred because they are specific. End-point and rate nephelometric methods are also available.

The chemical tests for blood use the pseudoperoxidase or peroxidase-like activity of the heme moiety to catalyze the reaction between a peroxide and the reduced form of a chromogen to produce an oxidized chromogen that has a blue or green color, depending on the system. For the Multistix reagent pad, the oxidant is diisopropylbenzene dihydroperoxide and the chromogen is tetramethylbenzidine. The Rapignost method uses cumene hydroperoxide and tetramethylbenzidine dihydrochloride. The Chemstrip system uses tetramethylbenzidine and 2,3-dimethyl-2,5-dihydroperoxyhexane. Hemoglobin or myoglobin produce solid shades of green to greenish-blue on the reagent pads. In all cases, intact RBCs are lysed on contact with the reagent pad.

If only a few to a moderate number of cells are present, a speckled green pattern on a yellow background is produced, although, with a grossly bloody specimen, the pad will be a dark, solid bluish green. Depending on the brand of reagent strip used, the range is 0.015 to 0.062 mg/dL hemoglobin, or 5 to 20 RBCs/μL.

False-positive results are associated with the presence of strong oxidants and microbial peroxidases. False-negative results are observed with high levels of ascorbic acid ($\geq$9 mg/dL for Multistix; 5 mg/dL or more for Rapignost; Chemstrip unaffected); high amounts of urinary nitrite ($\geq$10 mg/dL); and high salt and protein levels, which tend to decrease the lysis of the RBCs on the reagent pad.

The UA Perfect Automated Urinalysis System assay for blood is specific for hemoglobin. It depends on the strong pseudoperoxidase action of the heme nucleus found in the hemoglobin. In this system, a chromogen is oxidized by an organic peroxide under the influence of the heme to produce a measurable color. False-positive results may be caused by menstrual contamination, strong oxidizing detergents in the specimen container, or bacterial peroxidases. High levels of ascorbic acid ($\geq$100 mg/dL) or exposure to light may decrease hemoglobin values. A urinary pH of $\geq$4.0 may cause a false increase in hemoglobin values.

Bilirubin and Urobilinogen

Most of the bilirubin in the body is formed by the reticuloendothelial system as a breakdown product of the hemoglobin released from senescent RBCs. The heme ring is opened to form the linear tetrapyrrole biliverdin, which, in turn, is converted to bilirubin, an intensely orange-yellow, lipid-soluble, neurotoxic compound. At this point, the bilirubin has not been conjugated by the liver and is termed "indirect" bilirubin because it is not water soluble and does not react "directly" with an aqueous reagent, but requires an organic solvent or a coupling agent to react.

As it is released into the bloodstream by the reticuloendothelial cells, bilirubin becomes reversibly bound to albumin and is carried to the liver where the hepatocytes rapidly remove it from the albumin by a carrier-mediated active transport process. In the hepatocytes, the bilirubin is conjugated with glucuronic acid to produce water-soluble, nontoxic bilirubin mono- and diglucuronides. The glucuronides are termed "direct" bilirubin because they react with aqueous reagents "directly" without the addition of organic solvents or coupling agents.

The liver excretes the conjugated bilirubin as a constituent of the bile and it passes ultimately into the small intestine. In the intestinal tract, conjugated bilirubin is converted back to its unconjugated form and is reduced by the anaerobic flora of the gastrointestinal tract to several colorless tetrapyrroles, collectively termed urobilinogen. Most of this urobilinogen is then reduced to stercobilinogen, and in the large intestine, the two types of compounds are oxidized to urobilins and stercobilins, which are orange-brown and contribute to the characteristic color of the feces.

Normally a portion of the urobilinogen (~20%) is reabsorbed into the enterohepatic circulation and reenters the bloodstream. The liver removes most of this reabsorbed urobilinogen from the blood and reexcretes it into the bile, but a small amount (2–5%) remains in the bloodstream, is carried to the kidney, and passes the glomerular filtration barrier to be excreted in the urine at a level of 1 mg/dL or less.

Conjugated bilirubin appearing in the urine (bilirubinuria) means that there is an obstruction to the flow of bile from the liver. This can occur with gallstones in the common bile duct, carcinoma at the head of the pancreas, and inflammatory processes in the liver leading to intracanalicular pressure and regurgitation of bile. Bilirubin also appears in the urine with the Dubin-Johnson and Rotor types of congenital hyperbilirubinemia. Urinary bilirubin and urobilinogen together with fecal color are useful in the differential diagnosis of jaundice, as shown in Table 7-2.

The reagent strip methodology for bilirubin is based on a coupling reaction between bilirubin and a diazonium salt. Multistix reagent strips use diazotized dichloroaniline in a strongly acid medium, resulting in color ranges through various shades of tan. Rapignost reagent strips use a 2,4-dichlorobenzene-diazonium salt in an acid medium, also producing shades of tan. The Chemstrip reagent is dichlorobenzene-diazonium tetrafluoroborate with color changes from pink to red-violet.

False-positive results are primarily due to pigmented materials in the urine, including medications such as Pyridium that have a similar color at the low pH of the reagent pad and mask the result. False-negative results occur from testing specimens that are not fresh, because bilirubin is unstable and is destroyed in the light or is oxidized in the air to unreactive biliverdin. Sensitivity of the test is lowered with high concentrations of ascorbic acid and nitrite.

The UA Perfect Automated Urinalysis System assay for bilirubin is based on the coupling reaction of a diazonium salt with bilirubin in an acid medium containing a surfactant to yield a measurable color reaction. The assay is specific for bilirubin. False-positive results may occur in the presence of elevated hemoglobin (≥ 250 μg/dL) or protein (100 mg/dL), and false-negative results with high ascorbic acid (≥ 100 mg/dL), although false-negative results are usually due to specimens that either are not fresh or have been exposed to light. For urobilinogen, this system also uses the coupling reaction of a diazonium salt with urobilinogen in an acid medium containing a surfactant to yield a measurable color reaction.

The Ictotest is a confirmatory test based on a diazo method in which bilirubin is coupled to *p*-nitrobenzenediazonium *p*-toluene sulfonate to form a blue or purple color. It is about four times more sensitive to bilirubin than the reagent strip tests. Because the chemical principle of the Ictotest method and the reagent strip tests is similar, the tablet test is subject to the same interferences as those discussed with the reagent strip tests.

The urobilinogen reagent strip methodologies for Chemstrip and Rapignost both use an azo-coupling reaction of urobilinogen with a diazonium salt in an acid medium to form an azodye. Colors range from light pink to dark pink. For Chemstrip, the diazonium salt is 4-methoxybenzene-diazonium-fluoroborate; for Rapignost, it is fluorodiazonium-tetrafluoroborate. The Multistix method uses a modified Ehrlich reaction in which *p*-diethylaminobenzaldehyde, in conjunction with a color enhancer, reacts with uro-

TABLE 7-2
Urine and Fecal Findings in Jaundice

Finding	Normal	Obstruction to Bile Flow	Hemolysis, Hemolytic Anemia	Liver Damage, Hepatitis, Cholestasis
Urinary bilirubin	Absent	Increased, dark urine	Absent	Increased early
Urinary urobilinogen	Present	Neoplasm—low or absent; gallstones—variable	Increased	Decreased early; increased late
Fecal color	Dark	Pale; intermittent with gallstones in common bile duct; persistent with neoplasm in duct or pancreas	Dark	Pale early and dark late in hepatitis; pale with cholestasis

(From Schumann GB, Schweitzer SC: Examination or urine. In Henry JB: ed: *Clinical diagnosis and management by laboratory methods.* 18th ed. Philadelphia: WB Saunders Company, 1991.)

bilinogen in a strongly acid medium to produce a pink-red color.

For the Rapignost, Chemstrip, and Multistix methodologies, false-positive results for urobilinogen may occur with substances whose color masks the color change in the reagent pad (e.g., Pyridium). In addition, the Multistix reagent pad is not specific for urobilinogen; false-positive results occur from the presence of other Ehrlich-reactive substances such as porphobilinogen (PBG), sulfonamides, and *p*-aminosalicylic acid. False-negative results for all three methods may be caused by the urine preservative formalin (>200 mg/dL) and by improper specimen storage, so that urobilinogen is oxidized to urobilin.

As mentioned earlier, the urobilinogen pad on the Multistix reagent strip also reacts with PBG, which is a porphyrin precursor and an important intermediate compound in the formation of heme. Two molecules of delta-aminolevulinic acid (ALA) condense in a reaction catalyzed by ALA dehydratase to form PBG. If heme synthesis is disrupted, the porphyrin precursors or porphyrins accumulate according to the defect or defects in the pathway. Various inherited or induced disorders of porphyrin metabolism (discussed in Chapter 10) are characterized by increased urinary amounts of porphyrin precursors (PBG and ALA) or porphyrins (porphyrinuria). A positive Multistix test for urobilinogen may in fact be indicating the presence of PBG.

The Watson-Schwartz test, a modification of the original Ehrlich's reaction, is used routinely to screen for PBG in urine and can be used to differentiate PBG from urobilinogen and other substances that react with Ehrlich's reagent. Equal volumes (~2 mL) of urine and Ehrlich's reagent are mixed in a tube; approximately 4 mL of saturated sodium acetate is added, and the solution mixed again. A characteristic red or magenta color indicates a positive reaction. An extraction is next performed by vigorously shaking approximately 2 mL of chloroform with the red mixture.

After the separation of phases, a red aqueous phase (the top layer) indicates the presence of PBG or another Ehrlich-reactive substance. If the chloroform layer is red, increased amounts of urobilinogen are present. The aqueous layer is next transferred to a clean tube, and an equal volume of butanol is added. After vigorous shaking and separation of phases, a red aqueous layer (at the bottom) indicates PBG. If the red color is in the butanol phase (on top), urobilinogen or other Ehrlich-reactive substances are present.

A less complicated but less sensitive test is the Hoesch test, which is specific for PBG, although false-positive or questionable results can be caused by indoles or certain drugs (e.g., Pyridium). The Hoesch test is based on the "inverse" Ehrlich's reaction: Urobilinogen interference is eliminated by adding a small volume of urine to a relatively large volume of reagent so that an acid reaction is maintained. In this test, 2 mL of modified Ehrlich's reagent (Hoesch reagent) is placed in a tube, and only two drops of urine are added. A deep pink or red color develops at the urine/reagent interface if PBG is present.

Nitrite

The microorganisms involved in urinary tract infections (UTIs) are usually gram-negative enteric bacilli from the normal flora present in the intestinal tract. The most common causative agent is *E. coli* and, less commonly, species of *Proteus*, *Enterobacter*, and *Klebsiella*. In many cases the infecting organism contains the enzyme nitrate reductase, which is necessary to reduce nitrate to nitrite. Nitrates are normally consumed in the diet and are excreted in the urine without nitrite formation. Several factors affect the formation of nitrite: The infecting organism must be a nitrate reducer; urine must be present in the bladder a minimum of 4 hours for nitrate conversion; and adequate amounts of nitrate must be consumed in the diet.

Screening for nitrite in the urine is not a substitute for an adequate microbiologic workup in suspected cases of UTI. However, it does provide a rapid and economic (although indirect) means of identifying the presence of nitrate-reducing bacteria in the urine. Patients with UTIs may present with asymptomatic bacteriuria, and the nitrite test provides a means of identifying such patients.

The general method used in the reagent strips for nitrite testing involves the diazotization of nitrite with an aromatic amine to produce a diazonium salt, followed by an azo-coupling reaction with an aromatic chromogen. The azodye produced causes a color change from white to pink. For the aromatic amine, Chemstrip uses sulfanilamide, whereas Multistix and Rapignost both use *p*-arsanilic acid. The aromatic chromogen in the case of Rapignost is *N*-(naphthyl)-ethylenediammonium dihydrochloride; for Chemstrip and Multistix it is tetrahydrobenzoquinolinol.

False-positive results may occur with pigmented materials in the urine such as the drug Pyridium, as well as by improper collection and storage of the specimen followed by bacterial proliferation. False-negative results are related to ascorbic acid interference (≥25 mg/dL) and various factors that inhibit or prevent nitrite formation (e.g., insufficient time for conversion, lack of substrate, overlong exposure resulting in the conversion of nitrate to nitrite to nitrogen).

For the UA Perfect Automated Urinalysis System

assay for nitrite, an aromatic amine reacts with nitrite to form a diazonium salt that couples with an indicator to yield a colored complex. The test is specific for nitrite. False-negative results may be caused by low dietary nitrate, elevated ascorbic acid (>100 mg/dL), or a sample in which the nitrite has been converted to nitrogen (urinary stasis). Contact with bleach in the container may cause low values. False-positive results may be caused by samples that are not fresh or in which there has been excessive bacterial growth.

Leukocytes

The finding of significant numbers of leukocytes in the urine is evidence of an inflammatory process, including UTI. The leukocyte esterase test is an indirect measure of leukocytes and is one means of detecting UTIs. Esterase activity has been demonstrated in the azurophilic or primary granules of granulocytic leukocytes, including polymorphonuclear neutrophils (PMNs), monocytes (histiocytes), eosinophils, and basophils. Positive reactions occur most often with increased neutrophils present due to bacterial infection.

The esterase test uses fresh, clean-catch, or catheterized specimens to give a reasonably good indication of the presence of neutrophil esterases when approximately 10 or more cells per microliter is used as an indication of pyuria.[12] Contamination with vaginal fluid may result in positive results.

Increased numbers of WBCs may be observed in the urine with or without bacteriuria, although the most commonly observed cause of leukocyturia is a bacterial infection of the urinary tract accompanied by bacteriuria. Infections involving other agents such as trichomonads, yeasts, and chlamydia cause leukocyturia without bacteriuria.

Reagent pads for leukocyte esterase incorporate an ester together with a diazonium salt. Hydrolysis of the ester liberates the corresponding alcohol (containing an aromatic ring), which is then coupled with the diazonium salt to form an azodye that tints the pad various shades of purple or violet. The Multistix ester is a derivatized pyrrole amino acid ester that is split by the leukocyte esterase to liberate 3-hydroxy-5-phenyl pyrrole, which then reacts with a diazonium salt to produce a purple product. The Chemstrip and the Rapignost pads contain indoxylcarbonic acid ester, which is split by the esterase to liberate indoxyl.

False-positive results occur with pigmented substances—foodstuffs or drugs—that mask the color of the reagent pad (e.g., Pyridium, nitrofurantoin, beets). False-negative results occur with increased protein (500 mg/dL), glucose (≥3 g/dL), and specific gravity, as well as with the presence of drugs such as gentamicin or cephalosporin.

The UA Perfect Automated Urinalysis System assay for leukocyte esterase uses an amino acid ester that is hydrolyzed by the leukocyte esterase to liberate a chromophore that produces color. The assay is specific for LE. Elevated bilirubin (≥3.0 mg/dL), protein (100 mg/dL), or hemoglobin (250 μg/dL) may increase LE values. The presence of strong oxidizing agents in the urine container may give false-positive results. Abnormal urinary pH (≤pH 4.0 or ≥pH 9.0) may alter values. High levels of glucose (>3000 mg/dL) in the urine may cause false-negative results.

Specific Gravity

Although specific gravity is a physical property of the urine that was discussed in Chapter 6, it is included here because two manufacturers of urinalysis reagent test strips provide it as a chemical means of indirectly determining specific gravity. There is some disagreement concerning the use of reagent strips to determine specific gravity because they do not measure the "true" or total solute content but only ionic solutes.[1] On the other hand, it is actually the ionic solutes that are of diagnostic value because they are involved in the concentrating and secreting activities of the kidneys.

The reagent strip methodology involves a polyelectrolyte, a pH indicator, and an alkaline buffer. Ionic solutes in the urine cause hydrogen ions to be released by the polyelectrolyte. As the pH of the test pad decreases, the color of the indicator changes. The polyelectrolyte for the Multistix pad is poly (methylvinyl ether/maleic anhydride); the indicator is bromothymol blue. For the Chemstrip, the indicator is the same and the polyelectrolyte is EGTA (ethyleneglycol-bis [aminoethylether] tetra-acetic acid).

Highly buffered alkaline urines may cause low readings relative to other methods. A correction of 0.005 units may be added to readings if the urine pH is ≥6.5. Moderate quantities of protein (100–750 mg/dL) may cause elevated readings. The Chemstrip package insert states that urines with specific gravities above 1.025 are not reliably measured with current relative ionic concentration methodology. Test samples above 1.025 should be retested with a refractometer or urinometer.

The UA Perfect Automated Urinalysis System assay for specific gravity is based on the apparent pKa change of certain pretreated polyelectrolytes in relation to ionic concentration. In the presence of an indicator, colors range from deep blue-green in urine of low ionic concentration through green and yellow-green in urine of increasing ionic concentration. The assay allows determination of urine specific gravity from 1.000 to 1.035. Highly buffered urine samples (≥0.5 mol/L) may alter results. Elevated protein levels of 100 mg/dL or greater may increase the specific gravity reading. Urines with a pH of 4.0 may show increased specific gravity values, and a pH of ≥9.0 may lower it.

Ascorbic Acid

The Rapignost is the only reagent strip that includes a test pad for ascorbic acid (vitamin C). Because ascorbic acid is a reducing agent, large amounts of this compound may interfere with several of the reagent strip tests that depend on reactions with diazo reagents or peroxides (e.g., glucose, blood, bilirubin, nitrite, and LE). The most frequently observed interference is with the reagent strip test for blood, when RBCs are observed microscopically but the reagent pad is negative because of interference from ascorbate.

The reagent test pad for ascorbic acid contains an oxidized dye (2,6-dichloro-phenol-indophenol) that is reduced by the ascorbic acid, resulting in a color change from gray-blue to orange. There are no known test interferences.[10]

Quality Control

Reagent strips and reagents should be properly labeled with the date of opening or preparation, purchase date, expiration date, and appropriate safety information.[13] The reagent strips should be checked against known negative and positive control solutions on each shift and whenever a new bottle is opened. Reagents are checked daily or when tests requiring their use are requested. Results of all reagent checks are recorded.

According to the Clinical Laboratory Improvement Act (CLIA) of 1988, a minimum of two control specimens (negative or normal and positive or increased) must be run in every 24-hour period when patient specimens are run.[11] The control must be carried through the entire test procedure and treated in the same way as any unknown specimen to be affected by any or all of the variables that influence the unknown specimen. Commercial control materials can be purchased for most analytes, including specimens for the chemical screening of urine by reagent strips and tablets. Chemical and tablet tests must also be checked in the QC process.

Because the UA Perfect system is specific for each analyte, some commercial controls may be incompatible (nonreactive) with all or part of the system's assays.

Illustrative Case Studies

CASE 7-1

With a long history of chronic tonsillitis and adenoiditis, this 5-year-old boy was admitted for tonsillectomy and adenoidectomy. There is also a family history of Alport's syndrome (hereditary nephritis), with which the child had been diagnosed previously. Alport's syndrome is characterized by intermittent hematuria, impairment of renal function, proteinuria, leukocyturia, and casts of various types.

The admission urinalysis was consistent with the diagnosis of Alport's syndrome because it was significant for blood large; protein trace mg/dL; color amber; appearance hazy; WBCs 10–20/HPF; RBCs 50–100/HPF; and 1–5 RBC casts.

CASE 7-2

This patient, a 38-year-old man with a history of IDDM and DKA, came to the ER complaining of SOB, weakness, and malaise, which he had experienced for the previous 4 days. He also reported nausea, vomiting, and chills.

The admission urinalysis was significant for: glucose 500 mg/dL; ketones 15 mg/dL; blood moderate; protein trace mg/dL; WBCs 2–5/HPF; RBCs rare/HPF; casts 0–1 granular/LPF. ABGs were: pH 7.19 (7.38–7.46); pCO_2 19.0 mm Hg (32–46); HCO_3 7.3 mEq/L (21–29); base excess −18.7 (−2 to +2). The Chem 10 (a blood chemistry panel) indicated CO_2 11 mEq/L (24–35); anion gap 23 (1–11); and glucose 427 mg/dL (70–110). Hemoglobin A_{1c} was 13% (4.4–6.1%). The positive glucose and ketone results on the urine dipstick suggest DKA, which is borne out by the chemistry analyses and ABGs that fit the picture of DKA: metabolic acidosis, elevated blood sugar, and increased hemoglobin A_{1c} (indicating poor glycemic control for several days preceding the test).

continued

Illustrative Case Studies (continued)

CASE 7-3

After a day of abdominal pain (which radiated to her back and left shoulder), nausea, and vomiting, this 46-year-old woman came to the ER. She was known to have a 2-year history of pancreatitis, NIDDM (taking glyburide), and hypothyroidism (taking levothyroxine). Her admitting diagnosis was acute pancreatitis, and her initial blood work showed cholesterol 544 mg/dL (<200 desirable); glucose 417 mg/dL (70–110); amylase 370 U/L (25–115); lipase >1400 IU/L (0–150); and triglycerides 3810 mg/dL (35–135). Her admission urinalysis was significant for: glucose 500 mg/dL; ketones 40 mg/dL; and protein trace mg/dL. With pancreatitis, insulin production is compromised, so the urine glucose and ketones correlate with this as well as the NIDDM. Blood amylase and lipase results indicate acute pancreatitis.

An ultrasound study of the abdomen was negative for gallstones, but a focal hypoechoic area within the body of the pancreas was observed, suggesting inflammation or a mass. After supportive therapy and proper diet, the patient improved steadily and was discharged on a low-fat diet, Lopid (gemfibrozil), and insulin. The discharge diagnosis was acute pancreatitis secondary to hypertriglyceridemia.

CASE 7-4

After several days of nausea, vomiting, weight loss, and abdominal pain, this 9-year-old girl was brought to the ER. The admission diagnosis was new onset of IDDM and DKA. Her admission urinalysis was significant for glucose >1000 mg/dL; ketones 40 mg/dL; and pH 5.0.

Her admission blood work showed: glucose 603 mg/dL (70–110); and a bicarbonate of 10 mEq/L (22–26). She was placed on fluids and an insulin drip. The urine results and the chemistry analyses correlate with the diagnosis of IDDM and DKA.

After a short stay in the hospital, she and her mother were given instructions on how to manage her diabetes and she was discharged with a supply of insulin and a 2000-calorie American Diabetic Association (ADA) diet plan.

CASE 7-5

With a history of "gallbladder attacks," this 20-year-old woman was admitted through the ER complaining of abdominal pain. A laparoscopic cholecystectomy was performed, and a gallstone was found at the neck of the cystic duct. Her admission urinalysis showed bilirubin large; protein trace; color amber; appearance hazy; WBCs 0–2/HPF; RBCs 0–2/HPF; epithelial cells 3+; Ictotest positive. The positive bilirubin and Ictotest suggest that the obstruction in the biliary tree resulted in the regurgitation of bile into the circulation, with subsequent appearance of conjugated bilirubin in the urine.

CASE 7-6

After severe abdominal pain and vomiting for 2 days, this 29-year-old woman was admitted to the ER with a history of ethanol abuse, cirrhosis secondary to ethanol abuse, bulimia, and panic attacks. She appeared to be dehydrated and said that during the previous 2 days she had consumed a pint of vodka but had not eaten anything. She had tried to rehydrate herself with water, orange juice, and Pedialyte, but could not keep anything in her stomach. Her admission diagnosis was acute pancreatitis.

The admission urinalysis was significant for bilirubin moderate; ketones >80 mg/dL; blood moderate; protein >300 mg/dL; WBCs 5–10/HPF; RBCs 10–20/HPF; epithelial cells: few squamous, few renal, few transitional; casts TNTC hyaline, rare WBC; Ictotest positive. Blood chemistries were significant for AST 244 U/L (8–42); ALT 98 U/L (3–36); total protein 9.8 g/dL (6.4–8.2); albumin 6.5 g/dL (3.4–5.0); LD 288 U/L (100–190); uric acid 19.6 mg/dL (2.4–5.1); cholesterol 315 mg/dL (<200 desirable); BUN 46 mg/dL (5–25); sodium 132 mEq/L (135–145); potassium 3.5 mEq/L (3.5–5.3); chloride 70 mEq/L (101–111); CO_2 27 mEq/L (24–35); anion gap 35 (1–11); glucose 170 mg/dL

continued

Illustrative Case Studies (continued)

(70–110); creatinine 1.5 mg/dL (0.6–1.0). Serum amylase was 267 U/L (25–115), and lipase was 367 IU/L (0–150).

The urine results that correlate with the diagnosis include the positive bilirubin and Ictotest, whereas the positive ketones correlate with the lack of proper nutrition for the period just before hospitalization. The blood chemistries reflect multiple involvements, including the pancreatitis, cirrhosis, alcohol consumption, and bulimia.

CASE 7-7

With a history of delivering a premature, nonviable fetus the previous month, this 27-year-old woman was admitted through the ER for possible cocaine overdose. In the ER, she was apneic and bradycardic, but her condition improved after the administration of Narcan (naloxone). Her diagnosis was cocaine/ethanol intoxication with suicidal tendencies.

The admission urinalysis was significant for glucose 500 mg/dL; and ketones trace. Her blood alcohol was 169 mg/dL, and the urine drug screen was positive for cocaine. She was given supportive therapy with an adequate diet and was eventually discharged with a referral for suicidal tendencies. The urinalysis results suggest the effects of the alcohol and cocaine on glucose utilization.

CASE 7-8

This 61-year-old woman was admitted complaining of loss of appetite, nausea, vomiting, and SOB. She had been diagnosed with chronic renal failure and HTN 7 months previously, and was taking Procardia (nifedipine). Her admission diagnosis was end-stage renal failure of unknown etiology with uremia, HTN, and anemia. Her admission urinalysis was significant for: specific gravity 1.010 (1.003–1.030); blood moderate; protein >300 mg/dL; LE trace; color straw; appearance slightly hazy; WBCs 10–20/HPF; and RBCs 2–5/HPF. The urinalysis results that correlate with the diagnosis include the specific gravity, the blood and protein, the color, and the cells.

An arteriovenous fistula was prepared, and the patient was fitted with a PermACath for dialysis. While in the hospital, she was dialyzed 3× each week and her HTN was controlled with Dilacor. At various times during her hospitalization, creatinine levels in the blood ranged from 5.8 to 6.8 mg/dL (0.6–1.0) and the BUN ranged from 63 to 69 mg/dL (5–25). The elevated creatinine and BUN correlate with the diagnosis of end-stage renal failure. She was discharged to continue dialysis at a local dialysis center with Compazine (perchlorperazine) for nausea, Epogen (to stimulate RBC production after dialysis), and Dilacor (for HTN).

 Case Histories and Study Questions

CASE HISTORY 7-1

This patient is a 29-year-old woman with a long history of IDDM. She has been checking her blood sugar at home daily and administering her own insulin. She was admitted through the ER after 2 days of vomiting, upper abdominal pain, and right jaw pain. Her admission diagnosis was DKA and dehydration. The admission urinalysis (no microscopic) was significant for glucose >1000 mg/dL and ketones >80 mg/dL. Her condition was resolved with fluid and electrolyte therapy and insulin drip. Significant results from her admission blood work included CO_2 8 mEq/L (24–35); glucose 716 mg/dL (70–110). Blood gases showed: pH 7.28 (7.38–7.46); HCO_3 8 mEq/L (21–29); base excess −16 mEq/L (−2.0 to +2.0); and pCO_2 17 mm Hg (32–46).

Case Histories and Study Questions (continued)

Study Questions for Case History 7-1

1. What urinalysis results correlate with the diagnosis of DKA? Explain.
2. What results from the blood analyses, including the ABGs, correlate with this same diagnosis? Explain.

CASE HISTORY 7-2

This 71-year-old woman was transferred from a rural hospital complaining of SOB and showing evidence of pulmonary edema. There was no history of chest pains, nausea, vomiting or diaphoresis. Her admission diagnosis was CHF (acute exacerbation), MI (subendocardial), DM, and HTN. Medications included Lasix, morphine, nitroglycerin, and Procardia.

Laboratory tests were significant for increased CK, 544 U/L (21–215) with a CKMB of 29.2 ng/mL (0–4), which is a relative index of 54. During the first few days of her hospital stay, blood glucose ranged from 201 to 365 mg/dL (70–110); creatinine ranged from 1.9 to 3.7 mg/dL (0.6–1.0); and BUN ranged from 31 to 46 mg/dL (5–25). Admission urinalysis was significant for: glucose 100 mg/dL; blood moderate; protein >300 mg/dL (<90); WBCs 2–5/HPF; RBCs 10–20/HPF; epithelials/LPF few squamous, few renal; casts/LPF 5–10 granular, rare WBC. After aggressive treatment of the CHF, her condition improved moderately with Cardizem (then Procardia), Nipride, and Cardura. She received intravenous nitroglycerin and insulin. The discharge diagnosis was status postsubendocardial MI, triple-vessel cardiac disease, CHF, renal insufficiency, HTN, and DM. She was scheduled to return to the hospital eventually for a triple-vessel coronary bypass.

Study Questions for Case History 7-2

1. What renal condition do the urinalysis data suggest? Explain.
2. Do the analyses on blood correlate with this? Explain.
3. What is the pathophysiology behind the renal condition in question 1? Explain.

CASE HISTORY 7-3

This patient, a 46-year-old man, was admitted complaining of diarrhea (experienced during the entire previous month) and jaundice, together with gas and nausea for the previous 3 weeks. Because of a long history of alcoholism, his admission diagnosis was "probable cirrhosis," but further work showed a large, infiltrating mass in the liver that turned out to be hepatocellular carcinoma. The porta hepatis was entirely blocked, causing severe obstructive jaundice.

The admission urinalysis showed bilirubin large; color amber; casts/LPF 1–5 granular and 1–5 WBC; Ictotest positive. Blood chemistries showed total bilirubin 32.1 mg/dL (0–1.5); conjugated bilirubin 22.2 mg/dL (0–0.4); ALP 299 U/L (37–107); AST 302 U/L (8–42); ALT 46 U/L (3–36); total protein 4.9 g/dL (6.4–8.2); albumin 2.1 m/dL (3.4–5.0); and LD 272 U/L (100–190).

Study Questions for Case History 7-3

1. What urine results correlate with the diagnosis? Explain.
2. How do the blood analyses correlate with this? Explain.

REFERENCES

1. Brunzel NA. *Fundamentals of urine and body fluid analysis.* Philadelphia: WB Saunders, 1994.
2. Chemstrip Package Insert. Indianapolis, IN: Boehringer-Mannheim Corporation, 1995.
3. Chemstrip Micral Urine Test Strips Package Insert. Indianapolis, IN: Boehringer-Mannheim Corporation, 1995.
4. Hawthorne VM. Preventing the kidney disease of diabetes mellitus: Public health perspectives. Consensus statement. *Am J Kidney Dis* 1989;13:1–6.
5. Hindmarsh JT. Microalbuminuria. *Clin Lab Med* 1988;8: 611–616.

6. Kaplan LA, Pesce AJ, eds. *Clinical chemistry*. 2nd ed. St. Louis: CV Mosby, 1989.
7. Mogensen CE. Microalbuminuria as a predictor of clinical diabetic nephropathy. *Kidney Int* 1987;31:673–689.
8. Multistix Package Insert. Elkhart, IN: Bayer Corporation— Diagnostics Division (formerly Miles, Inc.), 1995.
9. Peters T. Albumin in urine. *Clinical Chemistry News* 1990;16: 10–12.
10. Rapignost Package Insert. Somerville, NJ: Behring Diagnostics, Inc., 1995.

11. Ringsrud KM, Linné JJ. *Urinalysis and body fluids: A color text and atlas*. St. Louis: Mosby–Year Book, 1995.
12. Schumann GB, Schweitzer SC. Examination of urine. In: Henry JB, ed. *Clinical diagnosis and management by laboratory methods*. 18th ed. Philadelphia: WB Saunders, 1991: 387–444.
13. Strasinger SK. *Urinalysis and body fluids*. 3rd ed. Philadelphia: FA Davis, 1994.
14. UA Perfect Automated Urinalysis System, Product Information. Tampa, FL: Chimera Research & Chemical, Inc., 1996.

BIBLIOGRAPHY

Ward KM. Microalbuminuria: Clinical laboratory aspects. *Clin Lab Sci* 1989;2:212–213.

Watts GF, Bennett JE, Rowe DJ, et al. Assessment of immunochemical methods for determining low concentrations of albumin in urine. *Clin Chem* 1986;32:1544–1548.

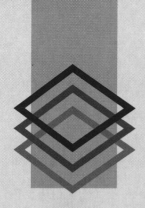

8

The Microscope

Introduction

The Microscope

Few would argue with Richardson's statement[15] that "Sight is, without a doubt, the grandest of our personal senses. With it we can rapidly perceive the number, size, shape, texture, color, and position of those objects around us." The capability of our eyes has been extended to the very remote with telescopes and to the very small with microscopes. The word *microscope* is derived from the Greek *mikros*, small, + *skopein*, to look.

Resembling a simple camera, the eye has a lens in front and a light-sensitive layer (the retina) covering its interior, rear portion. The structure of the lens includes an outer, transparent cornea; the iris, which changes the pupil diameter; and the lens proper. The lens is unique because its focal length can be varied (within certain limits) without being repositioned relative to the retina. When the shape of the lens is altered, the focal length is changed.

Within certain limits, objects appear larger as they are brought closer to the eye. The practical limit for this is the ability of the lens to focus the object clearly; this ability varies from person to person. This limit can be overcome by the use of an instrument we call the microscope.

Types of Microscopy

Although we are most familiar with the light microscope, there are several other types. One type is the electron microscope, both transmission and scanning, which can be found in a few reference laboratories and in many research institutions.

New categories of microscopes now under experimental development[21] offer prospects for revealing more detail in biologic specimens by extending the limits of resolution; providing specialized contrast mechanisms; permitting observation of specimens under unusual and generally more physiologic conditions; and providing more convenient or efficient viewing and recording of images. These instruments include the ion microscope, the neutron microscope, the photoelectron microscope, the scanning tunneling microscope, the atomic-force microscope, the nuclear magnetic resonance microscope, the acoustic microscope, "superresolving" instruments and confocal systems, and the video-enhanced light microscope. Although it is well to be aware of these developments, and although some of these systems may eventually find their way into the everyday work of the clinical laboratory, the traditional light microscope, with its many modifications as we know them, undoubtedly will continue to be the "workhorse" for many years to come.

The Light Microscope

Developmental History

A simple microscope consists, minimally, of a single, short-focus, positive (magnifying) lens. The ray diagram for this simple arrangement is shown in Figure 8-1. The magnifying lens probably originated with the ancient Assyrians; crude lenses of glass were found in the ruins of Nineveh, a city that was destroyed in 612 B.C. More refined lenses used as magnifying glasses or spectacles were known by the end of the 13th century.[11] Important observations were made with a simple microscope by Anton van Leeuwenhoek of Delft, Holland during the period 1671 to 1723. Subjects included bacteria, spermatozoa, and blood cells. Van Leeuwenhoek's microscope, which he made with his own hands, consisted of a single lens with two screws to focus the specimen. The magnification achieved was 40× to 280×.

Even though van Leeuwenhoek was successful in using a simple microscope for his historic work, this type of instrument has several limitations. At higher magnifications the lens must be very near the sample, and the eye must be very near the opposite side of the lens for objects to be seen. This is illustrated in Figure 8-2. Manipulation of the sample is severely limited because of the proximity of the lens and the observer's head. The introduction of the compound microscope overcame several of these limitations. As lens improvements gradually came along, it became the instrument of choice.

In its basic form, the compound microscope consists of a lens (or group of lenses) called the *objective*, and a second lens (or group of lenses) known as the *eyepiece* or *ocular*. The function of these lenses is shown in Figure 8-3. The objective lens produces an image of the sample, and the upper or "eye lens" of the eyepiece focuses the image of the specimen on the retina of the eye. This information is perceived by the eye and brain to be an enlarged image of the sample located about

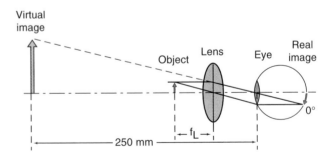

FIGURE 8-1 Ray diagram of a simple microscope. The object is imaged on the retina of the eye by the lens. This appears to the eye as if it were from an object at the position of the virtual image. (From Richardson JH. *Handbook for the light microscope: A user's guide*. Park Ridge, NJ: Noyes Publications, 1991.)

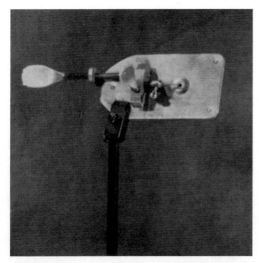
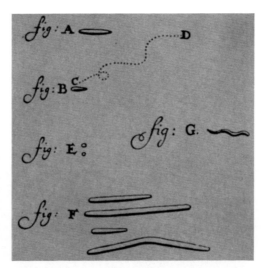

FIGURE 8-2 A. Leeuwenhoek used a microscope with a single biconvex lens to view bacteria suspended in a drop of liquid placed on a moveable pin. B. Although his microscope was capable of only 200 to 300-fold magnification, Leeuwenhocek was able to achieve these remarkable drawings of different bacterial types, which he submitted to the Royal Society of London. (From Volk, Gebhardt, Hammarskjold, Kadner. *Essentials of medical microbiology*. 5th ed. Philadelphia: Lippincott–Raven Publishers, 1996.)

250 mm below the eyepiece. This is a virtual image. The corresponding real image, which can be observed on a screen or recorded in photomicrography, is projected from the eyepiece at a distance of about 250 mm above it. These relationships are shown in Figure 8-4.

The oldest known descriptions and illustrations of a compound microscope come from Holland in the year 1625 for a microscope probably produced by Zacharias Janssen, a spectacle maker. In the second half of the 17th century, Marcello Malpighi in Italy and Robert Hooke in England were using the compound microscope for investigations in biology and in medicine. Hooke published an illustrated book, *Micrographia*, in 1665 that showed the existence of cellular structures in living organisms. The microscopes available at that time consisted of a tube with a simple objective lens mounted at one end and a simple eyepiece lens mounted at the other end. The ray diagram for this arrangement is shown in Figure 8-5.

It is interesting to note that van Leeuwenhoek used a single lens microscope for his historic observations, even though early compound microscopes were available at that time. Others tried but failed to confirm his observations both with simple and compound microscopes. Two reasons have been suggested for van Leeuwenhoek's unique success with the single-lens instrument. First, the crude compound microscopes

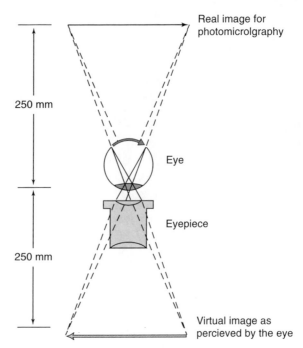

FIGURE 8-4 Schematic relationship between the virtual image as perceived by the eye and the real image that exists above the eyepiece; this latter image is the one used for photomicrography. (From Richardson JH. *Handbook for the light microscope: A user's guide*. Park Ridge, NJ: Noyes Publications, 1991.)

FIGURE 8-3 Ray diagram of a compound microscope; the object is just outside of the first focal plane of the objective (FOB); the intermediary image is just within the focal plane of the eyepiece FOC; compare with Fig. 8-1. (From James J. *Light microscope techniques in biology and medicine*. Dordrecht: Kluwer Academic Publishers, 1976.)

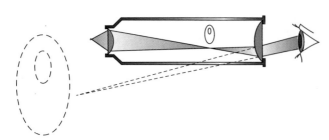

FIGURE 8-5 Ray diagram of a compound microscope. (From James J, Tanke HJ. eds. *Biomedical light microscopy*. Dordrecht: Kluwer Academic Publishers, 1976.)

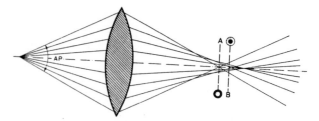

FIGURE 8-7 Spherical aberration. When the object is a luminous point emitting monochromatic light, a bright circle with darker border will be seen on a screen held in the object space at A; at plane B a bright ring with a darker center will be seen. AP-angular aperture of the lens. (From James J. *Light microscope techniques in biology and medicine*. Dordrecht: Kluwer Academic Publishers, 1976.)

available at that time produced only 30× to 40× magnification, and the images were of very poor quality. The single-lens instrument simply gave better images. Second, van Leeuwenhoek apparently was able to tolerate the requirement that the single-lens device be held pressed close to the eye (as mentioned earlier), and most other workers could not do this for very long. It has also been suggested that van Leeuwenhoek may have possessed exceptional visual acuity.

Because of aberrations (or image errors), a lens does not produce a perfect image of an object. Even though an improved stand and focusing mechanism for the compound microscope was produced by Cuff in 1744 (Fig. 8-6), the uncorrected lenses still produced highly distorted images even at relatively low power.

Aberrations only minimally affect the image produced by a single lens, but they are of critical importance in the compound microscope. The errors become more obvious as more lenses are included in the system. The major lens errors are spherical aberration, chromatic aberration, and curvature of field.

Spherical aberration (or aperture error) occurs because rays that pass through the outer portion of a lens come to a different focal point than rays that pass through the central area of a lens (Fig. 8-7). This results in an image that is blurred and cannot be sharply focused.

Chromatic aberration occurs because the refractive index of the lens material is not the same for different wavelengths of light. The focal point is nearer to the lens with shorter wavelengths, as illustrated in Figure 8-8. As a result, color fringes appear around very fine structures.

Curvature of field means the image of a flat plane perpendicular to the optical axis appears curved rather than flat. This is especially disturbing for photomicrography.

Toward the end of the 18th century, various combinations of positive and negative lenses made with different types of glass were used to produce lenses at least partially corrected for aberrations. The first successful achromatic microscopes of low magnification

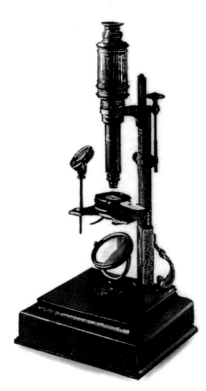

FIGURE 8-6 Microscope stand of Cuff, about 175° photograph made of an instrument from the collection of the National Museum of the History of Science in Leiden.

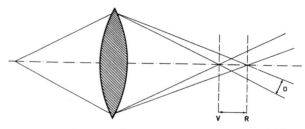

FIGURE 8-8 Chromatic aberration. As a consequence of different refractions of rays of various wavelengths coming from a luminous point emitting mixed light, dispersion occurs for which the distance D is a measure. On the optical axis, a spectrum of image points will be formed, with points for violet (V) and red (R) at the extremities. (From James J. *Light microscope techniques in biology and medicine*. Dordrecht: Kluwer Academic Publishers, 1976.)

were produced about 1800. These were spherically corrected for green light and chromatically corrected for red and blue-green light. From 1866 onward, Carl Zeiss and Ernst Abbe combined their talents to design and produce highly corrected lenses. These achievements also depended on the production of special types of glass by Otto Schott in his factory near the Zeiss works at Jena, Germany. Such outstanding developments in microscope design and performance made possible many important discoveries, such as a precise analysis of cell division (Flemming, 1882); myofilaments in contractile fibrils of the muscle cell (Kölliker, 1887); and Koch's discovery of the tubercle bacillus (1882).

Standard Components

The components of any microscope are mounted on a stand (or frame and body). For the special application of viewing the bottom of culture vessels or Petri plates, an inverted stand is used. The more common arrangement for work with transmitted light is the upright stand. The stand serves to hold the basic components of the microscope in place. They are the same regardless of the stand: a source of illumination, a condenser to focus the light onto the specimen, a stage to hold the specimen for viewing, and the optical tube (or body tube) with its eyepieces and objectives. A general diagram is shown in Figure 8-9.

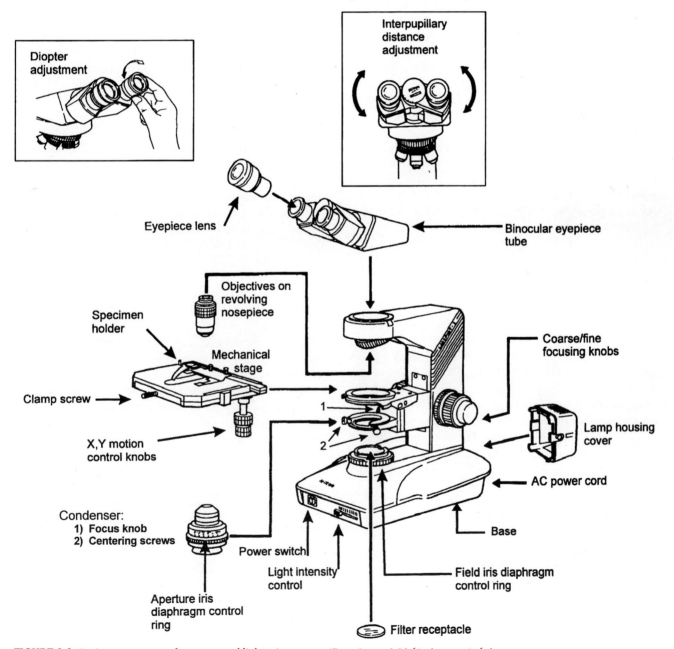

FIGURE 8-9 Basic components of a compound light microscope. (From James J. *Light microscope techniques in biology and medicine.* Dordrecht: Kluwer Academic Publishers, 1976.)

ILLUMINATION SYSTEM

The light source for modern instruments is usually mounted in the base together with a power transformer and controls to regulate brightness. There are two types of the most widely used source of illumination: a low-voltage incandescent lamp.

One type is an ordinary tungsten filament enclosed in an inert gas atmosphere by a soft glass envelope. After several hours of use, these sources gradually emit less light because the tungsten evaporates from the filament, deposits on the glass envelope, and gradually darkens it.

This darkening is avoided in the second type of incandescent lamp by the addition of a small amount of a halogen (such as bromine or iodine) admixed with the inert gas atmosphere. When the tungsten evaporates from the filament, it reacts to form a tungsten halide gas, which decomposes at the hottest part of the filament to reform the metal and release the halogen to react again. This prolongs the useful life of the lamp. The tungsten halogen lamps have a smaller sized, quartz glass envelope.

Light from the lamp is collimated by a collector or condensing lens (or system of lenses) and directed upward through the field diaphragm to the substage condenser. The field diaphragm serves to limit the diameter of the light beam entering the substage condenser as well as to reduce stray light.

SUBSTAGE CONDENSER SYSTEM

The purpose of the substage condenser system (or simply the condenser) is to distribute evenly and focus the light from the illumination source onto the specimen. The condenser is usually arranged on a focusing and centerable mount so the illumination can be properly aligned to the optical axis of the microscope. Proper illumination of the specimen is critical for the sharpness and general character of the image. It is the condenser that provides the necessary means to adjust the illumination of the sample. The condenser consists of at least two lenses, an iris diaphragm (termed the aperture diaphragm), and (usually) a carrier or holder for a removable filter.

The lenses of the condenser collect the light from the illumination system below and produce a cone of light converging at the sample plane. The angle of this cone of light is controlled and adjusted by the aperture diaphragm. Proper adjustment of the aperture diaphragm is critical in establishing the potential numeric aperture (N.A.) of the system, in minimizing glare and stray light, and in adjusting the contrast in the specimen. Refer to the section on The Objective Lens, later, for a brief discussion of N.A.

MECHANICAL STAGE

The stage supports the specimen to be viewed at right angles to the optical axis of the instrument. For transmitted light, the stage of course has an opening in the center to permit light to reach the specimen. In simpler designs, the stage is not moveable and the glass microscope slide on which the specimen is mounted is held in place on the stage by two metal clips. The slide is then moved around manually. Laboratory and research-grade microscopes have a mechanical stage with a quick-release spring clip device to hold the microscope slide firmly in place. The stage itself, with the mounted slide, can then be moved orthogonally in each direction by means of separate or coaxial control knobs. Some stages are equipped with vernier scales along one horizontal edge and one vertical edge to aid in relocating a particular field of view. For crystallographic and metallurgic studies, a round, revolving stage is used.

OPTICAL TUBE

The optical tube (or body tube) provides a light-tight support and correct spacing for the objective lenses and the eyepieces. To focus the specimen, either the tube is moved up and down in reference to the stand or the stage is moved while the optical tube remains stationary. Focusing is by means of coarse and fine single or coaxial adjustment knobs that drive gear mechanisms.

The length of the tube, or the mechanical tube length, must match the optical parameters of the objective design. Mechanical tube lengths vary from 140 to 250 mm. Some research model instruments have an adjustable, graduated draw tube that permits "fine tuning" the length of the optical tube to match the requirements for any specific objective lens.

The objective lenses are usually mounted in a revolving "nosepiece" to facilitate their selection and change during viewing. Advantages of this system include convenience and speed, as well as protection from dust. The revolving nosepiece requires that the objectives be parcentered and parfocal, as discussed briefly later.

The simplest eyepiece arrangement is on a monocular tube. More commonly, a binocular body is provided for two eyepieces to permit the use of both eyes simultaneously. In addition, the optical tube may be trinocular to permit the mounting of a camera.

The binocular body has two adjustments, one the interpupillary spacing adjustment, the other the interpupillary acuity adjustment. These adjustments are referred to again later in reference to microscope adjustments.

THE OBJECTIVE LENS

This element of the microscope produces the magnified primary image of the specimen and thus is perhaps the most important part of the entire system. Several parameters must be considered in achieving the optimum image for a given objective and instrument, including N.A., magnification, optical corrections, tube length, immersion fluid, coverglass (coverslip) thickness, flatness of field, parfocality, and working distance. In most instances, certain of these parameters are engraved on the barrel of the lens, including tube length required, coverglass thickness needed, magnification of the intermediate image, lens corrections, and the N.A.

A measure of the amount of light a lens can collect is the N.A., defined as: N.A. $= \eta \sin \alpha$, where η is the designated refractive index of the material between the sample and the lens and α is the half angle of the most oblique rays entering the lens. For an objective, "lens" means the front lens. The effective N.A. of the objective depends on the N.A. of the condenser. For maximum resolution with the system, the N.A. of the condenser should equal or at least be close to that of the objective.

The refractive indices of the materials in the light path between the objective lens and the sample also have a strong effect on the N.A. The controlling factor is the material that has the lowest refractive index. If air is a part of the light path, its refractive index of 1 controls the effective N.A. of the total system regardless of how high the N.A. of the lenses may be. Immersion media can be placed in between the objective lens and the coverglass/sample to improve the effective N.A. Media include water ($\eta = 1.33$), glycerin ($\eta = 1.440$), and oil ($\eta = 1.5$–1.6). The water immersion objective is essentially obsolete because the performance of oil immersion objectives does not depend on the coverglass thickness, and they also produce a more brilliant im-

age. The effect of oil immersion is shown in Figure 8-10.

As the N.A. of a lens increases, thereby increasing its potential resolving power, the actual resolving power that can be realized depends in large measure on the lens corrections. Gradually, over the years, lens designs have been produced that are increasingly successful in correcting lens aberrations. Lenses have been produced to correct simultaneously for spherical, chromatic, and curvature of field errors. An example of how two different types of glass are combined to correct for chromatic aberration is shown in Figure 8-11.

"Achromat" objectives are spherically corrected for green light, and chromatically corrected for red and blue-green light. The semiapochromatic or fluorite objectives are spherically and chromatically corrected for two colors. The objectives providing the best contrast and resolution are designated "apochromat" and are corrected chromatically for three colors and spherically for two. An objective lens corrected for curvature of field has the designation "plan."

Parfocality means that the distance between the sample and the intermediate image is made the same for each member of the objective lens set. Therefore, it is not necessary to refocus very much (if at all) when the objectives are changed one to another.

THE EYEPIECE

The eyepiece is a self-contained unit and is designed to fit into the upper end of the microscope body tube. The eyepiece has a lens at either end. The one at the upper end is the eye lens and the one below is the field lens. The eyepiece is designed to form a magnified image of the intermediate image produced by the objective lens. Eyepieces include the Huygens eyepiece, the Ramsden eyepiece, the compensating eyepiece, and the widefield eyepiece.

FIGURE 8-10 The effect of oil immersion. In situation I, without immersion, of three rays with an ever increasing angle toward the optical axis, only ray A reaches the objective in such a way that it can be presumed to take part in image formation, whereas ray C does not even reach the upper part of the object space, being totally reflected at the surface of the cover glass. In situation II, the same three rays reach the object space (virtually without being refracted) and both rays A′ and B′ probably can take part in image formation C′, reaching at least the upper part of the object space. It should be noted that the angles of ray A and B with the optical axis are greater than those of their counterparts A′ and B′). (From James J. *Light microscope techniques in biology and medicine*. Dordrecht: Kluwer Academic Publishers, 1976.)

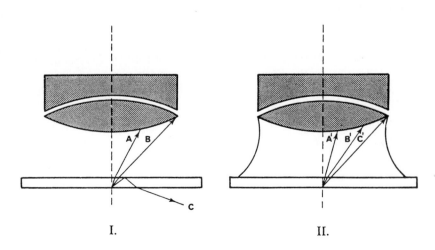

I.   II.

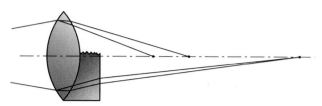

FIGURE 8-11 Correction of chromatic aberration for two colors by the combination of a positive and a negative lens of materials with different dispersion; both image points come to coincide, but it entails an increase in the focal distance of the refractive complex. (From James J. *Light microscope techniques in biology and medicine.* Dordrecht: Kluwer Academic Publishers, 1976.)

Types of Light Microscopy

BRIGHTFIELD

In this technique, the image of the specimen appears dark against a bright background. This illumination system has been used from the beginning of microscopy and is still the most commonly used. A major step forward with this approach to lighting the specimen was the development of a critical illumination technique by Köhler in the early 1900s. This method is used throughout the world and is reviewed in detail later under Adjustments.

Brightfield microscopy presents difficulties in visualizing translucent objects such as hyaline casts, mucus, and some cells. Contrast can be improved by adjusting the light intensity using the lamp voltage control built into the power supply. Contrast may also be adjusted by slightly opening or closing the aperture diaphragm on the substage condenser. However, as noted later, this adjustment should be used with discretion because closing the aperture down too far is detrimental to the effective N.A. of the system.

Once adjusted for Köhler illumination (discussed later), the condenser should be left in that position to maintain maximum resolution in the system. It is poor technique to rack the condenser up and down to alter contrast. By combining light source adjustments with *slight* changes to the aperture diaphragm, adequate contrast can usually be obtained.

Contrast can also be improved by the use of supravital stains such as the Sternheimer-Malbin stain supplied under various trade names by clinical and biologic supply houses. This stain and others are discussed in more detail in Chapter 9, "Microscopic Examination of Urine Sediment."

PHASE CONTRAST

The structural elements of the specimens we wish to resolve with the microscope differ only slightly in refractive index and therefore exert only a negligible influence on the light they transmit. This slight change is in the phase of momentary vibration state, which cannot be detected by the eye. Conventional brightfield illumination does not reveal brightness differences between the structural details of the specimen and its surroundings. The image lacks contrast and details remain invisible.

Small structural details can be revealed only by changing the *phase* image into an *absorption* image by means of staining. Other techniques such as darkfield, phase contrast, or Nomarski differential interference contrast can be used to obtain contrast. These methods take advantage of differences in optical density, refractive index, and phase differences produced in the specimen.

Many specimens, unless stained with supravital stains (or fixed and stained), are very difficult to study because not enough contrast is produced by the object (e.g., a hyaline cast) or components in the object (e.g., cellular features). Here the refractive indices involved are too similar to the surrounding medium as well as the glass microscope slide and coverglass for a good-quality image to be produced without reducing the light intensity to almost the vanishing point.

With phase contrast microscopy, subtle differences in refractive index and the subtle changes in phase these produce are converted into clearcut variations of light intensity and of contrast. Many workers prefer to examine the urine sediment unstained with phase contrast microscopy. However, it is well to keep in mind that certain highly refractive objects such as fat or some crystals are more easily identified using brightfield rather than phase contrast microscopy.

Objects viewed under the microscope retard light waves and produce phase changes to different degrees depending on their unique shape, refractive index, and absorbance properties. When some of the light waves are slowed while passing through an object, the intensity observed is lowered. Waves that are retarded exactly one half of a wavelength completely cancel out an unaffected light wave. The best contrast is achieved when light retardation is one fourth of a wavelength.

Components added to a brightfield microscope achieve this in phase contrast microscopy. Areas of the specimen appear light and dark with haloes of various intensities. With phase contrast, unstained specimens, especially living cells and components that have a low refractive index, are imaged in more detail than is possible with brightfield microscopy. On the other hand, certain objects and structures produce such bright haloes that visualization of detail and dimension is actually worsened.

The components necessary to convert a brightfield instrument to phase contrast must be added to both the condenser and the objective. For a particular objective, a corresponding annular diaphragm, resembling a target, is fitted to the condenser and produces a ring of light. The specimen is illuminated by this ring of light. The objective is fitted with a phase-shifting element that is the reverse of the condenser ring—that is, the central ring retards light by one fourth of a wavelength, producing a ring of reduced intensity. The light and dark rings must be centered for maximum contrast.

This can be achieved by removing an eyepiece and looking down the optical tube at the back lens of the objective (a focusing telescope helps here) and adjusting the condenser ring (the light ring) with the centering screws until the image shows the rings are centered—that is, the light ring is superimposed on the dark ring. Alternatively, one can view the object under phase contrast and simply adjust the centering screws until maximum contrast is achieved for a suitable test object (e.g., a hyaline cast). Each combination of light and dark rings needs to be adjusted separately for proper centering and maximum viewing contrast. A schematic view of a phase contrast system is shown in Figure 8-12.

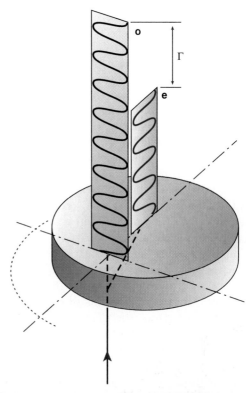

FIGURE 8-13 Schematic view of the development of a path difference when a light ray traverses a doubly refracting material, o = ordinary ray; e = extraordinary ray ;γ = path difference. (From James J, Tanke HJ, eds: *Biomedical light microscopy*. Dordrecht: Kluwer Academic Publishers, 1991.)

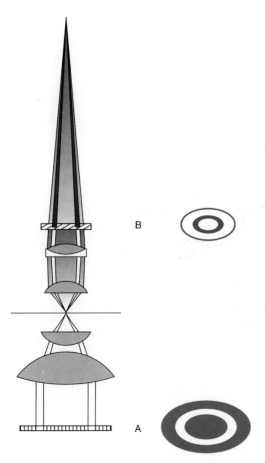

FIGURE 8-12 Schematic view of the practical realization of the phase contrast principle; A, phase annulus under the condenser, B, the corresponding phase plate in the objective. (From James J. *Light microscope techniques in biology and medicine*. Dordrecht: Kluwer Academic Publishers, 1976.)

POLARIZING

For the end view of a beam of unpolarized light, the wave theory of light propagation holds that vibration is occurring in all directions perpendicular to the direction of travel. Plane-polarized light vibrates in only one plane. Materials that produce plane polarized light are termed *polarizers*. Polarizing microscopy has widespread applications in the clinical laboratory, as well as in pharmaceuticals, forensics, pathology, geology, and other fields.

Some substances are able to refract light in two directions, one following the original light path, the other rotated 90° to the original. This relationship is pictured in Figure 8-13. Many such *birefringent* or optically active substances are found in the clinical laboratory, such as crystals, fibers, bones, or minerals. Birefringence can be negative or positive.

Negative birefringence is rotation to the left or counterclockwise (when looking toward the light source); positive birefringence is rotation to the right or clockwise. Monosodium urate crystals are negatively birefringent, and calcium pyrophosphate crystals are positively birefringent.

To convert a brightfield microscope to a polarizing one, two filters are required. One, called the polarizing filter, is located at some point below the condenser. If not built into the instrument, it can simply be perched as needed on top of the light port in the base of the microscope. The polarizer is constructed to permit light vibrating in an east–west direction perpendicular to the light path to pass to the specimen.

The other filter, the analyzer, is mounted in the microscope between the objective and the eyepiece. It is constructed to permit the passage of light that is vibrating in a north–south direction perpendicular to the light path. When the two filters are "crossed," the field appears black unless an optically active material is present to rotate the plane of the polarized light.

To identify crystals based on negative or positive birefringence, various compensator filters are used. The most common one in the clinical setting is the first-order red compensator. When this filter is placed between crossed polarizers, the field is no longer black but red-violet. The filter splits plane polarized light into two rays, slow and fast. The direction of the vibration of the slow ray is inscribed on the filter plate. The use of the compensator is discussed further in chapters dealing with the microscopic examination of the sediment from urine and other body fluids.

INTERFERENCE CONTRAST

There are two types of interference contrast microscopy—modulation contrast (Hoffman) and differential interference contrast (Nomarski). In these techniques, differences in the optical path through the specimen are converted to intensity differences. Both procedures achieve specimen images of high contrast and resolution without the haloing seen with phase contrast microscopy. Optical sectioning is possible with the methods because the image at each depth of field level is unaffected by material above or below the plane of focus. Images have a three-dimensional appearance. The technique is excellent for unstained specimens and is especially good for wet mounts.

Hoffman[10] introduced modulation contrast microscopy in 1977. Three modifications of brightfield microscopy are required: a special slit aperture placed below the condenser, a polarizer to control contrast placed below this slit aperture, and a special amplitude filter, called a modulator, placed in the back of each objective. A diagram illustrating this system is shown in Figure 8-14.

By removing the slit aperture, the instrument can be converted back to brightfield, darkfield, polarizing, or fluorescence techniques. Light from the first polarizing filter passes through the slit aperture, which is partially covered by the second polarizing filter. Rotat-

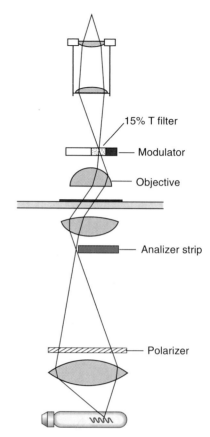

FIGURE 8-14 Schematic representation of the ray path in a light microscope adapted for modulation–contrast microscopy after Hoffman. (From James J, Tanke HJ, eds: *Biomedical light microscopy.* Dordrecht: Kluwer Academic Publishers, 1991.)

ing the slit aperture with its polarizer achieves variations in contrast and a reduction of scattering effects such as flare and fringes at specimen edges.

The light proceeds to the specimen and interacts with it, and the location at which the light enters the objective depends on diffraction within the specimen. The light passes through different parts of the modulator located at the back of the objective. The modulator is divided into three regions of different size and light transmission. The modulator determines the intensity gradients of light to dark observed in the three-dimensional image but does not effect a change in light phase. As stated by Hoffman,[10] "When light intensity varies above and below an average value the light is said to be modulated—thus the name modulation contrast."

With the technique known as differential interference contrast microscopy (Nomarski), intensity differences in the specimen image are produced through the use of birefringent crystal prisms (modified Wollaston prisms) as beam splitters. The prism placed before the specimen plane splits the light into two beams. These beams follow different paths through the specimen; a second prism placed after the objective recombines the

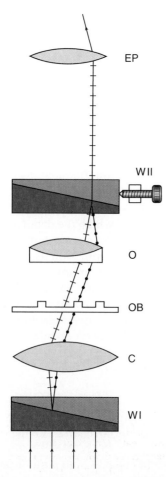

FIGURE 8-15 Scheme of the course of interfering rays in differential interference contrast. W I and W II = Wollaston-prisms; C = condenser; OB = object; O = objective; EP = eyepiece. A polarizer in front of W I and analyzer behind W II are not shown. (From James J. *Light microscope techniques in biology and medicine*. Dordrecht: Kluwer Academic Publishers, 1976.)

two beams of light into one. The light then passes into a polarizing (or analyzer) filter before entering the eyepieces.

It is the analyzer that produces the interference image observed by changing the direction of vibration of the recombined rays so that they interfere with each other. With this technique, it is possible to change the background field of view from black or dark gray to various colors such as yellow, blue, and so forth. Because in reality two images are formed but the eye does not resolve them, the specimen image observed appears to be in relief, or three-dimensional. The light path for this method is illustrated in Figure 8-15.

DARKFIELD

Darkfield microscopy produces a bright specimen image against a dark or black background. This procedure is used with unstained specimens. In the clinical laboratory it has been the preferred approach for the identification of spirochetes under the microscope.

For this procedure, a special condenser directs the light through the specimen only from oblique angles by means of a "darkfield stop" in the base of the condenser. Light passing through the specimen interacts with it (by refraction, reflection, or diffraction), which results in light entering the objective. The image is of a shining specimen on a black background. If there is no specimen, a black field of view is observed because no light is entering the objective.

FLUORESCENCE

In this technique, light of a selected wavelength is presented to the specimen. If a fluorescent substance is present that absorbs that particular excitation illumination, it emits a portion of that energy after a finite but short period of time as light (fluorescence) at a different, longer wavelength. The emitted light is transmitted to the eyepiece for viewing.

The procedure requires two filters. The first, called the excitation filter, selects the wavelength of the excitation light presented to the specimen. The second filter, called the barrier or emission filter, permits a specific wavelength of fluorescent light from the specimen to pass to the eyepiece. Some biologic materials are naturally fluorescent, but most applications of this technique require staining the specimen with fluorescent dyes called fluorophores. Each fluorescent substance or fluorophore has a unique excitation as well as emission wavelength.

Two types of optical systems are available. An older method is transmitted fluorescence microscopy, in which the excitation light is presented to the condenser, focused, and passed through the specimen to continue on up the optical tube to the analyzer and eyepieces. These systems require that an immersion medium be placed between the top lens of the condenser and the bottom of the microscope slide. A more convenient and recent modification is the reflected illumination system (or epi-illuminator), where the light impinges on the specimen from above through the objective lens. This is shown in Figure 8-16. A beam-splitting dichroic mirror in the system has a high reflectance for the light passed by the excitation filter. However, the mirror is transparent to the fluorescence coming from the specimen and allows it to pass upward through the barrier filter to the eyepieces.

Fluorescence microscopy is very sensitive to small quantities of fluorescent dyes or fluorophores attached to antibodies, antigens, bacteria, viruses, and the like. Thus, the method is frequently used with exquisite selectivity and sensitivity in microbiologic and immunologic procedures in the clinical laboratory.

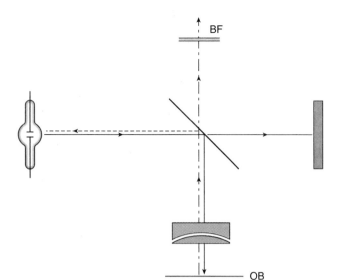

FIGURE 8-16 Schematic view of the course of the rays in a vertical fluorescence illuminator with dichroic mirror. OB = object plane; BF = barrier filter; at right, a dark layer absorbing unused excitation light that has passed the dichroic mirror. (From James J. *Light microscope techniques in biology and medicine.* Dordrecht: Kluwer Academic Publishers, 1976.)

OTHER TYPES

A very interesting, emerging method that has found use in biology and medicine is confocal microscopy, which is sometimes combined with fluorescent techniques. In this system,[23] both the illumination and detection optics are focused down on a single volume element of the specimen—that is, they are confocal. The illumination beam diverges above and below the plane of focus so that elements away from the focal plane receive a much lower flux of illumination. A complete image is built up by sequentially adding the volume elements within the focal plane. A confocal microscope is particularly effective when operating in fluorescence.

Routine Procedures

Adjustments

Two main types of illumination have been used over the years in setting up the microscope for optimal viewing. The first, so-called "critical" or Nelson illumination, produces an image of the lamp filament (or the ground glass in front of the lamp condenser) superimposed on the image of the specimen. With this system, it is necessary to rack the substage condenser just slightly downward to spread out the image of the filament and make it more diffuse so as to avoid interfering with the specimen image. Uneven illumination from the image of the coiled filament/ground glass can be a problem.

A second method of illumination, now the preferred system throughout the world, was developed by Köhler early in the 19th century and bears his name. The object of Köhler illumination is to permit the use of coiled filament lamps (the standard type) while avoiding uneven illumination.

With Köhler illumination, adjustments are made so that the image of the lamp filament does not appear in the field of view but is actually focused in the plane of the aperture diaphragm. This produces a bright, evenly lit field of view against which the detail of the specimen is plainly recognizable. Köhler illumination also results in as wide a cone of illumination as possible from the condenser to achieve maximum resolution of fine detail. In Köhler illumination, the field diaphragm controls the area of the focused specimen being viewed, but has no effect on intensity or resolution. The following procedure, for a binocular microscope, includes eyepiece adjustments together with steps to achieve Köhler illumination.

1. Turn on the microscope lamp, and adjust the intensity to a comfortable level with the voltage control.
2. Bring the ×10 objective into position, and secure a specimen slide on the mechanical stage. Position the specimen under the objective with the stage adjustment knobs.
3. Adjust the interpupillary distance until binocular vision is obtained. Focus the specimen with the coarse and fine adjustment knobs.
4. Perform the diopter adjustment by first bringing the specimen into sharp focus while viewing only with the right eye. Now, using only the left eye, focus the specimen by rotating the diopter adjusting ring located on the left eyepiece. If the left eye is dominant, reverse eyepieces and the procedure.
5. To obtain Köhler illumination, first close down the field diaphragm, then move the substage condenser up or down by means of the height adjustment knob to bring the image of the field diaphragm into sharp focus onto the already-focused image of the specimen. Once adjusted in this manner, the condenser should be left in that position to maintain Köhler illumination.
6. By means of the condenser centration knobs, adjust the image of the field diaphragm so that it occupies the center of the field of view.

7. Open the field diaphragm until its image just disappears from the field of view.
8. Lift out an eyepiece, and while observing the image of the aperture diaphragm at the back of the objective, adjust the diaphragm until it is two-thirds to three-fourths open. Then replace the eyepiece.
9. Readjust both the field and the aperture diaphragms each time an objective is changed.

While viewing a specimen, minor adjustments of the aperture diaphragm can be used advantageously to reduce stray light and glare, as well as to enhance contrast. However, the aperture diaphragm should not be used to reduce the brightness of the image field. This results in a loss of resolving power. It is better to adjust the brightness of the image field by means of the lamp voltage control, or, for photomicrography, by means of neutral density filters.

CARE AND PREVENTIVE MAINTENANCE

Modern clinical microscopes are precision instruments and should be handled and used with care and respect. A microscope should be carried firmly with both hands (one underneath the base). Routine cleaning and maintenance ensures long-term mechanical and optical performance. Dust, dirt, or other particulate matter should be removed from lenses with a soft, "camel hair" brush, or blown away with an ear or nose syringe. Some residues can be removed with lens paper after breathing on the lens surface to deposit a thin film of moisture. Manufacturer-recommended lens cleaners can also be used with the lens paper.

After using an oil immersion objective, the immersion oil should be wiped off with lens paper followed by lens cleaner and additional lens paper. Gauze, facial tissue, or lab wipes should not be used to clean lens surfaces because scratching can occur. Proper covering and storage of the microscope minimizes the accumulation of dust. The National Committee for Clinical Laboratory Standards Document POL1-T2[14] contains a section on general microscopy as well as an excellent summary of the care of the microscope.

REFERENCES

1. Hoffman R. The modulation contrast microscope: Principles and performance. *J Microsc* 1977;110:205–222.
2. James J. *Light microscopic techniques in biology and medicine*. Dordrecht, The Netherlands: Kluwer Academic Publishers, 1976.
3. National Committee for Clinical Laboratory Standards. *Physician's office laboratory guidelines: Tentative guideline*. NCCLS Document POL1-T2, Vol. 12, No. 5. 2nd ed. Villanova, PA: National Committee for Clinical Laboratory Standards, 1992.
4. Richardson JH. *Handbook for the light microscope: A user's guide*. Park Ridge, NJ: Noyes Publications, 1991.
5. Slayter E, Slayter H. *Light and electron microscopy*. Cambridge: Cambridge University Press, 1992.

BIBLIOGRAPHY

Abramowitz MJ. The polarizing microscope. *American Laboratory* 1990;22(9):72.
Abramowitz MJ. Darkfield illumination. *American Laboratory* 1991;23(11):60.
Abramowitz MJ. Fluorescence filters. *American Laboratory* 1990;22(3):168.
Abramowitz MJ. Köhler illumination. *American Laboratory* 1989;21(4):106.
Abramowitz MJ. Microscope objectives. *American Laboratory* 1989;21(10):81.
Abramowitz MJ. The first order red compensator. *American Laboratory* 1989;21(11):110.
Brunzel NA. *Fundamentals of urine and body fluid analysis*. Philadelphia: WB Saunders, 1994.
Herman B, Lemasters J, eds. *Optical microscopy: Emerging methods and applications*. San Diego, CA: Academic Press, 1993.
Herman F, Jacobson K, eds. *Optical microscopy in biology*. New York: John Wiley & Sons, 1990.
James J, Tanke HJ, eds. *Biomedical light microscopy*. Dordrecht, The Netherlands: Kluwer Academic Publishers, 1991.
Lacey AJ, ed. *Light microscopy in biology: A practical approach*. Oxford: IRL Press at Oxford University Press, 1989.
Ringsrud KM, Linné JJ. *Urinalysis and body fluids: A color text and atlas*. St. Louis: Mosby–Year Book, 1995.
Schumann GB. *The urine sediment examination*. Baltimore: Williams & Wilkins, 1980.
Schumann GB, Schumann JL. *A manual of cytodiagnostic urinalysis*. Salt Lake City, UT: Cytodiagnostics Company, 1984.
Schumann GB, Schumann JL, Marcussen N. *Cytodiagnostic urinalysis of renal and lower urinary tract disorders*. New York: Igaku-Shoin, 1995.
Schumann GB, Weiss MA. *Atlas of renal and urinary tract cytology and its histopathologic bases*. Philadelphia: JB Lippincott, 1981.
Smith RF. *Microscopy and photomicrography: A working manual*. Boca Raton, FL: CRC Press, 1990.
White JG, et al. Development of a confocal imaging system for biological epifluorescence applications. In: Herman B, Jacobson K, eds. *Optical microscopy for biology*. New York: Wiley-Liss, 1990.

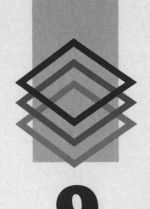

Microscopic Examination of Urine Sediment

9

ABBREVIATIONS USED IN THIS CHAPTER

2° = secondary

ABGs = arterial blood gases

AFB = acid-fast bacillus (bacilli)

AIDS = acquired immunodeficiency syndrome

AIN = acute interstitial nephritis

ATN = acute tubular necrosis

BAL = bronchoalveolar lavage

BP = blood pressure

BUN = blood urea nitrogen

C&S = culture and sensitivity

C-section = cesarean section

CAD = coronary artery disease

CAP = College of American Pathologists

CFU = colony-forming units

CHF = congestive heart failure

CK = creatine kinase

CKMB = creatine kinase isoenzyme 2 (CK-2)

(continued)

ABBREVIATIONS USED IN THIS CHAPTER

CLIA = Clinical Laboratory Improvement Act

CSF = cerebrospinal fluid

CT = computed tomography

ER = emergency room

HIV = human immunodeficiency virus

HPF = high power field

HTN = hypertension

ICU = intensive care unit

IDDM = insulin-dependent diabetes mellitus

IM = intramuscular

INH = isoniazid

IUP = intrauterine pregnancy

IV = intravenous

IVP = intravenous pyelogram

LE = lupus erythematosus

LPF = low-power field

MI = myocardial infarction

NCCLS = National Committee for Clinical Laboratory Standards

NIDDM = non–insulin-dependent diabetes mellitus

OIF = oil immersion field

PEG = percutaneous endoscopic gastrostomy

R/O = rule out

RBC = red blood cell

RCF = relative centrifugal force

RPM = rotations per minute

RTE = renal tubular epithelial cell

SIADH = syndrome of inappropriate secretion of antidiuretic hormone

SLE = systemic lupus erythematosus

SM = Sternheimer-Malbin

SOB = shortness of breath

TNTC = too numerous to count

UIP = usual interstitial pneumonia

UTI = urinary tract infection

WBC = white blood cell

Introductory Case Study

The patient, a 38-year-old woman, had been diagnosed with SLE a month before coming to California. An illegal immigrant, she was being held by the Immigration and Naturalization Service at the County Detention Facility. She was first seen in the hospital ER complaining of flank pain, fever, and dysuria. The urinalysis was significant for blood large; protein > 300 mg/dL; nitrite neg; leukocyte esterase trace; WBCs 20–50/HPF; RBCs 20–50/HPF; bacteria 4+; casts/LPF 1–5 WBC/mixed, 0–1 granular, and rare hyaline. The patient was treated in the ER for pyelonephritis, and was returned to the County Facility.

During the next several weeks, the patient was seen several times for combined UTI and lupus exacerbation problems with very similar urinalysis results, especially the proteinuria. On occasion, she was admitted to the hospital. In later admissions, mixed cellular and cellular/granular casts began to appear in the urine sediment. The generalized picture was pyelonephritis, glomerulonephritis (related to the SLE, so-called lupus nephritis), and the nephrotic syndrome (without lipiduria, fatty casts, and the like). At various times the urine C&S was positive for *Escherichia coli* or *Enterococcus* sp., and at times a direct Gram stain on the urine sediment showed gram-positive cocci resembling streptococci and gram-positive rods resembling corynebacteria. It also became apparent that she was allergic to potatoes. Even though she was carefully watched and her diet controlled, she might have been surreptitiously obtaining potato products (e.g., chips), so that in some instances her symptoms were a combination of her UTI problems, lupus nephritis, and food allergies. Further, there may have been periods of noncompliance in taking her medications.

During the 4-month period she was being seen at the hospital, her medications included a variety of antibiotics for the UTIs and prednisone for her lupus. The last time she was admitted to the hospital (before being sent to another state), her chief complaint was fever, weakness, and facial swelling.

The photomicrographs of the urine sediment for this case (Figs. 9-1 to 9-8) illustrate the combined effects of the pyelonephritis and lupus nephritis. The figures include examples of mixed cellular casts, waxy casts, clumps of WBCs, and coarsely granular casts. The peripheral blood smears for this patient showed LE cells on several occasions. One unusual photomicrograph from a peripheral blood smear obtained from this patient is included here (Fig. 9-9), showing an LE cell in the process of formation.

Continued

Introductory Case Study (continued) ━━━━━

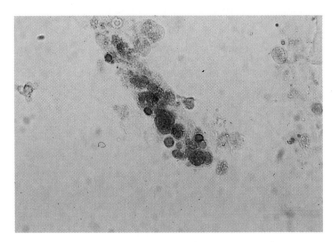

FIGURE 9-1 Mixed WBC/RBC/RTE cell cast. Urine sediment; SM stain; ×400.

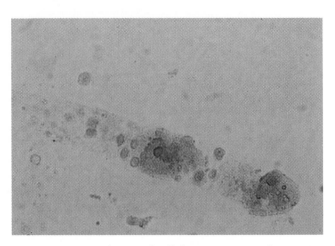

FIGURE 9-4 Granular/mixed cellular cast. Urine sediment; SM Stain ×400.

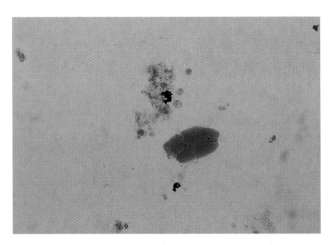

FIGURE 9-2 Fragment of granular/waxy cast. Urine sediment; SM stain; ×200.

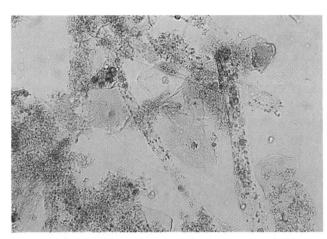

FIGURE 9-5 Granular/cellular casts, squamous epithelials, and amorphous background. Urine sediment; SM stain; ×200.

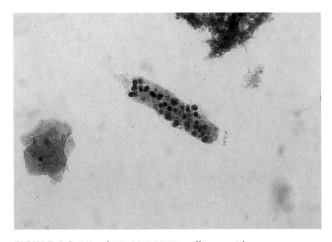

FIGURE 9-3 Mixed WBC/RBC/RTE cell cast with squamous epithelials. Urine sediment; toluidine blue stain; ×200.

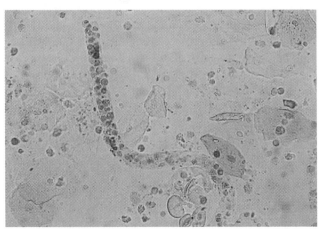

FIGURE 9-6 Mixed RBC/WBC cast with mixed cellular background. Urine sediment; SM stain; ×200.

Continued

Introductory Case Study (continued)

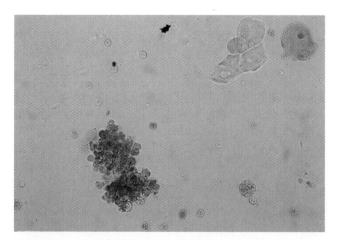

FIGURE 9-7 Clump of WBCs with mixed cellular background. Urine sediment; SM stain; ×200.

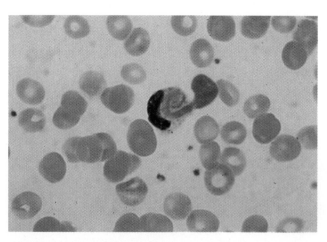

FIGURE 9-9 Peripheral blood; LE cell in process of formation. Peripheral blood smear; Wright's stain; ×1000.

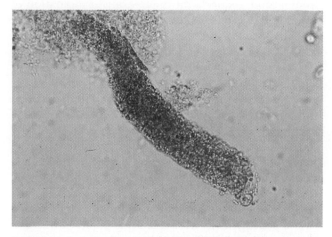

FIGURE 9-8 Coarsely granular cast. Urine sediment; SM stain; ×400.

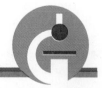

Significance of Formed Elements in Urine

In previous chapters, we discussed the physical examination and the chemical examination of urine. The microscopic examination of the urinary sediment is the third part of the routine urinalysis.

The urine specimen has been referred to as a liquid tissue biopsy of the urinary tract—painlessly obtained.[10,11] Of the laboratory procedures used for the detection of renal or urinary tract disease, the microscopic examination of urine is the most common.[25] The pellet from a centrifuged urine specimen contains all the insoluble material (formed elements) accumulated in the urine, starting with glomerular filtration and continuing on through the renal tubules and lower urinary tract, with the additional possibility of external contamination. The formed elements may include body cells of various types, casts of precipitated protein (some containing inclusions) formed in the renal tubules, microorganisms, parasites, crystals and amorphous deposits of chemicals, and various miscellaneous and exogenous items.

For many years, the microscopic analysis of the urine sediment has been a part of every "routine urinalysis." However, since approximately the mid-1980s, some workers have concluded that the microscopic analysis may not be necessary or cost efficient on every urine specimen tested.[2,13,14] Conversely, others have concluded that eliminating the urine microscopic analysis from routine urinalysis risks missing important information.[1,17,28] For example, one study[28] demonstrated that important cellular components can be present in urine specimens with negative dipstick results.

In many laboratories the microscopic analysis of the urine sediment is performed only when abnormal findings are seen in the physical and chemical analysis of the urine, or when indicated by the patient's condition or clinical history. Parameters considered significant vary among institutions but usually consist of various combinations of color, turbidity, protein, blood, nitrite, leukocyte esterase, or glucose. The NCCLS states that "The decision to perform microscopic examinations must be made by each individual laboratory based on its specific patient population."[19] It goes on to suggest that the microscopic analysis should be performed when requested by the physician, when determined by laboratory protocol, or when any abnormal physicochemical result is obtained. Because some of the formed elements found in the urine sediment usually have no clinical significance and others are considered normal unless present in increased amounts, the sediment analysis must include both the identification and the quantitation of the elements present.

The urine microscopic examination is the most time-consuming part of the routine urinalysis and, until rather recently, was also the least standardized component. Increasingly, many laboratories now use some sort of standardized system for the examination of the urine sediment. Normal or reference values for formed elements in the urine are often different from one laboratory to another because of variations in preparing the specimen for examination and in the standardized procedures and equipment that are available. Although the requirement for a sediment analysis on every urine remains controversial, most laboratorians agree that an accurate urine sediment examination is an essential medical laboratory test for symptomatic patients.[25]

Methodology and Quality Assurance

Specimen Requirements

Urine specimens are discussed in detail in Chapter 4, and only a brief review related to the microscopic examination of sediment is presented here.

COLLECTION

According to the NCCLS,[19] the specimen of choice for a microscopic evaluation is the first morning urine, even though a randomly collected specimen is often more convenient to the patient and is probably suitable for most screening purposes. The first morning specimen is the most concentrated for the day so that recovery of small amounts of abnormal constituents is maximized, and cells and casts that tend to disintegrate in urine of low specific gravity are better preserved. The first morning urine is also the most acidic, which means that cells and casts that tend to disintegrate at an alkaline pH are protected. Ideally, the urine should also be a midstream, clean-catch specimen to avoid contamination as much as possible.

HANDLING

Urine specimens should be examined within 2 hours of voiding, or they should be refrigerated and examined as soon as possible. Specimens are unacceptable for microscopic examination if they are left unrefrigerated for more than 2 hours. At the time of examination, requests for microscopic examination of urine should be accompanied by information about the type of specimen, the time of collection, as well as the results of testing for chemical and physical parameters.

Although refrigeration retards the development of bacteria and minimizes the shift to an alkaline pH because of ammonia production, cooling the specimen may result in the formation of amorphous or crystalline deposits. The amorphous deposits especially may interfere with the microscopic examination. Although the NCCLS does not recommend any chemical preservatives for routine urinalysis, their use may be helpful in certain instances. Formalin preserves various formed elements in the sediment and is present in several commercially available urine preservatives. Because formalin interferes with several of the chemical tests on dipstick reagent strips, it is possible to divide a well-mixed urine specimen into two parts, one part receiving formalin for the preservation of cells and casts, the other remaining unaltered for chemical testing.

Specimen Preparation

STANDARDIZATION

Essential for accuracy and precision in routine urinalysis, standardization reduces the ambiguity and subjectivity inherent in the procedure itself. Standardization is necessary for an accurate and precise routine urinalysis and begins with the arrival of the specimen to the laboratory, all specimens being processed according to a strict protocol.[25] According to the NCCLS,[19] the following specific factors must be standardized:

Volume of urine examined. Twelve milliliters of urine is the amount recommended for examination. If a volume less than 12 mL is submitted and processed, a corresponding factor must be applied to all numeric sediment counts.

Time of centrifugation. To ensure equal sedimentation of all specimens, the recommended time of centrifugation is 5 minutes.

Speed of centrifugation. The recommended RCF (relative centrifugal force) is 400. To calculate RCF from rotations per minute (RPM) for a specific centrifuge, use the following formula: RCF = 1.118×10^{-5} (upper) $\times$ r $\times$ N^2, where r = the radius in centimeters (at the bottom of the tube) and N = RPM.

Volume of sediment examined. Standardized commercial systems provide a slide with chambers of a given volume that hold a specific amount of concentrated sediment.

Reporting format. Every person at a given institution who performs a microscopic examination should use the same terminology, reporting format, and reference ranges. Decisions about which formed elements should be reported and quantitated should be made by the individual laboratory based on the patient population and professional skill level of the people performing the testing.

COMMERCIAL SYSTEMS

Several commercial systems have been developed to standardize the urine sediment analysis and improve the accuracy and precision of the procedure as performed by the laboratorian using light microscopy. Three rather similar standardized systems are the UriSystem (Fisher Scientific, Pittsburgh, PA); the KOVA system (ICL Scientific, Fountain Valley, CA); and the Count-6 or Count-10 systems (V-Tech, Inc., Palm Desert, CA). Each system provides centrifuge tubes and caps, transfer pipettes, a supravital stain, and a choice of standardized slides. Each system is designed to permit easy decanting of supernatant urine and consistent retention of a defined volume of undisturbed, concentrated sediment in the centrifuge tube. Similarly, each is designed to provide a consistent volume of resuspended sediment for microscopic analysis rather than using a "drop" of sediment under a coverslip on a microscope slide.

Standardized systems have been compared with "in-house" techniques[6] as well as among themselves.[15] In terms of accuracy, precision, and sensitivity, there can be little doubt that the commercial systems are better than "in-house" systems. Studies also show that lab-

oratories need to reevaluate their normal ranges for urine sediment analysis when converting to standardized systems or when switching between systems. Given the benefits gained by the use of a standardized system, coupled with its competitive cost, the use of glass slides and coverslips seems obsolete.[25]

The recently developed Cen-Slide 1500 System (Urohealth, formerly DAVSTAR, Costa Mesa, CA) uses a collection-dispensing container, the Cen-Slide tube, which is a centrifuge tube with a counting chamber at the tip; a specially designed centrifuge; a rack to permit proper settling after centrifugation; and a Cen-Slide microscope holder. The centrifuge automatically spins the samples for 20 seconds at the proper speed and then flicks the tubes to disperse the sediment evenly in the counting chamber. The Cen-Slide Holder correctly positions the tip of Cen-Slide Tube under the microscope objective for viewing.

As reviewed by Monferdini et al., the R/S 2000 (DiaSys, Waterbury, CT) consists of a glass optical counting chamber that is mounted on the microscope and attached to an aspiration pump.[16] The aspiration pipette is placed manually into the centrifuge tube after sedimentation (and decanting, if desired). Resuspension of the sediment occurs quickly because of the turbulence created during the aspiration of 180 μL. After passing through the viewing area of the optical slide, the sediment settles rapidly with even dispersion of formed elements. After analysis of the sediment, the tubing and optical slide are flushed automatically with 700 μL of saline and the system is ready for another specimen.

Examination of the Sediment

PROCEDURES

Each laboratory uses variations on a theme for examining the urinary sediment. In general, for each type of formed element in the urinary sediment, 10 fields are examined and the average number or "grading" is reported based on these 10 fields. An example is outlined in the following:

Low-Power Examination (10× objective)
    Casts. Each type of cast is graded and enumerated separately, and reported as the average number of casts observed per LPF.
    Squamous epithelial cells. Reported as few, moderate, or many; or as 1+, 2+, and so forth, per LPF.

Crystals. Normal crystals are reported as few, moderate, or many per LPF (note some laboratories use high power for this). Abnormal crystals are reported as the average number seen per LPF but should be confirmed before they are reported.

Mucus. This can be reported as scant, moderate, or heavy.

High-Power Examination (40× objective)

Red blood cells. Graded and reported on the basis of the average number seen per HPF. Abnormal forms such as dysmorphic cells are reported.

White blood cells. Graded and reported on the basis of the average number seen per HPF. The WBCs are usually neutrophils, but if unusual types such as lymphocytes or eosinophils can be identified, they should be reported.

Epithelial cells. Renal tubular epithelial cells (RTE; identified as to type), transitional epithelial cells, and oval fat bodies may be reported as few, moderate, or many; or as 1+, 2+, and so forth, per HPF.

Miscellaneous. This category includes structures such as microorganisms, parasites, sperm (reported for men only), and the like. These categories may be graded as few, moderate, or many, or described numerically such as 1+, 2+, 3+, and so forth.

TABLE 9-1
Typical Reference Values for Urinary Sediment

Formed Element	12:1 Concentration
RBCs	0–3/HPF
WBCs (neutrophils)	0–8/HPF
Hyaline casts	0–2/LPF
RTCs	Few/HPF
Transitional epithelials	Few/HPF
Squamous epithelials	Few/LPF
Bacteria and yeast	Neg/HPF
Abnormal crystals	None/HPF

(From Schumann GB, Schumann JL, Marcussen N. *Cytodiagnostic urinalysis of renal and lower urinary tract disorders.* New York: IGAKU-SHOIN Medical Publishers, Inc., 1995.)

The term "too numerous to count" (TNTC) may be used when markedly increased numbers of formed elements are observed, although each laboratory has a certain "cut-off" value for the use of this term. For example, the rule might be to use TNTC if the number of WBCs/HPF is greater than 20, or 30, and so forth. As part of quality assurance, the microscopic results should be correlated with the physical and chemical findings to identify discrepancies that can then be investigated for both technical and clerical errors. Each laboratory develops its own reference values for urinary sediment based on its patient population and "system" of urinalysis (Table 9-1).

METHODS TO INCREASE CONTRAST

Supravital Stains

A mixture of crystal-violet and safranin, also known as the Sternheimer-Malbin (SM) stain, is commonly used in many laboratories. This stain is absorbed well by WBCs, epithelial cells, and casts, providing better delineation of structure. Nuclei and cytoplasm are stained contrasting colors. It is available commercially as Sedi-Stain (Clay-Adams, Sparks, MD), Kova-Stain (ICL Scientific), and others. The stain (one or two drops) is mixed with the concentrated urine sediment (usually 1 mL) before examination.

A 0.5% solution of toluidine blue is also a good supravital stain to differentiate between the nucleus and cytoplasm in various cells. For example, it aids in distinguishing between cells of similar size, such as leukocytes and small renal collecting duct cells.

Acetic Acid

Although it is not a stain, acetic acid can be used to aid in the identification of white blood cells. Small WBCs with nuclei and granulation not readily apparent may be difficult to differentiate from RBCs and certain epithelial cells. Adding one or two drops of a 2% solution of acetic acid enhances the nuclear pattern of WBCs and epithelial cells and lyses the RBCs.

Lipid Stains

Globules of neutral fat or triglycerides floating free in the urine or contained within cells or casts may be difficult to distinguish from other objects but stain orange or red with lipid stains like Sudan III or Oil Red O. Only neutral fats stain with these reagents; cholesterol and cholesterol esters do not stain but can be confirmed with polarizing microscopy.

Gram Stain

Usually carried out in the microbiology department, a direct Gram stain of a dry preparation of the urine sediment on a microscope slide provides immediate information on bacteria found in the urine, differentiating them as gram negative or gram positive. These slides can be viewed with the oil immersion objective and the bacteria characterized as cocci, rods, and so forth.

Hansel's Stain

Patients with acute interstitial nephritis resulting from hypersensitivity to medication have increased numbers of eosinophils in the urine sediment. It is important to identify this condition so that the offending drug can be withdrawn before permanent renal damage occurs. Although Wright's stain or Giemsa's stain can be used, many workers prefer Hansel's stain specifically to identify eosinophils in the urine. The stain consists of methylene blue and eosin-Y in methanol (Lide Labs, Florrisant, MO).

Microscopy Techniques

To delineate the more translucent formed elements of the urine (such as hyaline casts, crystals, and mucus) using brightfield microscopy, it is usually necessary to reduce the light intensity. For this problem, the use of phase contrast microscopy or interference contrast microscopy can greatly aid in the identification of such translucent objects. Stains can be used to facilitate the differentiation of leukocytes, epithelial cells, cellular casts, and the like.

Objects that are birefringent (optically active) rotate the plane of polarized light. When such objects are viewed with crossed polarizing filters, they appear to be sources of light against a dark or black background. Polarizing microscopy can be used in differentiating RBCs, which are not birefringent, from the ovoid form of calcium oxalate, which is birefringent. Lipid droplets containing cholesterol show a characteristic "Maltese cross" pattern when viewed with polarized light, whereas other lipids do not. Starch also shows the Maltese cross pattern, but crystals or objects that might be confused with starch do not. Casts are not birefringent (although cholesterol-containing lipid droplets in the casts are), but fibers containing cellulose, which might be confused with casts, are strongly birefringent.

Quality Assurance

As with most other laboratory procedures, quality assurance in urinalysis requires the continual monitoring of every aspect of the process as it relates to the patient, the physician, and the laboratory. Quality assurance is more than just quality control. It also encompasses standardization, technical competence, and continuing education.[25] Some of the commercially available urinalysis control materials contain stabilized RBCs and WBCs (or simulated WBCs [plastic particles]) so that specimen preparation and microscopic examination

may be monitored and evaluated. Stabilized casts and epithelial cells (or simulated ones) are apparently not yet available in commercial control materials.

Schumann and Schweitzer[25] advocate in-house controls (urine specimens chosen by the supervisor and run by each shift) as an excellent means of monitoring the precision of both the macroscopic and the microscopic urinalysis. They suggest the use of in-house urine specimens as "known controls" on a daily basis, with known specimens slipped into the workload as "unknown controls" on a monthly basis.

Proficiency surveys (interlaboratory comparison testing on a periodic basis) have been a standard requirement for College of American Pathologists (CAP) accreditation for many years and are also required by the Clinical Laboratory Improvement Act (CLIA) of 1988.[5] Urinalysis proficiency surveys often include Kodachrome slides for the identification of sediment components, such as casts, cells, and artifacts. One approach to using the slides is for each technologist in the laboratory to identify the sediment components independently. After results are shared, one answer is submitted to the survey agency. Although this format has limitations, it does allow evaluation of competence in microscopic identification. In addition, arriving at an answer by consensus provides an opportunity to maintain and improve the competence of personnel.[5]

Cytocentrifugation and Cytodiagnostic Urinalysis

Observing stained or unstained specimens of urine sediment has traditionally been the way to screen asymptomatic patients who show macroscopic urinalysis abnormalities. Early detection of hematuria and urinary tract infections can be achieved by using standardized systems and microscopic enhancements such as phase contrast microscopy. However, many elements found in urine sediment are difficult to interpret using unstained brightfield microscopy, including mononuclear cells, inclusion-bearing cells, pathologic casts, RTEs and fragments, premalignant and malignant urothelial cells, and malignant cells of nonurothelial origin.

Cytodiagnostic urinalysis is primarily used to narrow the clinician's diagnosis of inflammatory, infectious, degenerative, or neoplastic conditions involving the kidney as well as the lower urinary tract.[23] Like all medical laboratory tests, cytodiagnostic urinalysis should be considered after a clinical history and physical examination. It is not a screening test but is meant for patients with signs, symptoms, or histories of urinary tract disorders.

Developments since the early 1980s have expanded the role of urinary cytology to include diagnosis of renal disease as well as lower urinary tract neoplasms. Urinary cytology is safe for the patient, economical, noninvasive to minimally invasive with regard to specimen collection, and able to detect and monitor numerous renal and lower urinary tract disorders.[28]

To carry out cytodiagnostic urinalysis, cytocentrifugation must be used to prepare the specimens for examination. An appropriate amount of a concentrated urine sediment is placed in a specially designed cartridge fitted with a microscope slide, then placed in a cytocentrifuge (e.g., Cytospin, Shandon Southern Instruments, Sewickley, PA) for slow-speed centrifugation. A dry, circular monolayer of sediment components remains on the slide after centrifugation, and the slide can be permanently fixed using an appropriate reagent before staining. For cytology studies, Papanicolaou stain is preferred, although Wright's or Giemsa's stain can also be used. The end result is a preparation of formed elements with their structural details greatly enhanced by staining. The slides are permanent, and can be viewed with oil immersion and retained in the laboratory for study and reference.

Formed Elements in Urinary Sediment

A variety of formed elements may be found in normal urine sediment. Small numbers of elements usually considered to be pathologic (RBCs, WBCs, casts) can be perfectly normal. As a means of monitoring disease progression or resolution, the components found in urine sediment can be identified and enumerated. To determine at what point the amount of each formed element present indicates a pathologic process, it is necessary to be familiar with the expected normal or reference range for each component.[5] A few RBCs, WBCs, epithelial cells, and hyaline casts may be observed in the urine sediment from normal, healthy individuals. Their number varies and depends on the standardized slide system and procedure used for the microscopic examination. Because of changes that occur in unpreserved urine, specimen collection and storage strongly affect what formed elements are observed during the microscopic examination.

Blood Cells

ERYTHROCYTES (RED BLOOD CELLS)

As viewed with the 40× objective, RBCs appear as enucleate, smooth, biconcave, moderately refractile, pale discs that are usually about 7 μm in diameter. When they are observed from different angles, they may have an hourglass shape (viewed from the side) or appear as discs with a central pallor if viewed from above. In hypertonic solution, they become smaller and crenated as water is lost from the cell. In hypotonic urine, erythrocytes swell and release their hemoglobin to become "ghost cells."

Bleeding may be assumed to be renal in origin when increased numbers of erythrocytes are found in the urine together with RBC casts. Aberrant or dysmorphic erythrocytes are specific for glomerular bleeding. Increased numbers of erythrocytes[25] in the urine may be present in:

1. Renal disease, including glomerulonephritis; lupus nephritis; interstitial nephritis associated with drug reactions; calculus; tumor; acute infection; tuberculosis; infarction; renal vein thrombosis; trauma including renal biopsy; hydronephrosis; polycystic kidney; and occasionally acute tubular necrosis and malignant nephrosclerosis
2. Lower urinary tract disease, including acute and chronic infection; calculus; tumor; stricture; and hemorrhagic cystitis after cyclophosphamide therapy
3. Extrarenal disease, including acute appendicitis; salpingitis; diverticulitis; and tumors of the colon, rectum, and pelvis; acute febrile episodes; malaria; subacute bacterial endocarditis; polyarteritis nodosa; malignant hypertension; blood dyscrasias; and scurvy
4. Toxic reactions due to drugs, such as sulfonamides, salicylates, methenamine, and anticoagulant therapy
5. Physiologic causes, including exercise

On occasion, RBCs may be confused with oil droplets, yeast cells, air bubbles, ovoid calcium oxalate crystals, or even WBCs (in hypertonic urine). Oil droplets and air bubbles exhibit a great variation in size and are highly refractile. Yeast cells usually show budding and do not stain with supravital stains. Acetic acid or toluidine blue may be used to accentuate the nuclei in WBCs. Acetic acid lyses the RBCs while leaving all other components unchanged.

The microscopic observation of RBCs in the urinary sediment should be correlated with the results of both the physical and chemical examinations.[5] The color and turbidity of the specimen or the color of the sediment may correlate well with a positive result for blood on the dipstick. Sometimes a specimen gives a positive chemical test for blood but no RBCs are visible on microscopic examination. Lysis of the RBCs in the specimen or in the body liberates hemoglobin (which reacts on the reagent strip), leaving behind the stroma or cell membranes, which appear as faint, colorless circles often called "shadow cells" or "ghost cells." Subdued light should reveal the presence of these cell membranes, but they are more obvious with phase contrast microscopy. False-positive chemical tests for blood are also possible with substances like myoglobin, microbial peroxidases, and strong oxidizing agents.

The opposite problem may occur: a sediment may reveal RBCs, but the chemical screen is negative. The most common reason for such a false-negative result is ascorbic acid. If this cause is ruled out, then perhaps the elements are not RBCs after all but some entity that resembles RBCs, such as yeast or an unusual form of calcium oxalate crystals.

Illustrations of RBCs are given in Figures 9-10 and 9-11 and are seen in Case Studies 9-2 and 9-7, as well as in Chapter 10 (Case Study 10-13). Crenated RBCs are shown in Figure 9-10, and dysmorphic RBCs are seen in Figure 9-11.

LEUKOCYTES (WHITE BLOOD CELLS)

Neutrophils

Under the 40× objective, neutrophilic leukocytes appear as granular spheres about 12 μm in diameter. In fresh urine specimens, nuclear detail is fairly well defined even with brightfield microscopy. As the cells age and begin to disintegrate, nuclear lobes begin to fuse and neutrophils then may be difficult to distinguish from collecting duct RTEs. In dilute hypotonic urine, neutrophils swell as they take in water, lysing rapidly at room temperature. The refractile cytoplasmic granules within the swollen cells exhibit brownian movement, giving rise to the descriptive name "glitter cells."

Increased numbers of leukocytes in the urine (pyuria or leukocyturia), principally neutrophils, are associated with almost all renal diseases and inflam-

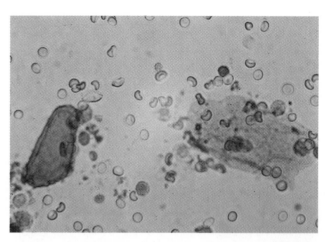

FIGURE 9-11 RBCs and mixed cellular background; urine sediment. SM stain; ×400.

matory conditions of the genitourinary tract. Bacterial infections include pyelonephritis, cystitis, prostatitis, and urethritis. Nonbacterial disorders include glomerulonephritis, LE, interstitial nephritis, and tumors. Calculus disease at any level may give rise to increased numbers of urinary leukocytes because of either stasis-induced ascending infection or localized mucosal inflammatory response.[25] Increased numbers of leukocytes in the urine may be observed with fevers and after strenuous exercise.

Cellular lysis and disintegration may lead to a positive chemical screening test for leukocyte esterase, even though few if any WBCs are evident microscopically. Further, some cells such as lymphocytes contain no leukocyte esterase. In the case of leukocyturia with a negative leukocyte esterase screening test, it is important to determine whether the cells are granulocytic leukocytes and whether the reagent strips are functioning properly.

Neutrophils are illustrated in Figures 9-12 to 9-14 and are seen in Case Studies 9-1, 9-4, and 9-5, as well as in Chapter 10 (Case Study 10-15).

Eosinophils

If clinically indicated, leukocyturia should be further analyzed for the presence of eosinophils.[25] A cytocentrifuge preparation is stained with Hansel's secretion stain (methylene blue and eosin-Y in methanol, Lide Labs). This stain is considered superior to Wright's stain and other stains in detecting eosinophils in urine. Eosinophiluria is a good predictor of acute interstitial nephritis (AIN) associated with drug hypersensitivity and is occasionally observed with chronic UTIs. Because untreated AIN can lead to permanent renal damage, it is important to detect it early so that the offending drug (such as penicillin and its analogs) can be discontinued in time to permit recovery.

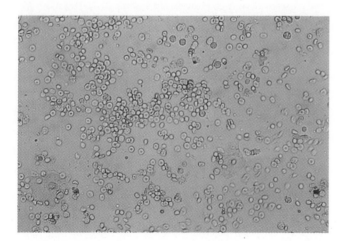

FIGURE 9-10 RBCs and mixed cellular background; urine sediment. SM stain; ×200.

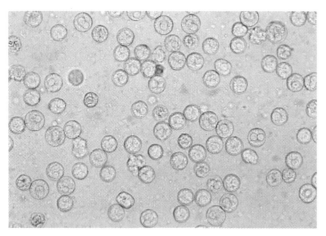

FIGURE 9-12 WBCs with bacteria; urine sediment. SM stain; ×400.

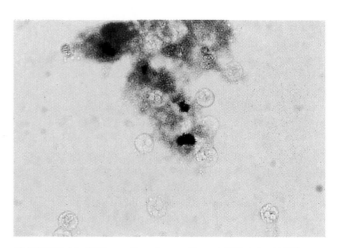

FIGURE 9-14 Glitter cells; urine sediment. SM stain; ×400.

Lymphocytes

Lymphocytes are present in inflammatory conditions such as acute pyelonephritis, although they are usually not recognized because neutrophils predominate. They can be identified by using cytocentrifugation followed by Wright's or Papanicolaou stain. Most of the lymphocytes found in the urinary sediment are small, about 6 to 9 μm in diameter. Leukocyturia is observed in patients experiencing renal transplant rejection, but lymphocytes predominate rather than neutrophils.

Monocytes and Macrophages (Histiocytes)

Both monocytes and macrophages are actively phagocytic and are seen in the urine sediment. Renal tubulointerstitial diseases resulting from infections or immune reactions draw monocytes and macrophages to the site of inflammation by chemotaxis. Monocytes

range in diameter from 20 to 40 μm, have a single large nucleus, contain abundant cytoplasm with azurophilic granules, and may contain large vacuoles. Macrophages are derived from monocytes, average 30 to 40 μm in diameter (although they can be as small as 10 μm or as large as 100 μm in diameter), have a single large nucleus, and their abundant cytoplasm may also be vacuolated. Macrophages that reside in interstitial tissues are often referred to as histiocytes. Macrophages and monocytes are more easily identified using supravital stains on the urine sediment or using Papanicolaou stain after cytocentrifugation.

Monocytes and macrophages that have ingested lipids, and renal tubular cells that have absorbed fats, are all termed "oval fat bodies." Polarizing microscopy or lipid stains may be used to confirm the identity of these cellular inclusions.

Histocytes are illustrated in Figures 9-15 and 9-16.

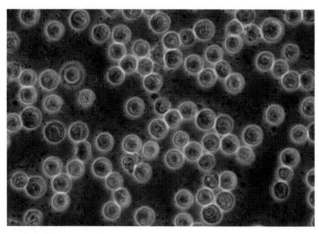

FIGURE 9-13 Same specimen and field of view as Figure 9-12. SM stain/phase contrast; ×400.

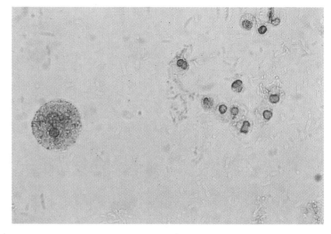

FIGURE 9-15 Histiocyte with WBCs and bacteria; urine sediment. SM stain; ×400.

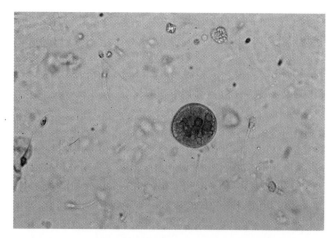

FIGURE 9-16 Histiocyte with sperm; urine sediment. SM stain; ×400.

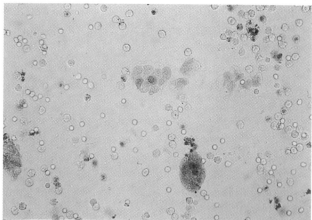

FIGURE 9-17 Binucleated RTE (proximal tubule) with WBCs, RBCs, and small transitional epithelials; urine sediment. Toluidine blue stain; ×200.

Epithelial Cells

In general, three types of epithelial cells are found in the urine sediment: renal tubular epithelial cells, transitional epithelial cells (or urothelial cells), and squamous epithelial cells, with squamous epithelial cells the most commonly seen. The appearance of a few epithelial cells in the urine is not unusual because they are derived from the linings of the genitourinary system, and unless they are present in large numbers or in abnormal forms, they represent normal sloughing of old cells.

RENAL TUBULAR EPITHELIAL CELLS

Using the Papanicolaou stain, renal tubular cells from the proximal and the distal convoluted tubules have been identified and may be semiquantitated. Proximal convoluted tubular cells are relatively large (20–60 μm), have granular cytoplasm, and are oblong or cigar shaped so that they may resemble granular casts.[23] The nucleus is small, often eccentric, and has a dense chromatin pattern. The cells can be multinucleated.

Distal convoluted tubular cells are approximately 14 to 25 μm in diameter, are round to oval in shape, and are smaller than the proximal tubule cells. The nucleus is small, dense, and usually eccentric and the cytoplasm is granular, much like that of proximal tubular cells.[23] Increased numbers of proximal and distal convoluted tubular cells are found in the urine as a result of acute ischemic or toxic renal tubular disease (acute tubular necrosis) associated with drug toxicity (nonsteroidal pain relievers, aminoglycosides), heavy metals, immunosuppressants, and mushroom poisoning. Renal tubular cells may contain inclusions such as lipids (oval fat bodies), hemosiderin from hemoglobin-

uria/myoglobinuria, melanin granules from melanuria, and bilirubin pigment, which also colors other elements of the sediment.

Renal tubular epithelial cells from the proximal and the distal convoluted tubules are illustrated in Figures 9-17, 9-18, and 9-79, and are seen in Case Study 9-5 as well as in Chapter 10 (Case Study 10-2).

COLLECTING DUCT EPITHELIAL CELLS

Epithelial cells from the small and large collecting ducts measure 12 to 20 μm and are cuboidal, polygonal, or columnar (never round) with a large, usually slightly eccentric nucleus. Progressing to the renal calyces, collecting duct cells become larger and more columnar. The urine sediment may contain increased numbers of collecting duct cells in all types of renal diseases, including nephritis, acute tubular necrosis, kidney transplant rejection, and salicylate poisoning.

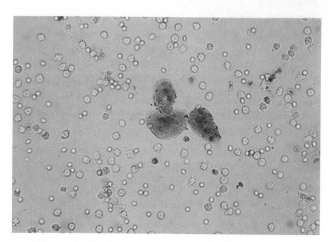

FIGURE 9-18 RTEs (proximal tubule) with WBCs and RBCs; urine sediment. Toluidine blue stain; ×200.

FIGURE 9-19 RTEs (collecting duct), bacteria, and urine sediment. SM stain; ×400.

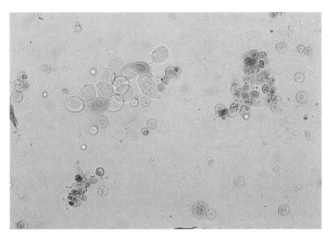

FIGURE 9-20 Transitional cells with mixed cellular background; urine sediment. SM stain; ×200.

Renal epithelial fragments of collecting duct origin have been described, whereas proximal and distal convoluted tubular cells are not found in fragment form.[25] Three or more renal cells of collecting duct origin constitute a renal epithelial fragment and indicate a more severe form of renal tubular injury with basement membrane disruption. These fragments indicate ischemic necrosis and are usually associated with renal tubular injury and pathologic casts.

Collecting duct cells are demonstrated in Figure 9-19.

TRANSITIONAL EPITHELIAL (UROTHELIAL) CELLS

"Urothelium, lining the surfaces of the renal pelvis, ureter, bladder, prostatic ducts, seminal vesicles and proximal urethra, is composed of large, superficial (umbrella-like) cells covering several layers of smaller, more basilar cells."[23] In men, urothelium also lines the proximal urethra, whereas in women, it does not extend past the base of the bladder.

The average thickness of normal urothelium is five to seven cell layers.[23] The cells vary considerably in size, from those found in the superficial layer, which are large, flattened, umbrella-like cells, to those in the intermediate layers, which are smaller and rounder, to those from the basal layer, which are elongated or columnar.

In the urine, urothelial (transitional) cells range from 40 to 200 μm in size.[25] They may absorb water and become rounded or pear shaped with a dense oval/round nucleus and abundant cytoplasm. They may appear flat and almost squamous like, and may be binucleate or multinucleate, as well as vacuolated. If they have tail-like projections, they are referred to as caudate cells.

A few urothelialcells are present in normal urine, reflecting normal desquamation. Increased numbers of transitional epithelial cells are often present in the urine in cases of UTI, and clusters or sheets of transitional cells are seen after urinary catheterization or other instrumentation procedures. Sheets of cells appearing without such procedures suggest transitional cell carcinoma anywhere from the renal pelvis to the bladder and indicate the need for cytologic investigation. Binucleated or multinucleated cells (reactive transitional cells) are seen with acute inflammatory processes within the urinary tract.

Transitional epithelial cells are illustrated in Figures 9-20 to 9-22 and are seen in Case Study 9-10, as well as in Chapter 10 (Case Studies 10-4, 10-10, 10-14, and 10-15).

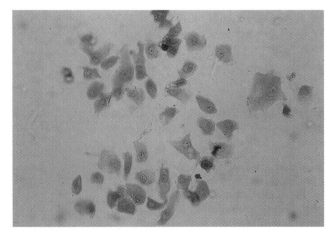

FIGURE 9-21 Reactive transitional epithelials; urine sediment. SM stain; ×200.

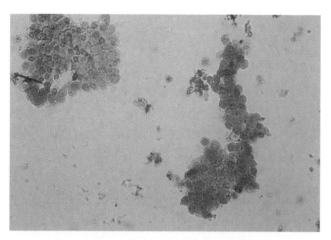

FIGURE 9-22 Two groups of transitional epithelial cells from a catheterized specimen; urine sediment. SM stain; ×200.

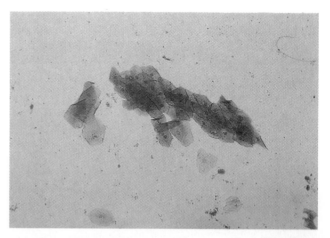

FIGURE 9-24 Squamous epithelial cells; urine sediment. SM stain; ×100.

SQUAMOUS EPITHELIAL CELLS

These are the most common and the largest of the epithelial cells observed in the urine. Lining the distal portion of the male urethra and the entire female urethra, they are large (40–60 μm), thin, and flat, although they may appear curled or rolled up into cylinders. In urine from women they often represent vaginal/perineal contamination and in urine from uncircumcised men they also suggest specimen contamination. They occur singly or in clumps or sheets, and are easily identified using the 10× objective.

Squamous epithelials are illustrated in Figures 9-23 and 9-24 as well as in Chapter 10 (Case Studies 10-13 and 10-15).

Casts

FORMATION AND GENERAL CHARACTERISTICS

As a gelatin desert takes on the shape of the mold in which it is formed, proteins in urine that congeal in the tubular lumen of a nephron (primarily in the distal convoluted tubule and collecting duct) form cylindrical "casts."

The basic matrix of a cast is considered to be a glycoprotein, known as Tamm-Horsfall protein, secreted by renal tubular cells at a fairly constant rate, and providing immunologic protection from infection.[28] Plasma proteins present in the filtrate can also be incorporated into the cast. Any component in the urine (e.g., cells, bacteria, crystals) can be incorporated into a cast. When the cast becomes detached from the tubular epithelial cells, it is flushed on down through the system to the urinary bladder.

Factors that enhance cast formation include an acid pH, increased concentration of solutes, urinary stasis, and increased concentration of proteins in the filtrate. Casts may be classified according to their matrix, inclusions, pigments, and the type of cells present. Table 9-2 summarizes the types and clinical significance of renal urinary casts.[23]

CAST MATRIX

Hyaline casts, which are translucent and nearly featureless, are difficult to see with brightfield microscopy unless the light intensity is markedly reduced. They are easily observed with phase-contrast microscopy. They are the most frequently seen cast and it is considered normal to observe up to two hyaline casts per LPF. Normal, transient increases in hyaline casts occur after

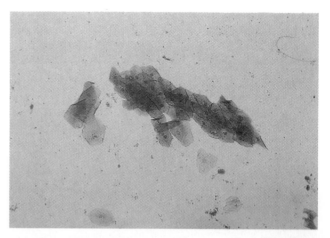

FIGURE 9-23 Squamous epithelials, WBCs, and one transitional epithelial; urine sediment. SM stain; ×200.

TABLE 9-2
Types and Clinical Significance of Renal Urinary Casts

Type of Cast	Clinical Significance
Physiologic	
Hyaline	Exercise, dehydration, fever, and nonspecific renal injury
Finely granular	Damaged glomeruli; leakage of proteins into urine (same as hyaline)
Pathologic	
Coarsely granular	Cellular degeneration; tubulointerstitial disease
Erythrocytic	Glomerulopathy; tubulointerstitial bleeding
Blood	Glomerulopathy; tubulointerstitial bleeding
Fibrin	Glomerulopathy; leakage of coagulation products into urine
Leukocytic	Tubulointerstitial inflammation
Neutrophilic	Acute nephritis; acute pyelonephritis
Lymphocytic	Chronic nephritis; acute allograft rejection
Eosinophilic	Allergic nephritis
Renal tubular cell	Acute renal failure, acute tubular necrosis (ATN); tubulointerstitial disease; acute allograft rejection
Waxy	Tubulointerstitial disease; chronic renal failure
Fatty	Nephrotic syndrome
Mixed	Tubulointerstitial disease
Broad	Chronic renal failure
Myeloma	Myeloma cast nephropathy
Bile	Liver dysfunction; tubulointerstitial disease
Candidal	Renal candidiasis
Bacterial	Acute pyelonephritis; acute nephritis
Crystal	Acute renal failure (ATN)
Lithiasis	Renal lithiasis

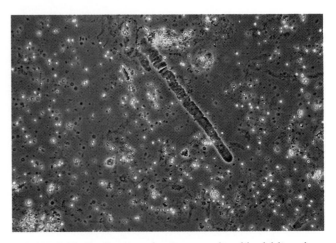

FIGURE 9-25 Hyaline cast showing accordion-like folding along part of its length; mixed background; urine sediment. SM stain/phase contrast; ×100.

pear homogenous and smooth, with sharp margins and blunt ends as well as cracks or convolutions along the lateral margins. Their appearance suggests they are brittle. Waxy casts are associated with tubular inflammation and degeneration, chronic renal failure, and renal allograft rejection. Waxy casts that are unusually broad are called renal failure casts and imply advanced tubular atrophy or dilation associated with end-stage renal disease. Waxy casts are illustrated in Figures 9-28 to 9-30 and are seen in Case Study 9-2, as well as in Chapter 10 (Case Studies 10-1 and 10-7).

INCLUSION CASTS

Coarsely and finely granular casts are often seen in the urinary sediment. They may occur with hyaline casts after periods of stress or strenuous exercise. Increased numbers of granular casts are associated with

strenuous exercise, dehydration, heat exposure, and emotional stress. Increased numbers are also associated with acute glomerulonephritis, pyelonephritis, chronic renal disease, and congestive heart failure.[28] Hyaline casts are illustrated in Figures 9-25 to 9-27 and are seen in Case Studies 9-3 and 9-5, as well as in Chapter 10 (Case Study 10-7).

Waxy casts are more refractile than hyaline casts and are therefore more easily visualized with bright-field microscopy. Waxy casts may represent the final phase of dissolution of finely granular casts. Because the breakdown of granules takes time, the presence of waxy casts suggests localized nephron obstruction and oliguria. With brightfield microscopy, waxy casts ap-

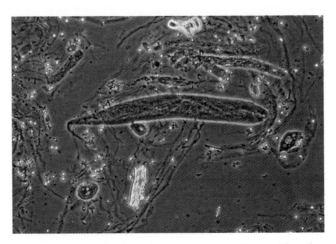

FIGURE 9-26 Hyaline/granular casts; one very large, with "cylindroid" tail; urine sediment. SM stain/phase contrast; ×100.

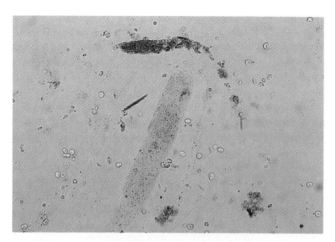

FIGURE 9-27 Large hyaline casts and smaller granular/cellular cast with RBCs in background; urine sediment. SM stain; ×200.

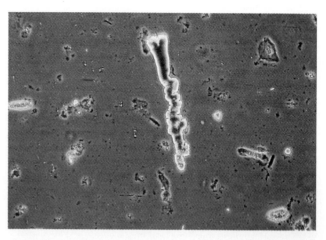

FIGURE 9-29 Same specimen and field of view as Figure 9-28, but with phase contrast; urine sediment. SM stain/phase contrast; ×100.

pyelonephritis, viral infections, chronic lead poisoning glomerulointerstitial disease, and renal allograft rejection. Granular casts are illustrated in Figures 9-31 and 9-32, and are seen in Case Studies 9-3, 9-5, 9-6, as well as in Chapter 10 (Case Studies 10-7, 10-11, and 10-13).

Fatty casts are formed when lipid material is incorporated into the protein matrix from lipid-laden renal tubular cells. As with freely floating lipid droplets, the fatty material can be neutral fat, cholesterol/cholesterol esters, or mixtures. Fatty casts are commonly seen when there is heavy proteinuria and are a feature of the nephrotic syndrome. Fatty casts are illustrated in Figures 9-33 and 9-34.

Other inclusion casts include those containing hemosiderin granules (derived from hemosiderin-containing renal tubular cells) as well as various types of crystals. Crystals can collect along mucus threads and create the appearance of a true cast. One should be able to visualize the hyaline matrix encompassing the crys-

tals if the object is a true cast. Crystal casts occur when the crystals actually precipitate within the tubules and may irritate or damage the tubular epithelium. Hematuria may irregularly be associated with crystal casts.

PIGMENTED CASTS

Hemoglobin casts appear yellow to brownish red, although the color may be pale and difficult to interpret. Hemoglobin casts are also known as blood casts and usually accompany erythrocyte casts and glomerular disease. They may be seen with tubular bleeding but rarely with hemoglobinuria. Myoglobin casts are similar in appearance to hemoglobin casts and are seen with myoglobinuria after acute muscle damage. Bilirubin usually stains most urine constituents a yellowish brown color, including any casts that are present (Case Study 9-2). Bilirubinuria and bilirubin casts are associated with obstructive jaundice. Pyridium (phenazopy-

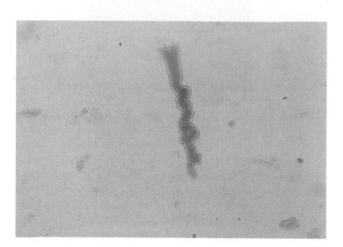

FIGURE 9-28 Waxy cast; urine sediment. SM stain; ×100.

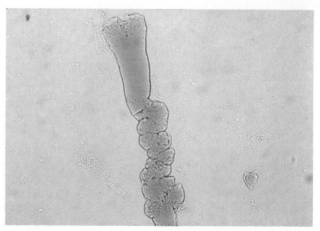

FIGURE 9-30 Same specimen and field of view as Figure 9-28, at higher magnification; urine sediment. SM stain; ×200.

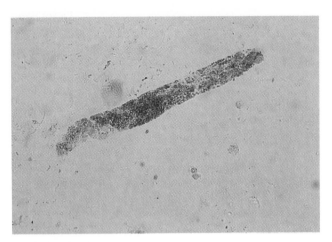

FIGURE 9-31 Granular cast; urine sediment. SM stain; ×200.

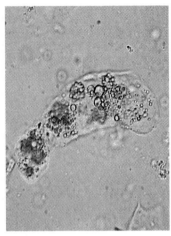

FIGURE 9-33 Fatty casts; urine sediment ×400. (University of Washington Department of Laboratory Medicine, with permis-

ridine) is a highly pigmented drug that stains casts and sediment elements a bright yellow to orange color.

CELLULAR CASTS

Finding erythrocyte (RBC) casts in the urine is diagnostic of glomerular disease or renal parenchymal bleeding. Damage to the glomerulus, most often because of immune injury, permits erythrocytes to escape into the tubule. With proteinuria and if conditions are optimal for cast formation, RBC casts form in the distal nephron.

To identify a cast as an erythrocyte cast, the outlines of the RBCs must be sharply defined in at least one area of the cast. Sometimes the cast is so fully packed with RBCs that the matrix cannot be seen. In contrast, slender, delicate casts may be seen with only a few RBCs visible in the matrix. The matrix is more visible with phase contrast microscopy. With stasis in the nephron, the cells in the cast may degenerate so

that the cast appears as a reddish brown, coarsely granular cast called a blood or hemoglobin cast (mentioned earlier, in the section on Pigmented Casts).

RBC casts are associated with acute glomerulonephritis, IgA nephropathy, lupus nephritis, subacute bacterial endocarditis, and renal infarction. In a few cases, tubulointerstitial disease may allow the transtubular entry of RBCs and their subsequent incorporation into casts, as with severe pyelonephritis. RBC casts have also been found in healthy individuals after their participation in contact sports (athletic pseudonephritis) such as football, basketball, or boxing. An RBC cast is illustrated in Figure 9-35 as well as in Chapter 10 the Introductory Case Study and Case Study 10-1. RBCs also occur with other cells in mixed cellular casts, as seen in the Introductory Case Study for this chapter.

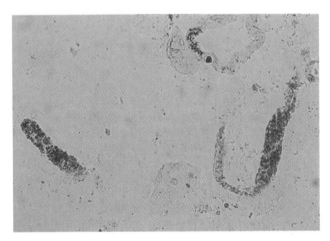

FIGURE 9-32 Granular casts; urine sediment. SM stain; ×200.

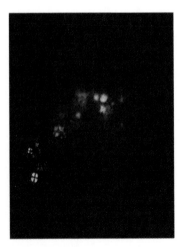

FIGURE 9-34 Fatty casts; POL; urine sediment; ×400. (University of Washington Department of Laboratory Medicine, with permission.)

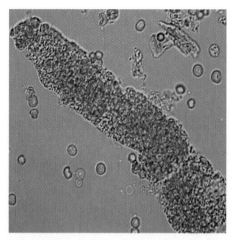

FIGURE 9-35 RBC cast; urine sediment; ×400. (University of Washington Department of Laboratory Medicine, with permission.)

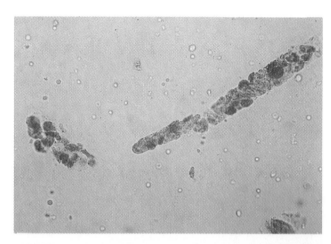

FIGURE 9-37 Mixed cellular cast; urine sediment. SM stain; ×200.

Leukocyte (WBC) casts are seen with renal inflammation or infection. The most commonly associated disease is pyelonephritis, in which the leukocytes enter the tubules from the interstitium and are accompanied by bacteriuria and varying degrees of proteinuria and hematuria. If the origin of the WBCs is glomerular (e.g., glomerulonephritis), then there will also be RBC casts and they will outnumber the WBC casts. If the WBCs in the cast have not started to degenerate, their multilobed nuclei and granular cytoplasm help in their identification. Partially disintegrated leukocytes may be difficult to distinguish from renal epithelial cells, so that identification may require the use of supravital stains or contrast microscopy. A WBC cast is illustrated in Figure 9-36 as well as in the Introductory Case Study for this chapter.

Renal tubular epithelial cells can become incorporated into casts in the same way as other cellular elements. If their characteristic nucleus and cell shape are apparent, identification should be possible. As they begin to degenerate, they are increasingly difficult to differentiate from WBCs, especially if the two types of cells are mixed in the same cast. As before, supravital staining or contrast microscopy aid in the identification. RTE casts are associated with acute tubular necrosis, viral (e.g., cytomegalovirus) disease, exposure to a variety of drugs, heavy metal poisoning, and ethylene glycol (antifreeze) intoxication. RTE casts are also associated with proteinuria, and granular casts often occur with them as well.

When two or more distinct cell types are present in casts, they are called mixed casts. Any combination of cells is possible. They may be enumerated and reported as cellular casts and their composition provided in the report. Mixed cellular casts are illustrated in Figures 9-37 to 9-39 and are seen in the Introductory Case Study

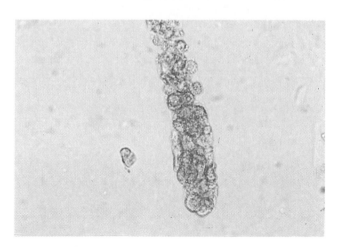

FIGURE 9-36 WBC cast; urine sediment. SM stain; ×400.

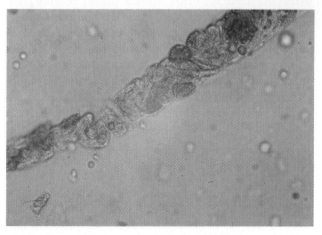

FIGURE 9-38 Mixed cellular cast (some RTE); urine sediment. SM stain; ×400.

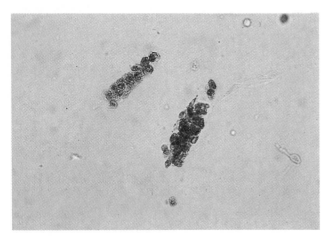

FIGURE 9-39 Mixed cellular cast; urine sediment. SM stain; ×200.

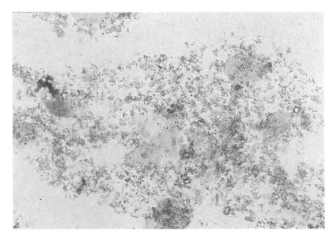

FIGURE 9-40 Amorphous urates; urine sediment. ×200.

for this chapter and Case Study 9-9, as well as in Chapter 10 (Case Studies 10-2, 10-5, and 10-6).

Crystals

As urinary solutes precipitate out of solution, either crystals or noncrystalline (amorphous) solids result. Crystals are not normally present in freshly voided urine but may appear while the urine stands, especially in the refrigerator. Only a few types of crystals are clinically significant, but because these few are indicative of a pathologic process, it is important that crystals be correctly identified and reported. The identification of crystals is based on their microscopic appearance in the urinary sediment together with information on the pH of the urine in which they were formed.

Factors that influence the formation and growth of crystals include the concentration of the solute in the urine, the pH of the urine, and the filtrate volume passing through the tubules. As the filtrate passes through the tubules, water is removed and solutes become more concentrated. If increased amounts of solutes are present because of dehydration (accompanied by reduced urine flow), dietary intake, or medications, supersaturation can occur and crystals may form, either while the urine is in the body or after the urine is voided. The factors affecting crystal formation and the formation of urinary calculi are interrelated, as discussed in Chapter 10.

ACIDIC URINE

Uric acid forms amorphous or noncrystalline salts of sodium, potassium, magnesium, or calcium in acidic urine. Under the microscope these amorphous urates

appear as small, yellow-brown granules that often interfere with the examination of the urine sediment. Refrigeration increases the precipitation of these amorphous urates and the urinary pigment uroerythrin often deposits on the surface of the particles, giving them a characteristic pink-orange color ("brick dust") observed macroscopically during the physical examination. Amorphous urates can be cleared by adding alkali to the sediment or warming it to approximately 60°C. Amorphous urates are illustrated in Figure 9-40 and are shown in many of the Case Studies.

Uric acid crystals occur in a variety of shapes and are usually yellow to orange-brown. They are typically flat and four sided, although other shapes include rhombic plates or prisms, oval forms with pointed ends (lemon shaped), wedges, barrels, rosettes, irregular plates, and cubes. With polarized light, uric acid crystals are birefringent and produce a variety of interference colors. Uric acid crystals appear in the urine of healthy individuals, although they are seen in the

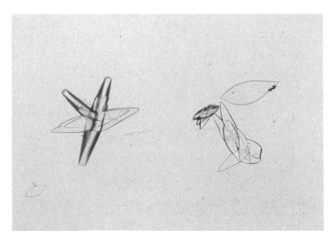

FIGURE 9-41 Uric acid crystals; urine sediment. ×100.

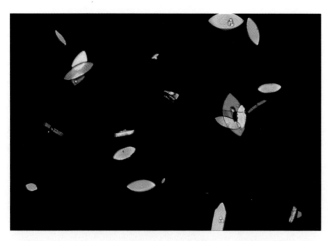

FIGURE 9-42 Uric acid crystals; urine sediment. POL; ×100.

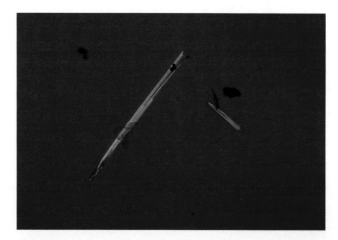

FIGURE 9-44 Na urate in urine sediment; POL with red compensator. ×400.

urine of gout patients and in other conditions associated with increased purine metabolism (e.g., cytotoxic drugs). Uric acid crystals are illustrated in Figures 9-41 to 9-43.

Acid urates occur as small brown spheres in pairs or clusters of three in slightly acid urine. If they are acidified on the microscopic slide, they slowly revert to uric acid plates.

Monosodium urate crystals appear as light yellow, slender needles or rods, singly or in small clusters. Their ends are blunt. They can be recognized using compensated polarized light, as illustrated in Figure 9-44. Refer to Chapter 14 for their appearance in synovial fluid.

Oxalic acid is one of the metabolites of ascorbic acid. The most common type of oxalic acid crystals observed in urine is the dihydrate form, which is octahedral (or "envelope"). The monohydrate crystals are small, ovoid, and dumbbell shaped when viewed from the side. The crystals are birefringent, so polarized light aids in differentiating them from RBCs or yeast cells. The concentration of calcium in the urine determines which type of crystal is formed.[4] Lower amounts of calcium result in the monohydrate form, and higher calcium concentrations precipitate the dihydrate form.

Calcium oxalate crystals are found in both acidic and in neutral urine, and are often found in the urine from normal, healthy individuals. Finding calcium oxalate crystals may simply be related to an oxalate-rich diet (e.g., tomatoes, spinach, rhubarb), but calcium oxalate crystals may also be associated with urolithiasis. Calcium oxalate accounts for 67% of the renal calculi in the United States. Increased numbers of calcium oxalate crystals may be induced after ingestion of ethylene glycol or in severe chronic renal disease. Calcium oxalate crystals are illustrated in Figure 9-45 as well as in some of the Case Studies.

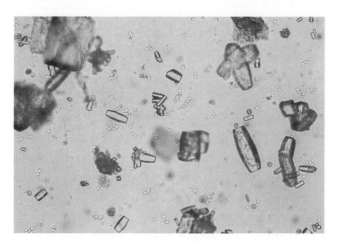

FIGURE 9-43 Uric acid crystals, barrel shape; yeast in the background; urine sediment. ×200.

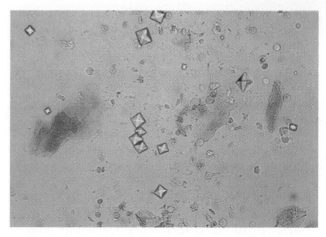

FIGURE 9-45 Calcium oxalate crystals; urine sediment. ×200.

Bilirubin crystals in the urine can take various forms: fine needles, granules, or plates. They are always yellow-brown and indicate the presence of large amounts of bilirubin in the urine. Bilirubin crystals are expected only if the chemical screen for bilirubin is positive, and they are frequently present in the urine of patients with liver disease. Urinary bilirubin is always the conjugated (direct) form rather than the unconjugated (indirect) form. Bilirubin crystals are not be always reported because they usually form in the urine after voiding. Bilirubin crystals are illustrated in Figure 9-46. Note that formed elements in the urine (e.g., casts) are often stained a yellowish brown by bilirubin present in the urine, as illustrated in Case Study 9-2.

Cystine crystals are colorless, six-sided (hexagonal) plates, sometimes with uneven sides, and often laminated or layered. Cystine crystals are associated with cystinuria, an inborn error of metabolism, and tend to be deposited in the tubules as calculi, resulting in renal damage. Because the crystals are associated with a disease process, they are counted in the urine microscopic examination and reported as the average number observed in 10 LPFs, but only reported if chemical confirmation is available.

Chromatographic procedures may used for definite identification, although presumptive confirmation for cystine may be carried out with the cyanide-nitroprusside test. In this procedure, cyanide reduces cystine to cysteine, and then the free sulfhydryl groups are reacted with nitroprusside to form a characteristic purple color. Illustrations of cystine crystals are provided in Figure 9-47 and in Chapter 10 (Case Study 10-12).

Although they may be observed in patients with severe liver disease, tyrosine and leucine crystals in the urine are usually associated with inborn errors of

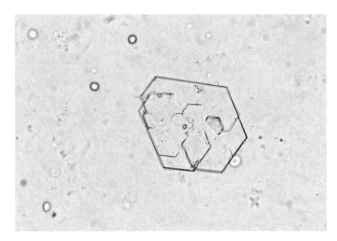

FIGURE 9-47 Cystine crystal; urine sediment. ×200.

metabolism. With these syndromes, the increased concentration of the amino acids in the blood leads to overflow aminoaciduria. Before they are reported, tyrosine and leucine should be confirmed by chromatographic methods. Tyrosine crystals appear as colorless (or yellow) fine, silky needles that may aggregate together in clusters or sheaves. They are illustrated in Figure 9-48.

Leucine crystals are very refractile, oily-appearing, yellow to brown spheres with radial and concentric striations. Leucine crystals are illustrated in Figure 9-49. Case Study 10-6 (liver failure) shows presumptive leucine crystals.

Cholesterol crystals appear as clear, flat, rectangular plates with notched corners. Cholesterol crystals are always accompanied by large amounts of protein and other evidence of lipiduria, such as free-floating lipid droplets, fatty casts, or oval fat bodies. They are seen with the nephrotic syndrome and in conditions result-

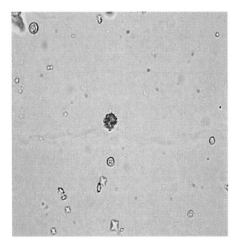

FIGURE 9-46 Bilirubin crystals; urine sediment; ×400. (University of Washington Department of Laboratory Medicine, with persmission.)

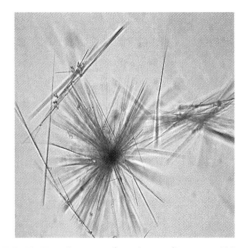

FIGURE 9-48 Tyrosine crystals; urine sediment; ×400. (University of Washington Department of Laboratory Medicine, with permission.)

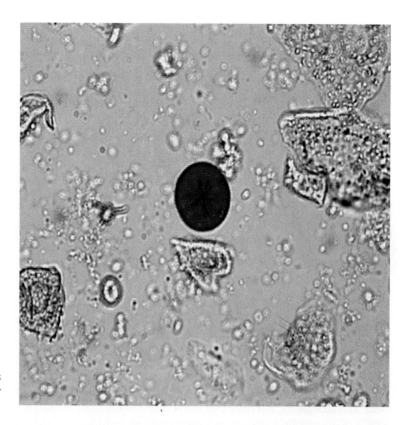

FIGURE 9-49 Leucine crystals; urine sediment; ×400. (University of Washington Department of Laboratory Medicine, with permission.)

ing in chyluria (tumors, filariasis resulting in rupture of lymphatic vessels into the renal tubules). Cholesterol crystals are birefringent and show interference colors.

The radiographic contrast medium diatrizoate meglumine (Renografin) forms crystals that are very similar to cholesterol crystals and behave in much the same way in polarized light. However, with diatrizoate meglumine, unlike cholesterol, the urine specific gravity is usually very high (e.g., greater than 1.040) and the crystals are not associated with proteinuria or lipiduria.

Cholesterol crystals, obtained from "kidney fluid," are illustrated in Figures 9-50 to 9-52. Although it is not visible in these photomicrographs, the crystals are accompanied in this specimen by lipid droplets containing cholesterol.

Numerous medications are excreted by the kidneys, and high concentrations in the urine can bring about precipitation. Termed "iatrogenic," the crystals result from the actions of a physician through the prescription of the drug. Ampicillin crystals appear as long, colorless, thin prisms or needles and indicate large doses

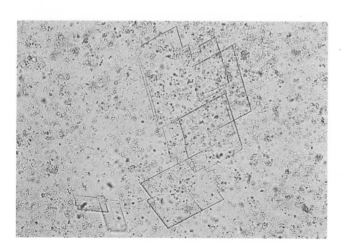

FIGURE 9-50 Cholesterol crystals, from "kidney fluid". ×200.

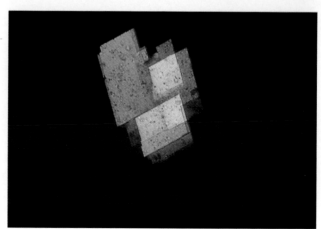

FIGURE 9-51 Same specimen and field of view as Figure 9-50, but with POL ×200.

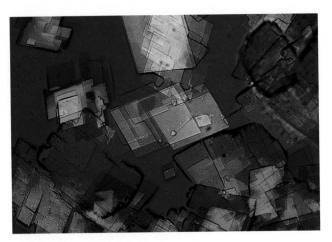

FIGURE 9-52 Cholesterol crystals with POL and red compensator, from "kidney fluid". ×100.

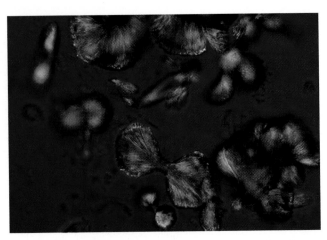

FIGURE 9-54 Sulfonamide; urine sediment; POL with red compensator. ×400.

of ampicillin. They are rarely observed. Sulfamethoxazole (e.g., Bactrim or Septra) is more commonly seen and appears as brown rosettes or spheres with irregular radial striations.

Sulfadiazine crystals are yellow to brown and appear as bundles of needles that resemble sheaves of wheat. Sulfonamide crystals are illustrated in Figures 9-53 and 9-54.

ALKALINE URINE

Amorphous phosphates are found in alkaline (and neutral) urine and cannot be distinguished microscopically from amorphous urates. They are differentiated from amorphous urates based on the urine pH, solubility characteristics, and to some extent, their macroscopic appearance. Large amounts of amorphous phos-

phates create a cloudy urine, but the precipitate is white rather than pink as with amorphous urates. Unlike amorphous urates, they are soluble in acid and do not dissolve when heated to 60°C. Just as with amorphous urates, amorphous phosphates make the microscopic examination of the sediment a chore and are best avoided by analyzing specimens within 2 hours of collection, thereby avoiding refrigeration, which leads to amorphous phosphate formation.

Triple phosphate (ammonium-magnesium phosphate) crystals are colorless and appear in various forms, although the most common and characteristic form is the type referred to as "coffin lid" (a six-sided prism). Crystals are often imperfectly formed and exhibit great size variation. The crystals are present in the urine of normal, healthy individuals and are observed with UTIs characterized by an alkaline pH. Triple phosphate crystals are illustrated in Figures 9-55 and 9-56.

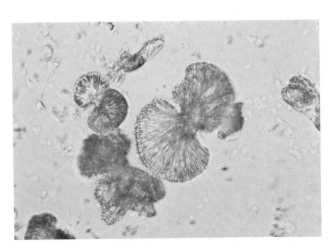

FIGURE 9-53 Sulfonamide crystals; urine sediment. ×400.

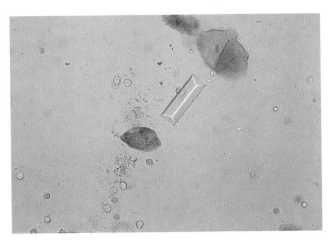

FIGURE 9-55 Triple phosphate crystal; WBCs; squamous epithelial cells; urine sediment. ×200.

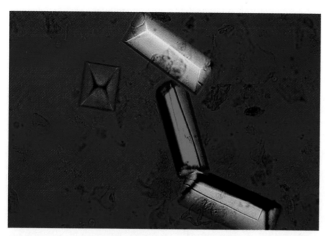

FIGURE 9-56 Triple-phosphate crystals; urine sediment. POL with red compensator; ×200.

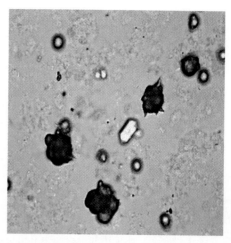

FIGURE 9-58 Ammonium biurate crystals; urine sediment; ×400. (University of Washington Department of Laboratory Medicine, with permission.)

Calcium phosphate crystals, sometimes called stellar phosphates, appear as colorless, thin prisms arranged in a rosette or star-shaped pattern. The prisms tend to have one end tapered or pointed, whereas the other end appears squared off. Calcium phosphate crystals appear microscopically as irregular, granular sheets or plates. Calcium phosphate crystals are illustrated in Figure 9-57.

Ammonium biurate crystals appear as yellow-brown spheres with striations on the surface, and irregular projections or spicules may also be present, giv-

ing rise to the term "thorn apple." Because they usually are seen in urine specimens that have been stored for a long period of time, they generally have no clinical significance. Ammonium biurate crystals are illustrated in Figure 9-58.

Calcium carbonate crystals appear as very small, colorless granular crystals that may be confused with bacteria because of their size and occasional rod shape. Calcium carbonate crystals are usually found in pairs (dumbbell shape) and can be positively identified through the production of carbon dioxide gas (effervescence) when acetic acid is added to the sediment.

Microorganisms and Parasites

Depending on the method of urine collection, and how soon after collection the examination takes place, bacteria may or may not be significant. A direct Gram stain on a well-mixed, uncentrifuged urine may be prepared and the observation of bacteria with the oil immersion lens suggests that more than 100,000 organisms/mL are present—that is, a significant bacteriuria exists.[25] Because the vagina and gastrointestinal tract normally contain bacteria, contamination from these sources often explains the presence of bacteria in the urine. The most commonly encountered bacteria are gram-negative rods because the enteric organisms are most often found in UTIs. Leukocytes are usually seen in the urine sediment with significant bacteriuria. Bacteria may be reported as few, moderate, or many per HPF. Bacteria in the urine sediment or on direct Gram-stained smears from urine are illustrated in Figures 9-59 to 9-61, as well as in several of the Case Studies.

Yeasts may cause UTIs, although yeast in the urine sediment often represents vaginal infection and subse-

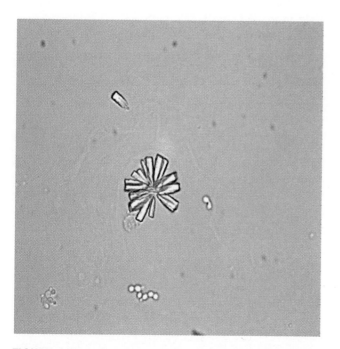

FIGURE 9-57 Calcium phosphate crystals; urine sediment; ×400. (University of Washington Department of Laboratory Medicine, with permission.)

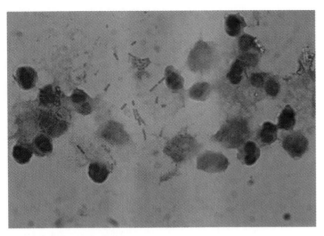

FIGURE 9-59 *Escherichia coli* with leukocytes; urine sediment. Gram stain; ×1000.

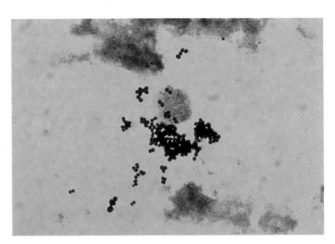

FIGURE 9-61 Staphylococci; direct Gram's stain on urine sediment. ×1000.

quent contamination of a poorly collected urine specimen. Conditions that enhance the development of a yeast infection include diabetes mellitus, pregnancy, and use of oral contraceptives. The most common yeasts found in urine sediment are *Candida* species. Immunosuppressed patients may have true kidney infections caused by yeasts.

Yeast cells are ovoid, colorless, refractile cells and may be confused with RBCs. Unlike RBCs, yeast cells usually are smaller, have a relatively thick cell wall, exhibit considerable variation in size, form buds and pseudohyphae, do not dissolve in acetic acid, and do not usually stain with supravital stains, although they are strongly gram positive and also stain well with Wright's stain. Yeast observed in urine sediment as well as on direct Gram-stained smears from urine are illustrated in Figures 9-62 to 9-64.

It is rare to find amebae in the urine, but they may reach the bladder from the lymph system or more likely

from fecal contamination of the urethra. RBCs and WBCs usually accompany the pathogenic *Entamoeba histolytica*.[25] In patients with schistosomiasis due to *Schistosoma haematobium*, typical ova are shed directly in the urine accompanied by erythrocytes from the bladder wall mucosa. The parasite most frequently observed in the urine is the protozoan *Trichomonas vaginalis*. It is primarily responsible for vaginal infections but may also infect the urethra, periurethral glands, bladder, and prostate.

Wet preparations of direct swabs from the vagina or urethra are usually examined for trichomonads, although the organism may often be seen as a contaminant in urine from female patients. *Trichomonas* cells average about 15 μm in length, have four anterior flagella, an anterior undulating membrane, and a sharp, protruding posterior axostyle. In wet preparations, trichomonads exhibit a characteristic flitting, jerky, nondirectional motility that aids in their identification.

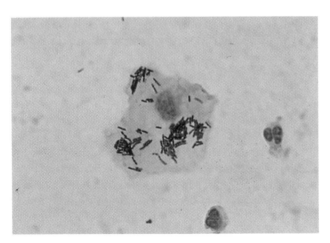

FIGURE 9-60 Gram-positive rods; squamous epithelial cells; leukocytes; urine sediment. Gram stain; ×1000.

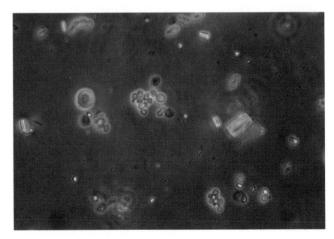

FIGURE 9-62 Yeast; phase contrast; urine sediment. ×400.

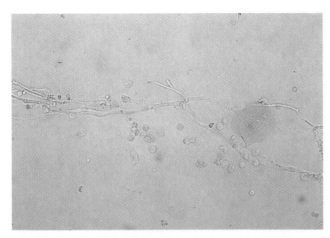

FIGURE 9-63 Yeast pseudohyphae with WBCs; urine sediment. SM stain; ×200.

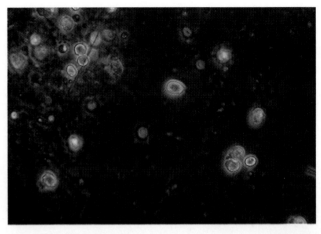

FIGURE 9-65 *Trichomonas vaginalis* with mixed cellular background; urine sediment. Phase contrast; ×400.

They can be mistaken for large leukocytes, renal tubular epithelial cells, or small transitional epithelial cells, and are best observed with phase contrast microscopy, which provides clear visualization of the flagella and undulating membrane. Trichomonads are illustrated in Figure 9-65.

As a result of fecal contamination, ova from the intestinal parasite *Enterobius vermicularis* (pinworm) may be found in the urine sediment. Pinworm ova from urine sediment are illustrated in Figure 9-66.

Miscellaneous Formed Elements

Threads or strands of mucus (a fibrillar protein) are often a component of the urine sediment but are difficult to visualize with brightfield microscopy unless the light intensity is drastically reduced. Mucus is readily observed with phase contrast or interference contrast microscopy. At least some of the mucus found in urine originates from the renal tubules because immunohistochemical tests have demonstrated the presence of Tamm-Horsfall protein in the mucus strands.[5] Some mucus found in the urine also originates in the genitourinary tract, particularly from the vaginal epithelium as a contaminant in urine from women. Although mucus strands may occasionally be mistaken for hyaline casts, a careful search for the cylindrical structure of casts and their rounded ends should permit correct identification.

Little clinical significance is attached to the presence of mucus in the urinary sediment, although it may be increased with some inflammatory conditions and irritation to the genitourinary tract. Mucus is illustrated in many of the Case Studies, particularly with the use of phase-contrast microscopy.

Lipid droplets may occur in urine sediment as free-floating globules, as lipid globules within oval fat bod-

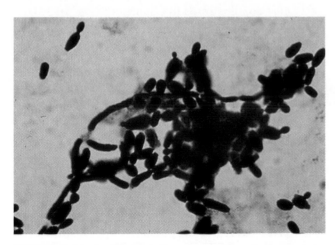

FIGURE 9-64 *Candida tropicalis*; urine sediment. Gram stain; ×1000.

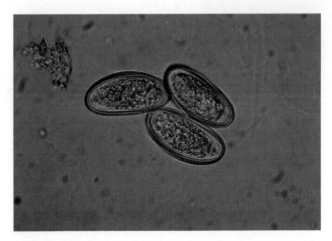

FIGURE 9-66 Pinworm ova (*Enterobius vermicularis*); urine sediment. SM stain; ×400.

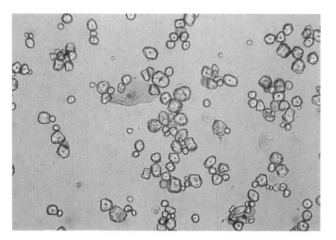

FIGURE 9-67 Starch granules; urine sediment. ×200.

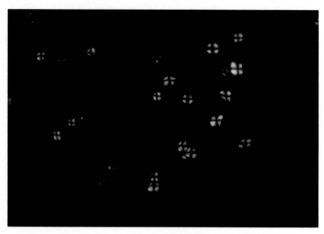

FIGURE 9-68 Starch granules; urine sediment. POL; ×200.

ies (e.g., lipid-laden renal tubular epithelial cells), or in fatty casts. With brightfield microscopy, the globules are highly refractile, are of varying sizes, and may have a light yellow or brown color. Droplets that are neutral fats without cholesterol are isotropic in polarized light, whereas lipid globules containing cholesterol and cholesterol esters are anisotropic in polarized light, showing up brightly against the dark background (crossed filters) with a Maltese cross pattern, and showing interference colors with a first-order red compensator.

Lipiduria is observed with a variety of renal diseases and may occur after severe crush injuries. It is most often observed with the nephrotic syndrome in combination with severe proteinuria, hypoproteinemia, hyperlipidemia, and edema. Lipid droplets showing the Maltese cross pattern for cholesterol are illustrated in Figures 9-33 and 9-34 (a fatty cast).

Spermatozoa are occasionally seen in the urine sediment from both men and women. Their presence is not routinely reported in some laboratories but may be an important finding in fertility studies or in cases of possible sexual abuse. The sperm head is about 4 to 6 μm long and the thin, threadlike tail is about 40 to 60 μm in length. Various forms may be seen and they may occur clumped in the sediment. Sperm are illustrated in Figure 9-16 as well as in a few of the Case Studies.

Starch granules are a frequent contaminant in the urine introduced by the use of powdered examination gloves or starch-containing body powders. The granules may be confused with cells or lipid globules. With brightfield microscopy, starch appears as irregular, generally round granules that may vary greatly in size, have a central depression/dimple/slit, show faint striations, appear highly refractile with polarized light, and show interference colors with a first-order red compensator. Starch is illustrated in Figures 9-67 and 9-68.

Cotton, hair, and other fibers may be introduced into the urine specimen at the time of collection or by laboratory personnel during specimen processing or examination. Disposable diaper fibers may be easily confused with waxy casts but unlike the casts, the diaper fibers are birefringent with polarized light. A fiber and a cast are illustrated in Chapter 10 (Fig. 10-16).

Illustrative Case Studies

CASE STUDY 9-1

This 43-year-old man was seen in the outpatient clinic complaining of weakness and anorexia experienced during the preceding month with episodes of "throbbing stomach pains" and occasional diarrhea. The patient is known to be HIV positive with a history of tuberculosis, pulmonary candidiasis, esophagitis, and gastritis. He has been taking Rifampin and INH for his tuberculosis and Megace for anorexia (AIDS related). His urinalysis was significant for ketone, trace; urobilinogen, 4.0; nitrite, positive; leukocyte esterase, small; WBCs, 5–10/HPF; RBCs, 2–5/HPF; bacteria, 3+; and Ictotest, positive.

continued

The urine was sent to Microbiology for C&S and for Gram's stain, which indicated TNTC gram-negative rods resembling enterics. The diagnosis given was a urinary tract infection, and he was given Bactrim and released to continue his previous medications. Results for the C&S on the urine showed a colony count greater than 100,000 CFU/mL of E. *coli.* A photomicrograph of the urine sediment (Fig. 9-69) and the direct Gram stain on the urine (Fig. 9-70) illustrate the UTI.

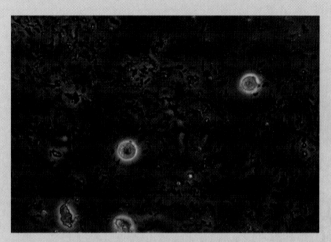

FIGURE 9-69 Bacteria and WBCs. Urine sediment; phase contrast/SM stain; ×400.

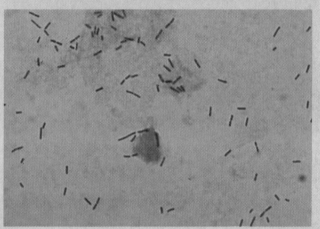

FIGURE 9-70 Direct Gram stain on urine, showing gram-negative rods; ×1000.

CASE STUDY 9-2

This 42-year-old woman was admitted through the ER presenting with a chief complaint of swelling in her abdomen and lower extremities worsening during the preceding 3 weeks. She also complained of being very tired and unable to lift herself; shortness of breath; pruritus; vomiting one to two times a day for 2 weeks; anorexia for 2 weeks; and jaundice (yellowing of the "whites" of her eyes). She was admitted with a diagnosis of alcoholic liver disease with ascites (new onset) R/O peritonitis, and anemia of chronic disease. Her history is significant for alcohol abuse, at least a six-pack of beer/day for the past 20 years.

Diagnostic paracentesis was negative for infection, as were blood cultures. Urinalysis was significant for bilirubin moderate; blood moderate; leukocyte esterase moderate; appearance cloudy; WBCs/HPF 20–50; RBCs/HPF 10–20; epithelial cells 1+; bacteria 4+; Ictotest positive. The urine C&S indicated a colony count of greater than 100,000 CFU/mL of E. *coli.* While in the hospital she was given 10 units of packed red cells for her anemia and 4 units of fresh frozen plasma for coagulopathy. She was treated for her ascites and edema, alcoholism, malnutrition, and urinary tract infection.

continued

Examples of the formed elements seen in the urine sediment for this patient are given in Figures 9-71 and 9-72 illustrating the UTI, but with waxy casts suggesting also a long period of depressed renal function. Some of the elements seem to be slightly "bile" stained, correlating with the positive bilirubin and Ictotest results.

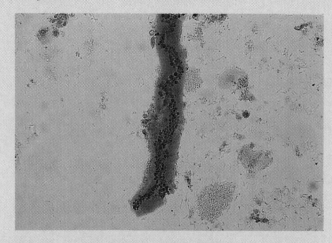

FIGURE 9-71 A pseudocast of RBCs adhering to a mucus strand is superimposed on a large waxy cast. Background of bacteria, WBCs, and squamous epithelials. Urine sediment; SM stain; ×200.

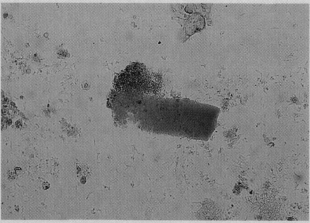

FIGURE 9-72 Small waxy cast with WBCs and bacteria. Urine sediment; SM stain; ×200.

CASE STUDY 9-3

A 32-year-old man was brought to the ER after taking a shower, falling in the hallway, and being found unresponsive on the floor about 30 minutes later. On the way to the hospital, his BP was 250/180 and he had gurgling respirations. His admission diagnosis was altered mental status R/O cerebral bleed. He was intubated and taken to the CT scanner, which showed a very large cerebral hemorrhage. It was decided that the patient needed an emergency craniotomy for evacuation of the blood. He was taken to surgery where the clot was evacuated by craniotomy. He was placed in the ICU, continued on the ventilator, and observed for the greater part of 3 weeks. He regained semiconsciousness, opening his eyes spontaneously and moving his right limbs spontaneously. He is paralyzed on the left side (right hemiplegia).

The patient's history is positive for alcohol abuse because he is a bartender and a heavy drinker as well. He is known to have been drinking heavily around the time of his accident. On admission, the urinalysis was significant for blood small; protein > 300 mg/dL; appearance hazy; WBCs 10–20/HPF; RBCs 2–5/HPF; epithelial cells/HPF few renal, few transitional; bacteria/HPF 1+; casts/LPF 10–20 hyaline, 10–20 granular, 0–1 WBC, rare mixed granular/WBC. Figures 9-73 and 9-74 illustrate the findings on this urine sediment, which relate mainly to the effects of alcohol abuse as well as all of the trauma connected with the cerebral hemorrhage and surgery.

continued

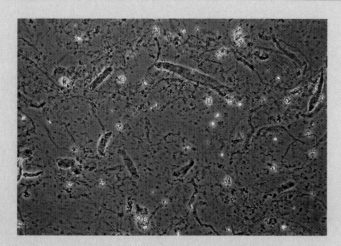

FIGURE 9-73 Mucus; hyaline casts; dirty background. Urine sediment; SM stain/phase contrast; ×100.

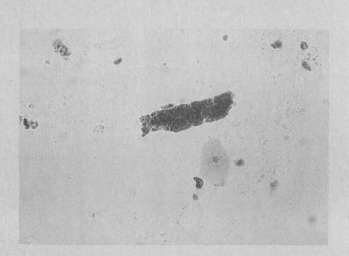

FIGURE 9-74 Coarsely granular cast. Urine sediment; SM stain; ×200.

CASE STUDY 9-4

The family of this patient, a 78-year-old woman, found her at home confused, nauseous, and vomiting. She told them she had not been eating very much, and they brought her to the ER. Her history is significant for NIDDM, controlled with Micronase (Glyburide); HTN; CAD; and peripheral vascular disease. Her CT scan was normal.

The admission urinalysis was significant for protein > 300 mg/dL; leukocyte esterase trace; appearance cloudy; WBCs TNTC/HPF; RBCs 0–1/HPF; epithelial cells rare; bacteria 4+. Perhaps because of some interference, the leukocyte esterase results do not agree closely with the microscopic observations, even though quality control results were acceptable for the shift during which this urinalysis was carried out. The urine Gram stain indicated TNTC gram-negative rods/OIF resembling enterics and > 25 gram-positive rods/OIF resembling diphtheroids. The C&S on the urine resulted in a colony count greater than 100,000 CFU/mL of E. *coli*.

The patient was treated with IV antibiotics and her mental status cleared soon after the start of this therapy. She was discharged home with oral antibiotics for the UTI. Figures 9-75 and 9-76 illustrate the UTI.

continued

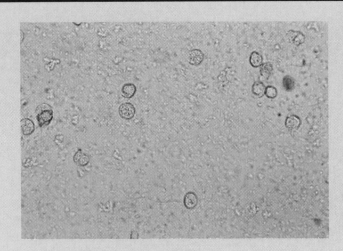

FIGURE 9-75 Bacteria and WBCs. Urine sediment; SM stain; ×400.

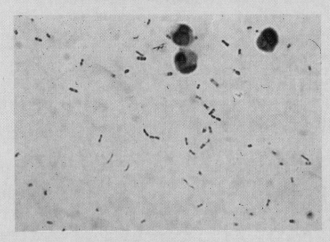

FIGURE 9-76 Gram stain of urine showing bacteria and three leukocytes. ×1000.

CASE STUDY 9-5

A 38-year-old women, this patient was admitted to receive a 3-day course of amphotericin B treatments (IV) because she cannot take medications by mouth. Her admission diagnosis was end-stage AIDS, multidrug-resistant tuberculosis, cytomegalovirus retinitis, disseminated histoplasmosis, and candidiasis. After her treatments she was discharged to a hospice unit, status terminal AIDS.

Her admission urinalysis was significant for protein 30 mg/dL; appearance hazy; WBCs/HPF 20–50; RBCs/HPF 0–2; epithelials 1+ transitional, few renal; bacteria/HPF 2+; casts/LPF 5–10 hyaline, rare granular, rare resembling RTE. Examples of the formed elements observed in the urine sediment are shown in Figures 9-77 to 9-82 giving a picture of renal toxicity 2° to amphotericin B and a generalized inflammatory response. Figure 9-83 shows *Histoplasma capsulatum* in the peripheral blood of this patient.

continued

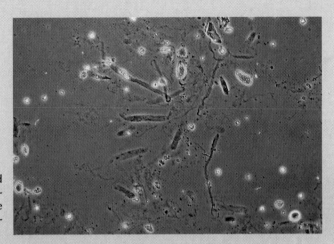

FIGURE 9-77 Hyaline casts, mucus, and two SM-stained, granular-appearing bodies which resemble RTE cells from the proximal convoluted tubule. Urine sediment; SM stain/phase contrast; ×100.

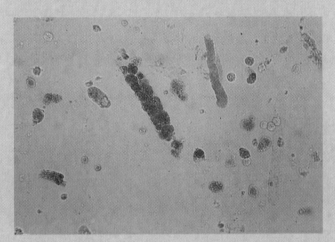

FIGURE 9-78 A granular cast, a mixed cellular cast, and partially degenerated RTE cells from the proximal distal tubule. Urine sediment; SM stain; ×200.

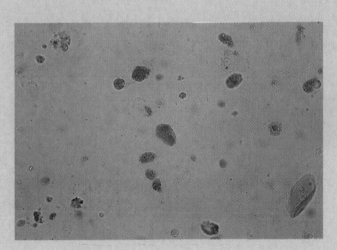

FIGURE 9-79 More examples of RTE cells from the proximal and distal tubules. Urine sediment; SM stain; ×200.

continued

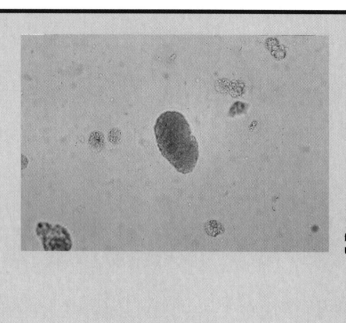

FIGURE 9-80 Leukocytes and an RTE cell from the proximal convoluted tubule. Urine sediment; SM stain; ×400.

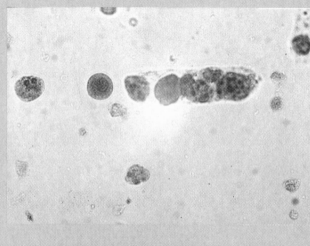

FIGURE 9-81 Fragment of mixed-cellular cast, a transitional cell, and an RTE cell resembling those from the distal convoluted tubule. Urine sediment; SM stain; ×400.

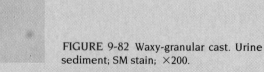

FIGURE 9-82 Waxy-granular cast. Urine sediment; SM stain; ×200.

continued

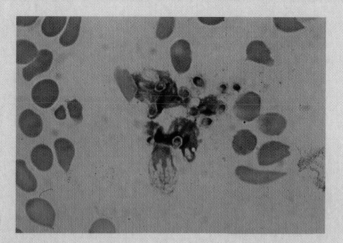

FIGURE 9-83 *Histoplasma*; peripheral blood. Wright's stain; ×1000.

CASE STUDY 9-6

Paramedics brought this patient, a 36-year-old man, to the ER because he was lethargic. According to a friend, the patient had become increasingly lethargic during the preceding week. Past medical history revealed IDDM (8 years), pulmonary cocci (cavitary cocci lesion in the right middle lobe diagnosed the year previous), and anemia. The patient had been taking Diflucan but ran out of the medication and did not make arrangements for more.

On admission, the patient was very lethargic, although responsive to verbal and tactile stimuli, and positive for Kussmaul breathing. Admission diagnosis was diabetic ketoacidosis. In the ER, the patient was started on an insulin drip and was admitted to the ICU for further evaluation. His admission urinalysis was significant for: glucose > 1000 mg/dL; ketones > 80 mg/dL; pH 5; appearance hazy; WBCs 0–2/HPF; RBCs 2–5/HPF; casts 1–5 granular/LPF. His admission blood chemistries were significant for CO_2 8 mEq/L (24–35); anion gap 26 (1–11); glucose 736 mg/dL (70–110); and his admission ABGs were significant for: pH 6.86 (7.38–7.46); pCO_2 9.4 mm Hg (32—36); pO_2 151 mm Hg (74–108); bicarbonate, 1.7 mEq/L (21–29); and base excess −32.2 mEq/L (−2.0 to +2.0). The admission diagnosis was diabetic ketoacidosis.

He was kept on insulin drip and copious fluids, and his blood sugar and electrolytes were followed every 2 hours. The next day, his status was much improved, he had become more alert, and his blood chemistries had improved. By the second day, his anion gap had closed to 7 and his electrolytes had normalized. By the third day, he was feeling well enough to go home and he was discharged with a 3-month supply of insulin and syringes with instructions to monitor his blood

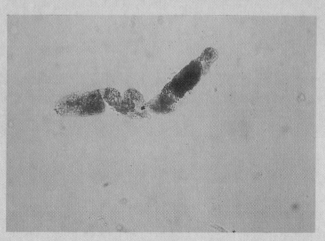

FIGURE 9-84 Granular cast. Urine sediment; SM stain; ×200.

continued

glucose before each meal and at bedtime, to keep records, and to bring the record to the clinic for a follow-up. At the next visit he was also to have his cocci serology checked to see if he needed to continue the Diflucan.

The appearance of the urine sediment for this patient is illustrated in Figures 9-84 and 9-85, and suggests a response to the stress of diabetic ketoacidosis.

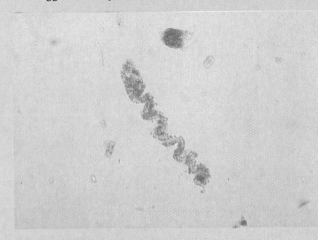

FIGURE 9-85 Granular cast. Urine sediment; SM stain; ×200.

CASE STUDY 9-7

This 65-year-old man was seen in the outpatient clinic complaining of gross hematuria ("blood and blood clots") in his urine that had been occurring during the previous 5 months. He has had a history of passing kidney stones for the past 22 years. The bleeding episodes come and go but he had no complaints of dysuria, frequency/urgency, or retention. A month before the current admission, an IVP showed a mass on his right kidney. The current admission was to conduct a cystoscopy with a ureteral pyelogram and brush biopsy of the affected area of the right kidney.

His admission urinalysis was significant for ketones trace; blood large; protein 100 mg/dL; nitrite positive; leukocyte esterase moderate; color brown; appearance slightly bloody; WBCs 5–10/HPF; RBCs TNTC/HPF; bacteria few. The brush biopsy was positive for malignancy, and 7 weeks later the patient was admitted to surgery for removal of the right kidney, ureter, and part of the bladder connected to the ureter. The pathology report indicated an invasive transitional cell carcinoma (papillary, solid) arising from the renal pelvis/calyceal urothelium and invading the adjacent renal parenchyma. The tumor was confined to the right kidney except for multifocal involvement of the ureter urothelium. The appearance of the urinary sediment at the time of the initial biopsy admission is shown in Figures 9-86 and 9-87.

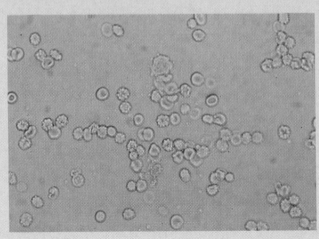

FIGURE 9-86 RBCs, some showing crenation. Urine sediment; SM stain; ×400.

continued

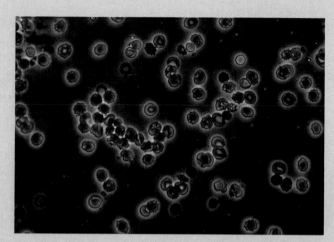

FIGURE 9-87 Same field of view as Figure 9-85, but with phase contrast. Urine sediment; SM stain; ×400.

CASE STUDY 9-8

This 57-year-old man initially presented to the hospital ER complaining of progressive shortness of breath, weight loss, and fever for the preceding 6 months. The patient had a history of tuberculosis, treated in southern California about 5 years ago, but on previous admissions reactivation of tuberculosis was ruled out. Repeated cocci serologies and CSF serologies were negative for cocci.

The patient was homeless and lived in alleys and under bridges in the local area. His history revealed a progressive decline in appetite and energy level, weight loss, fever and chills, night sweats, and vague abdominal pain of a nonradiating focal nature. He was initially SOB only when walking, but this had progressed to SOB even when he was at rest. Walking even less than a block made him extremely tired.

A BAL was significant for a finding of "usual interstitial pneumonia" (UIP), but tests for AFB, cocci, fungi, or *Pneumocystis carinii* were all negative. Cytologies were negative for malignancy. It was thought that the patient's problems ultimately stemmed from a secondary diagnosis of chronic alcoholism and that his generally poor nutritional status resulted in his current condition. He was chronically respirator-dependent (prognosis poor with UIP) and received PEG tube feedings to improve his nutritional status. He was transferred to a hospice facility in a neighboring county with a discharge diagnosis of respiratory failure, malnourishment contributing to respiratory failure, and syndrome of inappropriate secretion of antidiuretic hormone (SIADH) with hyponatremia 2° to chronic pulmonary disease.

The patient's discharge urinalysis was significant for: specific gravity < 1.005; blood moderate; WBCs 0–2/HPF; RBCs 20–50/HPF; epithelial cells few/HPF; bacteria few/HPF; casts 5–10 waxy, 0–1

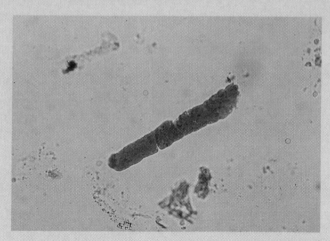

FIGURE 9-88 Waxy-granular cast. Urine sediment; SM stain; ×200.

continued

granular, rare mixed WBC/RTE, rare RTE, rare WBC/LPF. Examples of the sediment are illustrated in Figures 9-88 and 9-89, which relate to the patient's generally run-down condition, respiratory failure, and renal hypoxia.

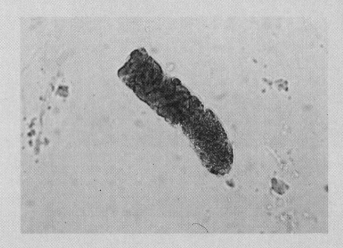

FIGURE 9-89 Granular/cellular cast. Urine sediment; SM stain; ×400.

CASE STUDY 9-9

This 90-year-old woman was seen in the ER because of altered mental status and complaints of epigastric-type pain. Before coming to the ER, she took some Pepcid for her stomach pain and Ambien (zolpidem tartrate) for insomnia. Still unable to sleep, she took more Ambien, and then got disoriented. Her CK was 337 U/L (19–76), and CKMB was 6.8%, a positive indicator for MI (ref. value < 4–6%). Her admission diagnosis was R/O MI. Her final diagnosis was CHF acute onset 2° to MI. Her admission urinalysis was significant for: blood large; protein > 300 mg/dL; WBCs 10–20; RBCs 5–10/HPF; epithelial cells 2+/HPF; bacteria few/HPF; casts rare RTE, 5–10 WBC, TNTC granular, and TNTC hyaline/LPF. The appearance of the urinary sediment on admission is shown in Figures 9-90 and 9-91, with casts reflecting the CHF and MI.

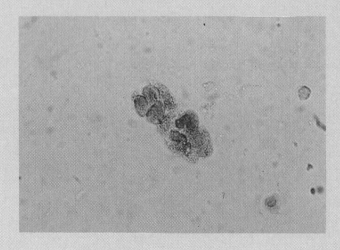

FIGURE 9-90 Partially degenerated mixed cellular cast (RTE/WBC). Urine sediment; SM stain; ×400.

continued

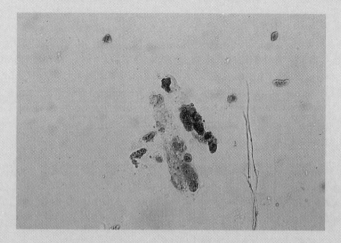

FIGURE 9-91 Cellular cast (RTE/WBC) and cellular/granular cast. Urine sediment; SM stain; ×200.

CASE STUDY 9-10

His mother brought this 1.5-year-old boy to the ER reporting that he had a fever, had been coughing, and appeared to be in respiratory distress. A diagnosis of pneumonia was made and the child was sent home with Pediazol (erythromycin ethylsuccinate and sulfisoxazole acetyl). The ER urinalysis was significant for: ketones 15 mg/dL; WBCs 2–5/HPF; RBCs 2–5/HPF; epithelials rare renal, few transitional, few squamous; bacteria negative/HPF; casts 5–10 granular/LPF. C&S was reported at a later date as negative. An example of the urine sediment is shown in Figure 9-92, showing a group of small transitional cells dislodged by catheterization.

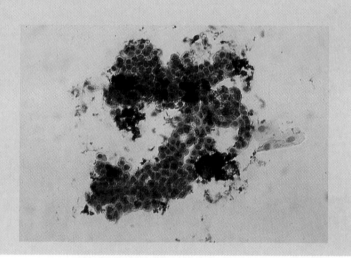

FIGURE 9-92 Group of small transitional cells. Urine sediment; toluidine blue; ×200.

Case Histories and Study Questions

CASE HISTORY 9-1

Coming through the ER complaining of severe abdominal pain (acute abdomen), this 20-year-old woman was admitted to R/O appendicitis, pancreatitis, pyelonephritis, abdominal abscess, or ruptured viscus. Because she was 36 weeks' (estimated) IUP, a low C-section was performed and the child was delivered. Her appendix was found to be

continued

ruptured, and it was removed at the same time. Blood cultures were positive for E. *coli*, sensitive to Cefotan (cefotetan disodium) and to gentamicin, which she was given. The urinalysis, obtained two days postsurgery, was as follows: glucose negative; bilirubin small; ketones 40 mg/dL; specific gravity 1.025; blood negative; pH 6.5; protein 30 mg/dL; urobilinogen 1.0 EU/dL; nitrite negative; leukocyte esterase trace; color orange; WBCs 5–10/HPF; RBCs rare/HPF; epithelial cells 1+/HPF; bacteria 1+/HPF; bacteria 1+; casts 1–5 granular; Ictotest negative. C&S was not requested on this urine. The urine sediment is illustrated in Figures 9-93 to 9-97.

Study Questions for Case History 9-1

1. What aspects of the urinalysis do you find significant?
2. What do you find significant about Figures 9-93 to 9-97?
3. What pathophysiologic aspects of this case are illustrated by the urine microscopics?

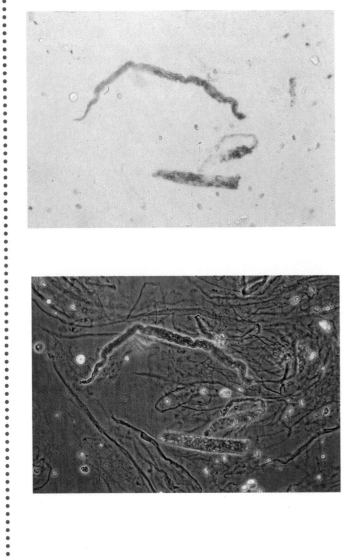

FIGURE 9-93 Urine sediment; SM stain; ×100.

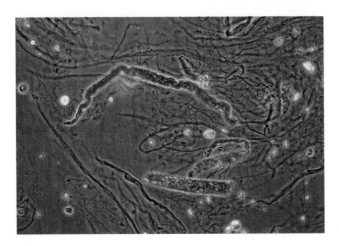

FIGURE 9-94 Same field of view as Figure 9-93 but with phase contrast. Urine sediment; SM stain/phase contrast; ×100.

continued

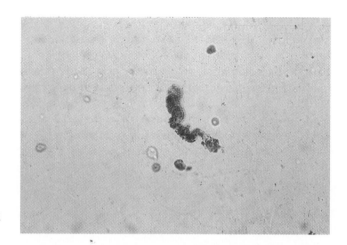

FIGURE 9-95 Urine sediment; SM stain; ×200.

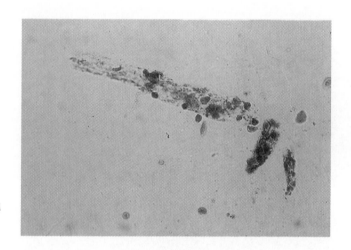

FIGURE 9-96 Urine sediment; SM stain; ×200.

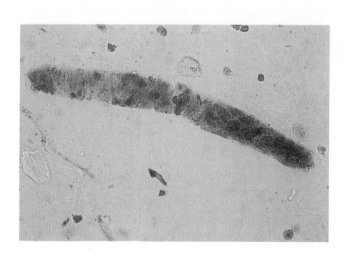

FIGURE 9-97 Urine sediment; SM stain; ×400.

continued

CASE HISTORY 9-2

An 82-year-old woman with a history of HTN treated with Vasotec (enalapril maleate), and of NIDDM, was seen in the outpatient clinic complaining of a blister on her lower lip that she said had been developing slowly for over a year. The blister was diagnosed as a mucocele (a mucus cyst), and an appointment was made to have it biopsied and excised at a future date. In the course of her examination, a routine urinalysis (without the microscopic) was requested and the urine was found to be significant for nitrite positive; and leukocyte esterase moderate. The results prompted the request for a C&S on the urine. The appearance of the urine sediment is shown in Figures 9-98 and 9-99, and the urine C&S subsequently indicated a colony count greater than 100,000 CFU/mL with an identification of E. *coli*.

Study Questions for Case History 9-2

1. What aspects of the urine sediment do you find significant?
2. What diagnosis would you give this case?
3. What type of treatment do you think this patient was given for the condition shown here?

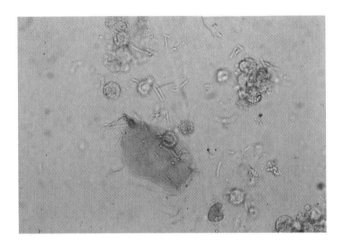

FIGURE 9-98 Urine sediment; SM stain ×400.

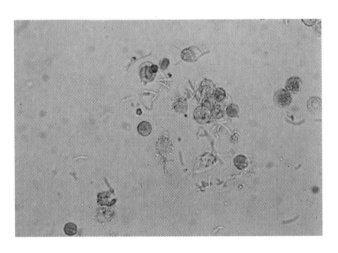

FIGURE 9-99 Urine sediment; SM stain; ×400.

continued

CASE HISTORY 9-3

With a medical history of HTN, IDDM, and CHF, this 57-year-old woman was attending a social event until the early morning hours, had been walking around complaining of SOB, and suddenly collapsed with a blood-tinged discharge coming from her mouth. She was rushed to the ER in a private car and on arrival was unresponsive to verbal or painful stimuli, and showed agonal respirations with a weak radial pulse. The impression was respiratory arrest, acute pulmonary edema, R/O MI. Subsequent laboratory work did not support the diagnosis of acute MI, suggesting instead acute pulmonary edema.

Her admission urinalysis produced the following results: glucose 250 mg/dL; bilirubin and ketones negative; specific gravity 1.010; blood small; pH 5.5; protein 100 mg/dL; urobilinogen normal; nitrite and leukocyte esterase negative; color amber; appearance hazy; WBCs 20–50/HPF; RBCs 0–2/HPF; epithelials few/HPF; bacteria 1+/HPF; casts TNTC granular/LPF. The appearance of her urinary sediment at admission is shown in Figures 9-100 to 9-102.

Study Questions for Case History 9-3

1. What urinalysis results do you find significant?
2. How would you characterize the casts found in Figures 9-100 to 9-102?
3. What pathophysiology of this case is most closely related to the urinary sediment findings?

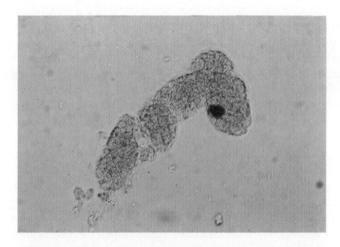

FIGURE 9-100 Urine sediment; SM stain; ×400.

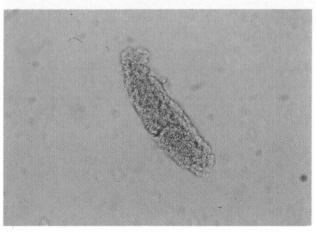

FIGURE 9-101 Urine sediment; SM stain; ×400.

continued

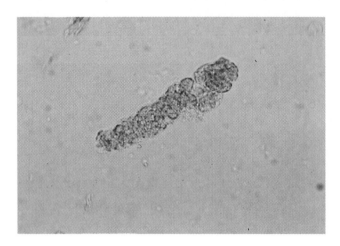

FIGURE 9-102 Urine sediment; SM stain; ×400.

CASE HISTORY 9-4

This 49-year-old man presented to the ER complaining of bilateral low abdominal pain that he had experienced for the preceding 5 months ("off-and-on") and worsening over the last 2 days. The pain was described as a "hot poker going through my abdomen" and associated with the abdominal pain was nausea, vomiting, and some coughing (nonproductive). The patient did not have diarrhea or any changes in appetite or weight. The patient had been diagnosed with AIDS the previous year and has disseminated tuberculosis. In the ER it was noticed that he also had a crusted, slightly erythematous rash on the toes of both feet.

On admission he was taking INH, rifampin, Bactrim DS, Megace, Flucon, MS Contin, and morphine elixir. The patient had been an intravenous drug abuser for many years but denies homosexuality. On initial presentation, the patient's chest x-ray study did not show any significant infiltrate. However, the abdominal x-ray study showed multiple air–fluid levels in the small bowel. The general impression on admission was ileus, probably related to narcotic abuse, including the morphine and MS Contin; AIDS; disseminated tuberculosis; and skin rash.

The patient was admitted for observation and also for treatment of ileus with nasogastric tube and administration of GoLYTELY. He continued to receive tuberculosis medications and his pain was controlled by the nonnarcotic, Toradol. His condition improved continuously and after 3 days he was discharged in stable condition with Bactrim DS, Diflucan (for fungal dermatitis), INH, and rifampin.

His admission urinalysis (microscopic not requested) was glucose, bilirubin, ketones, negative; specific gravity 1.020; blood negative; pH 7.0; protein 30 mg/dL; urobilinogen normal; nitrite and leukocyte esterase negative; color amber. A C&S was not requested. The appearance of the urine sediment is shown in Figures 9-103 to 9-106.

Study Questions for Case History 9-4

1. Are there any significant findings in the urinalysis?
2. How would you characterize the casts and cells observed in Figures 9-103 to 9-106?
3. What pathophysiologic picture is illustrated by the analysis of the urine sediment in this case?

continued

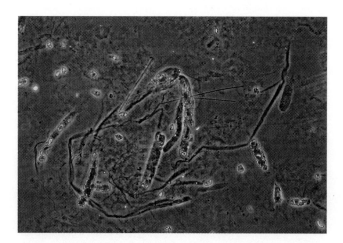

FIGURE 9-103 Urine sediment; SM stain/phase contrast; ×100.

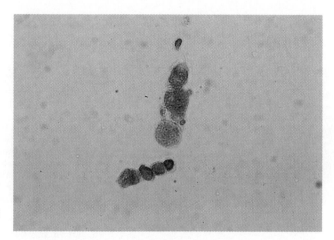

FIGURE 9-104 Urine sediment; SM stain; ×400.

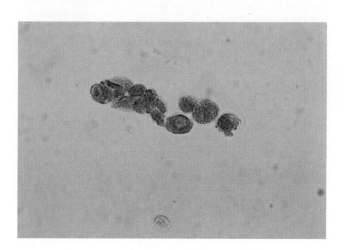

FIGURE 9-105 Urine sediment; SM stain; ×400.

continued

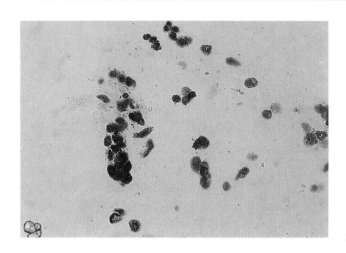

FIGURE 9-106 Urine sediment; SM stain; × s200.

REFERENCES

1. Allston CA. Macroscopic physicochemical testing [letter]. *Laboratory Medicine* 1989;20:341–342.
2. Bartlett R, Kaczmarczyk L. Usefulness of microscopic examination in urinalysis. *Am J Clin Pathol* 1984;82:713–716.
3. Brock DA, Hundley JM. Identifying calcium oxalate crystals in urine. *Laboratory Medicine* 1995;26:733–735.
4. Brunzel NA. *Fundamentals of urine and body fluid analysis*. Philadelphia: WB Saunders, 1994.
5. Ferris JA. Comparison and standardization of the urine microscopic examination. *Laboratory Medicine* 1983;14:659–662.
6. Haber MH. Pisse prophecy: A brief history of urinalysis. *Clin Lab Med* 1988.
7. Haber MH. Quality assurance in urinalysis. *Clin Lab Med* 1988; 431–447.
8. High SR, Rowe JA, Maksem JA. Macroscopic physicochemical testing for screening urinalysis. *Laboratory Medicine* 1988; 19:174–176.
9. Loo ST, Scottolini A, Luangphinith S, Adam A, Jacobs L, Mariani A. Urine screening strategy employing dipstick analysis and selective culture: An evaluation. *Am J Clin Pathol* 1984;81:634–642.
10. Mahon CR, Smith LA. Standardization of the urine microscopic examination. *Clin Lab Sci* 1990;3:328–332.
11. Monferdini D, Joinville M, Grove W. Improving urine sediment analysis. *Laboratory Medicine* 1995;26:660–664.
12. Nanji AA, Adam W, Campbell DJ. Routine microscopic examination of the urine sediment. *Arch Pathol Lab Med* 1984; 108:399–400.
13. Ringsrud KM, Linné JJ. *Urinalysis and body fluids: A color text and atlas*. St. Louis: Mosby-Year Book, 1995.
14. *Routine urinalysis and collection, transportation, and preservation of urine specimens: Tentative guideline*. NCCLS Document GP16-T. Villanova, PA: National Committee for Clinical Laboratory Standards (NCCLS), 1992.
15. Schumann GB, Schumann JL, Marcussen N. *Cytodiagnostic urinalysis of renal and lower urinary tract disorders*. New York: Igaku-Shoin Medical Publishers, 1995.
16. Schumann GB, Schweitzer SC. Examination of urine. In: Henry JB, ed. *Clinical diagnosis and management by laboratory methods*. 18th ed. Philadelphia: WB Saunders, 1991.
17. Szwed J, Schaust C. The importance of microscopic examination of the urinary sediment. *American Journal of Medical Technology* 1982;48:141–143.

BIBLIOGRAPHY

Benham L, O'Kell RT. Urinalysis: Minimizing microscopy. *Clin Chem* 1982;28:1722.
Fraser CG, Smith BC, Peake MJ. Effectiveness of an out-patient urine screening program. *Clin Chem* 1977;23:2216.
Free AH, Free HM. *Urinalysis in clinical laboratory practice*. Cleveland, OH: CRC Press, 1975.
Haber MH. *A primer of microscopic urinalysis*. 2nd ed. Garden Grove, CA: Hycor Biomedical, Inc., 1991.
Haber MH. *Urinary sediment: A textbook atlas*. Chicago: ASCP, 1981.
Schumann GB. The growing importance of urinary cytologic testing. *Laboratory Medicine* 1995;26:801–808.
Schumann GB. *Urine sediment examination*. Baltimore: Williams & Wilkins, 1980.
Schumann GB, Greenberg NF. Usefulness of macroscopic urinalysis as a screening procedure: A preliminary report. *Am J Clin Pathol* 1979;71:452.
Schumann GB, Schumann JL, Schweitzer S. The urine sediment examination: A coordinated approach. *Laboratory Management* 1983;21:45.
Schumann GB, Weiss MA. *Atlas of renal and urinary tract cytology and its histopathologic bases*. Philadelphia: JB Lippincott, 1981.
Strasinger SK. *Urinalysis and body fluids*. 3rd ed. Philadelphia: FA Davis, 1994.

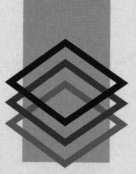

10 *Disease Correlations*

CHAPTER OUTLINE

Thrombotic Microangiopathies

    Classic (childhood) hemolytic–uremic syndrome

    Adult hemolytic–uremic syndrome

    Thrombotic thrombocytopenic purpura

    Sickle Cell Disease Nephropathy

Urinary Tract Obstruction (Obstructive Uropathy)

Urolithiasis (Renal Calculi, Stones)

Acute and Chronic Renal Failure

    Acute Renal Failure

    Chronic Renal Failure

METABOLIC DISEASES AND SCREENING TESTS

The Porphyrias

Aminoacidopathies

    Phenylketonuria

    Alkaptonuria (Ochronosis)

Tyrosinosis, Tyrosinemia, and Related Disorders

Maple Syrup Urine Disease (Branched-Chain Ketonuria)

Homocystinuria

Menaluria

Disorders of Carbohydrate Metabolism

    Diabetes Mellitus

    Galactosemia

    Mucopolysaccharidoses

    Hereditary Fructose Intolerance

    Deficiency of Fructose-1,6-diphosphate

    Fructosuria

    Pentosuria

DISEASES OF OTHER ORGAN SYSTEMS

Hepatorenal Syndrome

ILLUSTRATIVE CASE STUDIES

CASE HISTORIES AND STUDY QUESTIONS

ABBREVIATIONS USED IN THIS CHAPTER

2° = secondary

ABGs = arterial blood gases

ADH = antidiuretic hormone

AIDS = acquired immunodeficiency syndrome

AIP = acute intermittent porphyria

ALA = delta-aminolevulinic acid

ALP = alkaline phosphatase

ALT = alanine aminotransferase

AN = acute nephritis

ARF = acute renal failure

AST = aspartate aminotransferase

ATN = acute tubular necrosis

AU = asymptomatic urinary abnormalities

BAL = bronchoalveolar lavage

BNS = benign nephrosclerosis

BUN = blood urea nitrogen

C&S = culture and sensitivity

CA = cancer

CFU = colony-forming units

CHF = congestive heart failure

CK = creatine kinase

CKMB = creatine kinase isoenzyme 2 (CK-2)

COPD = chronic obstructive pulmonary disease

CPN = chronic pyelonephritis

CRF = chronic renal failure

CT = computed tomography

DI = diabetes insipidus

DM = diabetes mellitus

EP = erythropoietic porphyria

ER = emergency room

FSG = focal segmental glomerulosclerosis

GBM = glomerular basement membrane

GFR = glomerular filtration rate

GN = glomerulonephritis

HDL = high-density lipoprotein

HGA = homogentisic acid

HPF = high-power field

HSP = Henoch-Schönlein purpura

HTN = hypertension

ICU = intensive care unit

IDDM = insulin-dependent diabetes mellitus

IM = intramuscular

IUP = intrauterine pregnancy

IV = intravenous

IVP = intravenous pyelogram

LDH = lactate dehydrogenase

LDL = low-density lipoprotein

(continued)

ABBREVIATIONS USED IN THIS CHAPTER

LP(a) = lipoprotein "little a"

LPF = low-power field

MCD = minimal change disease

MCV = mean corpuscular volume

MGN = membranous glomerulonephritis

MI = myocardial infarction

MPGN = membranoproliferative glomerulonephritis

MPS = mucopolysaccharidoses

NIDDM = non–insulin-dependent diabetes mellitus

NL = nephrolithiasis

NS = nephrotic syndrome

OB = obstetrics

PBG = porphobilinogen

PKU = phenylketonuria

PN = pyelonephritis

PT = prothrombin time

PTT = partial thromboplastin time

R/O = rule out

RA = rheumatoid arthritis

RBC = red blood cell

RPGN = rapidly progressive glomerulonephritis

RTA = renal tubular acidosis

RTE = renal tubular epithelial cell

SLE = systemic lupus erythematosus

SOB = shortness of breath

TD = renal tubule defects

TIN = tubulointerstitial nephritis

TNTC = too numerous to count

U/L = international units per liter

UTOurinary Tract Obstruction (Obstructive Uropathy)

Urolithiasis (Renal Calculi, Stones)

Acute and Chronic Renal Failure

Metabolic Diseases and Screening Tests

The Porphyrias

Aminoacidopathies

Disorders of Carbohydrate Metabolism

Diseases of Other Organ Systems

Hepatorenal Syndrome

UO = urinary tract obstruction

UTI = urinary tract infection

VLDL = very–low-density lipoprotein

WBC = white blood cell

Introductory Case Study

This patient, a 6-year-old boy, was seen for a "recheck" by his physician concerning a previous admit involving a diagnosis of Henoch-Schönlein purpura (HSP) and hematuria. Three months earlier, the boy had stepped on a nail that penetrated his shoe and wounded his foot. He was seen in the ER and was given penicillin. The next day, he had a palpable red rash (not purple) over most of his legs, and he complained of joint and abdominal pain. He was brought to the ER, evaluated, given the diagnosis of HSP, and treated with prednisone. In this case, the most likely cause of the HSP was an allergic reaction to penicillin. With HSP, about 10% of the patients develop glomerulonephritis (GN), which may progress to renal failure.

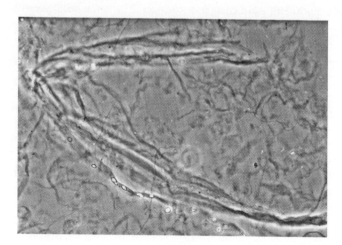

FIGURE 10-1 A slender RBC cast, with castlike objects not containing cells, and abundant mucus. Urine sediment; SM stain/phase contrast; ×200.

Continued

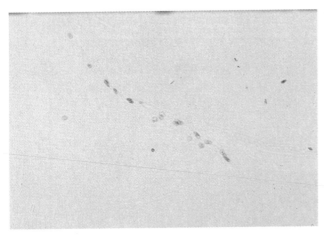

FIGURE 10-2 The same RBC cast as seen in Figure 10-1, moved slightly upward in the field of view. Urine sediment; brightfield microscopy; SM stain; ×200.

FIGURE 10-4 Same field of view as Figure 10-3, with bright field microscopy. Urine sediment; SM stain; ×100.

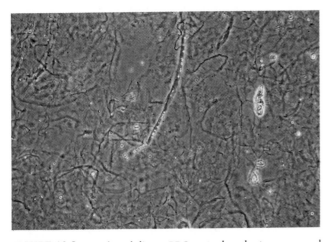

FIGURE 10-3 Another delicate RBC cast, abundant mucus, and background RBCs. Urine sediment; SM stain/phase contrast; ×100.

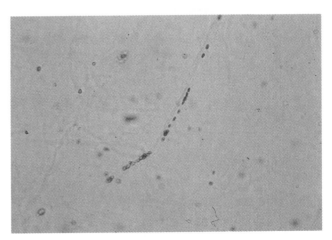

FIGURE 10-5 Same field of view as Figure 10-4, with higher magnification. Urine sediment; SM stain; ×200.

The recheck hospital visit described here produced a urinalysis significant for: blood trace; WBCs 0–2/HPF; RBCs 20–50/HPF; and casts 0–1 RBC/LPF. The urine sediment findings are illustrated in Figures 10-1 to 10-5, and show acute GN associated with the HSP. The delicate RBC casts are particularly noteworthy.

Diseases of the Urinary Tract

From ancient times, urine has been studied to diagnose human illness. A routine urinalysis may not only provide information about renal disease but may shed light on many metabolic diseases as well. The urinalysis may detect abnormalities before a patient manifests any clinical symptoms. Furthermore, the urinalysis provides a valuable tool for monitoring the progression of many diseases and evaluating the effectiveness of therapy.

Although renal diseases are responsible for a great deal of morbidity, they are not major causes of mortality.[9] In the United States, about 35,000 deaths are attributed yearly to renal disease, in contrast to about 750,000 to heart disease, 400,000 to cancer, and 200,000 to stroke. However, millions of people are affected annually by nonfatal kidney diseases such as infections of the kidney or lower urinary tract, kidney stones, and urinary tract obstruction.

As outlined by Coe, there are 10 syndromes that alone or in combination suggest the possibility of renal disease and become useful starting points for evaluating patients.[8] The following is a brief description of the 10 renal syndromes:

1. Acute nephritis (AN)—a glomerular syndrome dominated by the acute onset of hematuria (usually grossly visible), mild to moderate proteinuria, and hypertension. The classic example of AN is acute poststreptococcal GN.
2. Nephrotic syndrome (NS)—characterized by heavy proteinuria (more than 3.5 g/day), hypoalbuminemia, severe edema, hyperlipidemia, and lipiduria.
3. Asymptomatic urinary abnormalities (AU)—hematuria or proteinuria, or a combination of these two, usually a manifestation of subtle or mild glomerular abnormalities.
4. Acute renal failure (ARF)—dominated by oliguria or anuria with recent onset of azotemia. ARF can result from glomerular injury, interstitial injury, or acute tubular necrosis.
5. Chronic renal failure (CRF)—the end result of all chronic renal diseases, characterized by prolonged symptoms and signs of uremia.
6. Urinary tract infection (UTI)—characterized by bacteriuria and pyuria, may be symptomatic or asymptomatic, and may affect only the kidney (pyelonephritis [PN]), or only the bladder (cystitis).
7. Urinary tract obstruction (UO)—upper tract obstruction defined by intravenous or retrograde pyelography, lower tract obstruction suggested by slow urine stream, difficulty in emptying the bladder, hesitancy, overflow incontinence and dribbling.
8. Renal tubule defects (TD)—dominated by polyuria, nocturia, and electrolyte disorders (e.g., metabolic acidosis). They are either the result of other diseases that directly affect the tubules (e.g., medullary cystic disease), or they represent defects in specific tubular functions that may be inherited (e.g., cystinuria) or acquired (e.g., lead nephropathy).
9. Hypertension (HTN)—the average of blood pressure measurements taken on three separate occasions exceeds 145 mm Hg systolic or 95 mm Hg diastolic; principal entities usually sought are renal artery stenosis, mineralocorticoid excess, and pheochromocytoma.
10. Nephrolithiasis (NL)—renal stones are manifested by renal colic, hematuria, and recurrent formation.

Diseases of the Kidney

Diseases of the kidney may be classified into four types based on the four basic morphologic components initially affected: glomeruli, tubules, interstitium, and blood vessels.[9] In this traditional view, the early manifestations of disease affecting each of these four components tend to be distinct. However, because the structures of the kidney are anatomically interdependent, damage to one usually involves the others eventually. With disease progression, there is a tendency for all forms of chronic renal disease eventually to destroy all four components of the kidney, ending with CRF and so-called end-stage kidneys.

Vulnerability to disease varies with each structural component. Glomerular diseases are most often immunologically mediated; tubular and interstitial disorders are more likely due to toxic or infectious agents. Vascular diseases result in decreased renal perfusion, which subsequently brings about combined morphologic and functional changes in the kidney.

GLOMERULAR DISEASES

Glomeruli may be damaged by a variety of diseases, including immunologic, metabolic, and hereditary disorders. These are summarized in Table 10-1. In the case of primary glomerular diseases, it is the kidney that is primarily involved. In the secondary glomerular diseases (the systemic and hereditary disorders), the glomeruli become involved because of the progression of the primary disease. Table 10-2 summarizes the five major glomerular syndromes together with their clinical features. The primary glomerulonephritides as well as the secondary diseases affecting the glomerulus can result in these syndromes. Table 10-3 summarizes the major primary glomerulonephritides.

Morphologic Alterations

The various types of glomerular diseases are characterized by one or more of four distinct morphologic changes of the glomeruli. These basic tissue reactions include two classified as glomerular hypercellularity (e.g., cellular proliferation and leukocytic infiltration), glomerular basement membrane (GBM) thickening, and hyalinization with sclerosis. The histologic changes can be subdivided into diffuse (all glomeruli involved), global (the entire glomerulus involved), focal (only a certain proportion of the glomeruli involved), segmental (a part of each glomerulus involved), and mesangial (the mesangial region predominantly involved).

The so-called inflammatory diseases of the glomerulus are associated with cellular proliferation in the glomerular tuft. The cells may be mesangial, endothelial (capillary endothelium), and epithelial (podocytes).

TABLE 10-1
Glomerular Diseases

● ●

Primary Glomerulopathies
Acute diffuse proliferative glomerulonephritis
   Poststreptococcal
   Nonpoststreptococcal
Rapidly progressive (crescentic) glomerulonephritis
Membranous glomerulopathy
Lipoid nephrosis (minimal change disease)
Focal segmental glomerulosclerosis
Membranoproliferative glomerulonephritis
IgA nephropathy
Focal proliferative glomerulonephritis
Chronic glomerulonephritis

Systemic Diseases
Systemic lupus erythematosus
Diabetes mellitus
Amyloidosis
Goodpasture's syndrome
Polyarteritis nodosa
Wegener's granulomatosis
Henoch-Schönlein purpura
Bacterial endocarditis

Hereditary Disorders
Alport's syndrome
Fabry's disease

(From Cotran RS, Kuman V, Robbins SL. *Robbins pathologic basis of disease.* 5th ed. Philadelphia: WB Saunders, 1994.)

matrix. The loss of structural detail usually signals the end stage of the various forms of glomerular damage.

Pathogenesis of Glomerular Injury

Immunologic processes underlie most cases of primary GN as well as many of the cases of secondary glomerular involvement. Table 10-4 outlines the immune mechanisms for glomerular injury. Although cell-mediated and other immune mechanisms are involved, most attention has been given to antibody-mediated injury—circulating antigen–antibody complexes as well as complexes resulting from antigen–antibody reactions occurring within the glomerulus.

Acute Glomerulonephritis

Acute GN is characterized by inflammatory alterations in the glomeruli. Urinalysis findings include RBCs and RBC casts in the urine sediment, dysmorphic RBCs, hyaline and granular casts, and WBCs. Azotemia, oliguria, and mild to moderate HTN may also be part of the picture. Proteinuria and edema are observed but are not as severe as seen with NS.

ACUTE POSTSTREPTOCOCCAL GLOMERULONEPHRITIS (PROLIFERATIVE GLOMERULONEPHRITIS) This disease usually appears 1 to 4 weeks after a streptococcal infection of the pharynx or skin. Although it occurs most often in children 6 to 10 years of age, it can affect individuals at any age. Only certain strains of group A beta-hemolytic streptococci are nephritogenic, most cases being traced to types 1, 4, and 12, which have "M protein" in their cell walls.

Poststreptococcal GN is an immunologically mediated disease. The delay between the infection and the onset of nephritis represents the time required for anti-

In some types of acute GN, leukocyte infiltration may accompany cellular proliferation. Responding to local chemotaxis, the leukocytes (especially neutrophils and macrophages) easily infiltrate the glomeruli.

Two types of basement membrane thickening may be observed. In the type associated with diabetic glomerulosclerosis, the basement membrane itself becomes thickened with no obvious deposition of extraneous material. The second type of membrane thickening results from the deposition of amorphous, precipitated proteins on either side of or within the basement membrane. The most common type of thickening is due to extensive subepithelial deposition occurring with membranous GN (MGN). The deposits in most cases are thought to be immune complexes, although fibrin may also be present.

Glomerular hyalinization is characterized by the accumulation of a homogeneous, eosinophilic, extracellular material that causes the glomeruli to lose their structural detail and become sclerotic. The material is made up of precipitated plasma protein as well as increased amounts of basement membrane or mesangial

TABLE 10-2
The Glomerular Syndromes

● ●

Syndrome	Features
Acute nephritic syndrome	Hematuria, azotemia, variable proteinuria, oliguria, edema, and hypertension
Rapidly progressive GN	Acute nephritis, proteinuria, and acute renal failure
Nephrotic syndrome	>3.5 g proteinuria, hypoalbuminemia, hyperlipidemia, lipiduria
Chronic renal failure	Azotemia → uremia progressing over years
Asymptomatic hematuria or proteinuria	Glomerular hematuria; subnephrotic proteinuria

(From Cotran RS, Kuman V, Robbins SL. *Robbins pathologic basis of disease.* 5th ed. Philadelphia: WB Saunders, 1994.)

TABLE 10-3
Summary of Major Primary Glomerulonephritides

Disease	Most Frequent Clinical Presentation	Pathogenesis	Glomerular Pathology		
			Light Microscopy	Fluorescence Microscopy	Electron Microscopy
Poststreptococcal GN*	Acute nephritis	Antibody-mediated; circulating or planted antigen	Diffuse proliferation; leukocytic infiltration	Granular IgG and C3 in GBM* and mesangium	Subepithelial humps
Goodpasture's syndrome	Rapidly progressive GN	Anti-GBM COL4A3 antigen	Proliferation; crescents	Linear IgG and C3; fibrin in crescents	No deposits; GBM disruptions; fibrin
Idiopathic rapidly progressive GN	Rapidly progressive GN	Anti-GBM immune complex ANCA	Proliferation; focal necrosis; crescents	Linear IgG and C3 Granular	No deposits Deposits may be present
				Negative or equivocal	No deposits
Membranous GN	Nephrotic syndrome	Antibody-mediated; in situ Gp330 antigen	Diffuse capillary wall thickening	Granular IgG and C3; diffuse	Subepithelial deposits
Lipoid nephrosis	Nephrotic syndrome	Unknown, loss of glomerular polyanion	Normal; lipid in tubules	Negative	Loss of foot processes; no deposits
Focal segmental glomerulosclerosis	Nephrotic syndrome; nonnephrotic proteinuria	Unknown Ablation nephropathy ?Plasma factor	Focal and segmental sclerosis and hyalinosis	Focal; IgM and C3	Loss of foot processes; epithelial denudation
Membranoproliferative GN — Type I	Nephrotic syndrome	(I) Immune complex	Mesangial proliferation; basement membrane thickening; splitting	(I) IgG + C3; C1 + C4	(I) Subendothelial deposits
Membranoproliferative GN — Type II	Hematuria Chronic renal failure	(II) Autoantibody; alternative complement pathway activation		(II) C3 ± IgG; no C1 or C4	(II) Dense-deposit disease
IgA nephropathy	Recurrent hematuria or proteinuria	Unknown	Focal proliferative GN; mesangial widening	IgA + IgG, M, and C3 in mesangium	Mesangial and paramesangial dense deposits
Chronic GN	Chronic renal failure	Variable	Hyalinized glomeruli	Granular or negative	—

* GN, glomerulonephritis; GBM, glomerular basement membrane.
(From Cotran RS, Kuman V, Robbins SL. *Robbins pathologic basis of disease*. 5th ed. Philadelphia: WB Saunders, 1994.)

body formation. The presence of granular immune deposits in the glomeruli suggests an immune complex–mediated mechanism, although the streptococcal antigenic components responsible for the immune reaction have not been identified.

Morphologically, the glomeruli show hypercellularity resulting from the proliferation of endothelial and mesangial cells together with leukocyte (neutrophil and monocyte) infiltration. The cellular proliferation and infiltration are diffuse, involving all lobules of all glomeruli. Swelling of endothelial cells occurs and the combination of proliferation, swelling, and leukocyte infiltration obstructs the capillary lumina. Fibrin within the capillary lumina and the mesangium can be demonstrated with special stains. Interstitial edema may be observed and the tubules often contain RBC casts and may show evidence of degeneration.

In the typical case, a young child abruptly manifests malaise, fever, nausea, oliguria, proteinuria, and hematuria. The urine contains RBC casts. Periorbital edema and mild to moderate HTN are observed. Blood tests indicate an elevated antistreptolysin O titer, decreased serum complement, and the presence of cryoglobulins in the serum. With conservative therapy to maintain electrolyte and water balance, more than 95% of children with poststreptococcal GN recover totally. For adults infected in epidemics, the overall prognosis is good, but in only about 60% of sporadic cases do adult patients recover promptly. Chronic GN eventually develops in some adults

A similar form of GN occurs sporadically in association with nonstreptococcal agents such as other bacteria (e.g., staphylococcal endocarditis, pneumococcal pneumonia, and meningococcemia), viral disease (e.g., hepatitis B, mumps, varicella, and infectious mononucleosis), and parasitic infections (e.g., malaria, toxoplasmosis). For all of these conditions, the characteristics of immune complex nephritis are observed.

TABLE 10-4
Immune Mechanisms of Glomerular Injury

I. Antibody-Mediated Injury
  A. In situ immune complex deposition
    1. Fixed intrinsic tissue antigens
      a. Goodpasture's antigen (Anti-GBM* nephritis)
      b. Heymann's antigen (membranous GN*)
      c. Mesangial antigens
      d. Others
    2. Planted antigens
      a. Exogenous (drugs, lectins, infectious agents)
      b. Endogenous (DNA, immunoglobulins, immune complexes, IgA)
  B. Circulating immune complex deposition
    1. Endogenous antigens (e.g., DNA, tumor antigens)
    2. Exogenous antigens (e.g., infectious products)
  C. Cytotoxic antibodies
II. Cell-Mediated Injury
III. Activation of Alternative Complement Pathway

* GN, glomerulonephritis; GBM, glomerular basement membrane.
(From Cotran RS, Kuman V, Robbins SL. *Robbins pathologic basis of disease.* 5th ed. Philadelphia: WB Saunders, 1994.)

Rapidly Progressive (Crescentic) Glomerulonephritis

Rapidly progressive GN (RPGN) is a clinicopathologic syndrome in which damage to the glomeruli is accompanied by rapid and progressive decline in renal function. It frequently involves severe oliguria or anuria and usually results in irreversible renal failure within weeks or months. It is characterized histologically by the accumulation of cells in Bowman's space in the form of "crescents."

The crescents are formed by proliferation of parietal cells and by migration of monocytes and macrophages into Bowman's space, and sometimes neutrophils and lymphocytes as well. These cellular crescents eventually fill Bowman's space, compress the glomerular tuft, and may even close off the entrance to the proximal tubule. Fibrin strands are observed between the cellular layers in the crescents, and characteristic wrinkling of the GBM with focal disruptions in its continuity are evident on electron microscopy.

Rapidly progressive GN may occur after an infection (poststreptococcal), may be associated with systemic diseases (e.g., systemic lupus erythematosus [SLE]), and may be idiopathic. Although no single pathogenic mechanism can explain all cases, it is likely that the glomerular injury is immunologically mediated.[9] For RPGN associated with Goodpasture's syndrome, circulating anti-GBM antibodies can be detected by radioimmunoassay in more than 95% of cases. The anti-GBM antibodies cross-react with pul-monary alveolar basement membranes, producing the clinical picture of pulmonary hemorrhages associated with renal failure.

The renal manifestations of all forms involve hematuria with RBC casts in the urine, variable levels of proteinuria, and variable HTN and edema. Diagnosis is aided by assays for circulating anti-GBM antibodies. For RPGN associated with Goodpasture's syndrome, early intensive plasmapheresis combined with steroids and cytotoxic agents may bring dramatic remission. In other forms of RPGN, therapy is less successful, especially if not instituted before the development of oliguria, and patients may eventually require chronic dialysis or renal transplantation.

Nephrotic Syndrome

NS almost always occurs in patients with certain glomerular diseases, such as MGN (minimal change disease [MCD]), lipoid nephrosis, focal segmental glomerulosclerosis (FSG), and membranoproliferative GN (MPGN). NS may also be associated with many other forms of primary as well as secondary GN. The causes of NS are summarized in Table 10-5. The basis of the syndrome is increased permeability of the glomerular capillary walls resulting from either structural or physicochemical derangement.

The nephrotic syndrome is characterized by massive proteinuria (3.5 g/day or more), hypoalbuminemia with plasma albumin levels less than 3 g/dL, generalized edema, hyperlipidemia, and lipiduria. Serum albumin is depleted because of the heavy proteinuria and the inability of the liver's synthetic capacity to keep up with the loss. The loss of colloid osmotic pressure in the blood leads to the generalized edema, which is aggravated by sodium and water retention. The edema is characteristically soft and pitting, and is most prominent around the eyes (periorbital) and in the legs, but may be quite massive with pleural effusions and ascites.

The hyperlipidemia observed in NS in most cases consists of increased cholesterol, triglycerides, VLDL, LDL, LP$_{(a)}$, and apoproteins. HDL may be decreased in some patients. The hyperlipidemia appears to be partly caused by an increased synthesis of lipoproteins in the liver, the abnormal transport of circulating lipid particles, and decreased lipid catabolism. The lipids are able to cross the filtration barrier, resulting in lipiduria manifested as free-floating fat globules, oval fat bodies, or fatty casts. Waxy casts are also observed. Patients with NS are especially vulnerable to infections and to thrombotic complications owing to the loss of immunoglobulins, low–molecular-weight complement components, and the anticoagulant cofactors.

TABLE 10-5
Causes of Nephrotic Syndrome

	Prevalence* (%)	
	Children	Adults
Primary Glomerular Disease		
Membranous GN*	5	40
Lipoid nephrosis	65	15
Focal segmental glomerulosclerosis	10	15
Membranoproliferative GN	10	7
Other proliferative GN (focal, "pure mesangial," IgA nephropathy)	10	23
Systemic Diseases		
Diabetes mellitus		
Amyloidosis		
Systemic lupus erythematosus		
Drugs (gold, penicillamine, "street heroin")		
Infections (malaria, syphilis, hepatitis B, AIDS)		
Malignancy (carcinoma, melanoma)		
Miscellaneous (bee-sting allergy, hereditary nephritis)		

* GN, glomerulonephritis.

** Approximate prevalence of primary disease = 95% in children, 60% in adults. Approximate prevalence of systemic disease = 5% in children, 40% in adults.

(From Cotran RS, Kuman V, Robbins SL. *Robbins pathologic basis of disease.* 5th ed. Philadelphia: WB Saunders, 1994.)

Membranous Glomerulonephritis

MGN is a major cause of NS in adults. This disease is characterized by immunoglobulin-containing deposits along the epithelial (podocyte) side of the basement membrane, between the membrane and the overlying epithelial cells (which lose their foot processes). Well-developed cases show diffuse thickening of the capillary wall because of basement membrane material laid down over the immune deposits. Membrane thickening progressively encroaches on the capillary lumina, and sclerosis of the mesangium may occur, and the glomeruli may become totally hyalinized. The glomerular damage, resulting in leakage across the membrane, appears to result from complement activation, specifically the direct action of C5b-9, the complement membrane–attack complex.

Based on the uniform presence of immunoglobulins and complement in the subepithelial deposits, it is thought that MGN is a form of chronic antigen–antibody-mediated disease.[9] Although specific antigens can sometimes be implicated in secondary MGN, in most cases the antigens are not known. Secondary MGN has been associated with various disorders or etiologic agents such as SLE, diabetes mellitus (DM), thy-

roiditis, and exposure to metals (e.g., gold, mercury) or to drugs (e.g., penicillamine). However, in about 85% of patients, MGN is idiopathic.

For a patient who was previously healthy, MGN begins with the gradual onset of NS, although in a few cases (15%) there may be nonnephrotic proteinuria. Hematuria and mild HTN may be observed. Progression of MGN is associated with increasing sclerosis of the glomeruli, increasing blood urea nitrogen (BUN) and HTN, and a relative reduction in the severity of the proteinuria. Even though proteinuria continues in more than 60% of patients, only about 10% die or go into renal failure within 10 years, and renal insufficiency develops in no more than 40%.[9]

Minimal Change Disease (Lipoid Nephrosis)

MCD, a relatively benign disorder, is the most frequent cause of NS in children, with peak incidence between 2 and 6 years of age. By light microscopy, the glomeruli look essentially normal, but electron microscopy reveals the effacement of the podocyte foot processes. The foot processes are replaced by a rim of cytoplasm often showing vacuolization, swelling, and villous hyperplasia.

This alteration actually represents simplification of the epithelial cell architecture with flattening and swelling of foot processes, and is also present in other proteinuric states (e.g., MGN, diabetes). These alterations in morphology, when associated with normal glomeruli, characterize MCD in contrast to the other proteinuric states. The alterations seen in MCD are completely reversible after corticosteroid therapy and remission of the proteinuria.

The term "lipoid nephrosis" arises from the fact that the cells of the proximal tubules become filled with lipids as a consequence of the tubular reabsorption of lipoproteins present in the filtrate. Immunofluorescence techniques do not demonstrate immunoglobulin or complement deposits.

MCD sometimes follows a respiratory infection or routine prophylactic immunization. Corticosteroid therapy usually brings about a rapid improvement. These and other features of the disease point to an immunologic basis even though immune deposits are not found in the glomerulus. One hypothesis is that lipoid nephrosis involves some immune dysfunction, eventually resulting in the elaboration of a circulating cytokine-like material that affects visceral epithelial cells and causes proteinuria.[9] The changes in ultrastructure point to a primary visceral epithelial cell injury that results in loss of glomerular polyanions together with the glomerular charge barrier which, in turn, leads to the proteinuria.

With MCD, renal function remains adequate despite the massive proteinuria. Usually there is no HTN or hematuria. MCD is differentiated clinically from MGN based on its dramatic response to corticosteroid therapy. The nephrotic phase may recur, however, and some patients may become "steroid dependent." For children, the long-term prognosis is excellent, and even steroid-dependent disease resolves when children reach puberty. Long-term prognosis for adults is also excellent, although they are slower to respond to therapy.

Focal Segmental Glomerulosclerosis

FSG is characterized by sclerosis of some (focal) but not all glomeruli, and by the involvement of only a portion of the capillary tuft (segmental) in the affected glomeruli. The sclerotic glomeruli show hyaline masses and lipid droplets, collapse of basement membranes, and proliferation of the mesangium. With electron microscopy, nonsclerotic areas show the diffuse loss of foot processes characteristic of MCD, in addition to a pronounced, focal detachment of the epithelial cells with denudation of the underlying GBM. Immunofluorescence microscopy demonstrates the presence of IgM and C3 within the hyaline masses in the sclerotic areas.

The hyalinosis and sclerosis result from the entrapment of plasma proteins in extremely hyperpermeable foci and from the reaction of the mesangial cells to such proteins and to fibrin deposits.[9] The existence of a circulating systemic factor as the causative agent, such as a cytokine or a circulating toxin, is suggested by the fact that sometimes within 24 hours of renal transplantation, recurrence of proteinuria is observed in patients with focal sclerosis.

Laboratory findings routinely include hematuria and proteinuria. FSG may manifest as a primary (idiopathic) glomerular disease; may be associated with another glomerular disease, such as IgA nephropathy; or may be secondary to other disorders or etiologic agents (e.g., heroin abuse, AIDS, reflux nephropathy, and analgesic abuse nephropathy). Spontaneous remission in idiopathic FSG and a response to corticosteroid therapy are seldom seen. Progression of renal failure is variable, although children have a better prognosis than adults.

Membranoproliferative Glomerulonephritis

MPGN is characterized histologically by alterations in the basement membrane and proliferation of glomerular cells.[9] "Mesangiocapillary GN" is a frequently used synonym for MPGN because the proliferation is predominantly in the mesangium. Infiltrating leukocytes and parietal epithelial crescents are present in many cases. The glomeruli have a "lobular" appearance and the GBM is thickened, often focally. Ultrastruc-

tural and immunofluorescent features subdivide MPGN into types I and II. Two thirds of the cases are type I; these cases present evidence of immune complexes in the glomerulus and activation of both the classic and alternative complement pathways. Most of the cases of type II MPGN have abnormalities that suggest activation of the alternative complement pathway. Laboratory findings vary but frequently involve microscopic hematuria together with proteinuria, as well as decreased serum complement levels.

MPGN most often presents as NS in older children or young adults, although it may begin as AN or as mild proteinuria. Few spontaneous remissions are observed with either type, and the disease follows a slow, progressive course with CRF developing in approximately 50% of the patients within 10 years. In renal transplant recipients (type II especially), there is a high incidence of disease recurrence. Secondary MPGN is usually type I and may be associated with SLE, various infections (hepatitis B, schistosomiasis), chronic liver diseases, and certain malignancies. For an example of MPGN mixed with FSG associated with SLE, refer to Case Study 10-7.

IgA Nephropathy (Berger's Disease)

Berger's disease is probably the most common type of GN worldwide and is a frequent cause of recurrent gross or microscopic hematuria.[9] It is the most common cause of asymptomatic hematuria progressing to chronic GN.[33]

Berger's disease is characterized by the presence of prominent IgA deposits in the mesangial regions of the glomeruli that can be detected by immunofluorescence microscopy. IgA is the main immunoglobulin in mucosal secretions and is present in small amounts as the monomeric form in normal serum. Polymeric IgA1 (but not IgA2) can be demonstrated in the serum of patients with IgA nephropathy, as well as circulating IgA1 immune complexes in some cases. The evidence suggests a genetic or acquired abnormality of immune regulation leading to increased mucosal IgA synthesis in response to respiratory or gastrointestinal exposure to viruses, bacteria, or food proteins. The subsequent entrapment of IgA1 and IgA1 complexes in the glomeruli is followed by activation of the alternative complement pathway, with resultant damage to the glomeruli.

IgA nephropathy affects children and young adults and may occur within a day or two of mucosal infections of the respiratory, gastrointestinal, or urinary tract. In most cases, the hematuria lasts for several days, subsides, and then returns every few months. Mild proteinuria is usually observed and occasionally NS develops. The disease appears to be slowly progressive, with CRF developing in 50% of the patients over a period of 20 years. Increased risk of progression is associated with onset of the disease in old age, heavy proteinuria, HTN, and the presence of vascular sclerosis or crescents on biopsy. For an example of Berger's disease, refer to Case Study 10-1.

Chronic Glomerulonephritis

Chronic GN may be considered an end-stage pool of glomerular disease fed by streams of specific types of GN, as illustrated in Figure 10-6. In most cases, the development of chronic GN is subtle and progresses slowly to death in patients with uremia unless dialysis is used to maintain the patient or the patient receives a renal transplant. Sometimes the renal disease is discovered when a medical examination reveals proteinuria, HTN, or azotemia. At other times, a patient may present with nonspecific complaints such as loss of appetite, anemia, vomiting, or weakness.

The glomeruli appear as acellular, eosinophilic masses because of the characteristic hyaline obliteration of their morphology.[9] HTN is found with most patients, and the dominant clinical manifestations may be cerebral or cardiovascular. Patients dying in chronic GN also manifest pathologic changes outside the kidney that are related to the uremic state. These changes include uremic pericarditis, uremic gastroenteritis, secondary hyperparathyroidism with nephrocalcinosis and renal osteodystrophy, left ventricular hypertrophy due to HTN, and diffuse alveolar damage (pulmonary changes known as uremic pneumonitis).

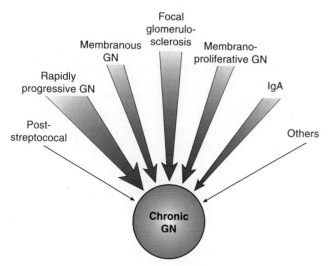

FIGURE 10-6 Primary glomerular diseases leading to chronic glomerulonephritis (GN). The thickness of the arrows relects the approximate proportion of patients in each group who progress to chronic GN. Poststreptococcal (1 to 2%); rapidly progressive (crescentic) (90%); membranous (50%); focal glomerulosclerosis (50 to 80%); MPGN (50%); IgA nephropathy (30 to 50%). (From Cotran RS, Kuman V, Robbins SL. *Robbins pathologic basis of disease*. 5th ed. Philadelphia: WB Saunders, 1994.)

Urinalysis reveals hematuria, proteinuria, and many varieties of casts, including broad casts. The urine specific gravity stays at about 1.010 (loss of concentrating ability), and the glomerular filtration rate (GFR) is decreased. With end-stage renal failure, serum analyses reveal elevated BUN, creatinine, and phosphorus, but decreased calcium.

Glomerular Lesions and Systemic Disease

This grouping refers to the glomerular involvement associated with many immunologically mediated, metabolic, or hereditary systemic disorders. For some (e.g., SLE and DM), the glomerular involvement is a major clinical manifestation.

SYSTEMIC LUPUS ERYTHEMATOSUS Systemic lupus erythematosus gives rise to a heterogeneous group of lesions and clinical presentations. Clinically, the findings include recurrent microscopic or gross hematuria, AN, NS, CRF, and HTN. Five patterns of histologic changes in the glomerulus are possible but are not unique to SLE. Glomerular damage occurs as a result of immune complex deposition (DNA and anti-DNA complexes) followed by complement activation. CRF is a frequent cause of death for SLE patients. For an example of SLE, refer to Chapter 9, Introductory Case Study.

HENOCH-SCHÖNLEIN PURPURA This syndrome is characterized by purpuric skin lesions on the extensor surfaces of the arms and legs as well as on the buttocks; abdominal pain, vomiting, and intestinal bleeding; arthralgia; and renal abnormalities. About one third of the patients exhibit renal abnormalities that include gross or microscopic hematuria, proteinuria, and NS.

Henoch-Schönlein purpura is most often encountered in children 3 to 8 years of age but is also expressed in adults, in which case the renal manifestations are usually more severe. Onset often follows an upper respiratory infection; about one third of patients exhibit atopy. The renal lesions may manifest as mild focal mesangial proliferation, diffuse mesangial proliferation, or relatively typical crescentic GN.[9] The course is quite variable, although hematuria may recur for many years after onset. Prognosis for most children is excellent. The prognosis for patients with the more diffuse lesions or NS is not as good, and renal failure occurs in patients with crescentic lesions. Refer to the Introductory Case Study for this chapter for an example of Henoch-Schönlein purpura.

BACTERIAL ENDOCARDITIS Bacterial endocarditis is associated with glomerular lesions that represent a type of immune complex nephritis initiated by bacterial antigen–antibody complexes. Clinically, various levels of hematuria and proteinuria are found, and an acute nephritic presentation may be observed as well as a rapidly progressive GN in a few cases. Milder expressions have a focal and segmental necrotizing GN, whereas more severe examples show a diffuse proliferative GN. The rapidly progressive forms show large numbers of crescents.

DIABETIC GLOMERULOSCLEROSIS Glomerulosclerosis associated with DM is a major cause of renal morbidity and mortality. End-stage kidney disease develops in as many as 30% of insulin-dependent type I diabetics, which accounts for 20% of deaths in patients younger than 40 years of age.[9]

"Diabetic nephropathy" is the term for the group of lesions that often occur concurrently in the diabetic kidney, including nonnephrotic proteinuria, nephrotic syndrome, and chronic renal failure. Diabetes also affects the arterioles, resulting in arteriolar sclerosis. Diabetes leads to increased susceptibility to the development of pyelonephritis, especially papillary necrosis, and it results in a variety of tubular lesions. The glomerular morphologic changes include thickening of the capillary basement membrane (observed in all diabetics), diffuse diabetic glomerulosclerosis, and nodular glomerulosclerosis.

It is thought that diabetic glomerulosclerosis is caused either by the insulin deficiency, the resultant hyperglycemia, or some other aspect of glucose intolerance. There is some evidence that tight control of blood glucose levels may help prevent the development and progression of diabetic nephropathy, and, as discussed in Chapter 7, tests for microalbuminuria (20–200 μg/minute) have been advocated as a way to gain an early warning of impending diabetic nephropathy and allow time to improve glycemic control.

AMYLOIDOSIS As a pathologic substance, amyloid is deposited between cells in various tissues and organs of the body in a wide variety of clinical settings.[9] Histochemically, amyloid appears as an amorphous, eosinophilic, hyaline, extracellular substance that progressively accumulates, encroaches on adjacent cells, and produces pressure atrophy of the cells.

Although the deposits have a uniform appearance and staining reaction, amyloid is not a chemically distinct entity. There are two major and several minor biochemical forms deposited by several different pathogenetic mechanisms. Approximately 95% of the amyloid material consists of fibrillar proteins, and the remainder is glycoprotein.

Although 15 biochemically distinct forms of amyloid proteins have been identified, two are most com-

mon. One, called amyloid light chain protein, is derived from plasma cells and contains immunoglobulin light chains; the second, designated amyloid-associated protein, is a nonimmunoglobulin synthesized by the liver. Indications are that, in most patients, some derangement in the immune apparatus underlies amyloidosis.

With renal involvement, amyloid is deposited in the glomeruli. The typical amyloid fibrils are seen within the mesangium and subendothelium, and occasionally within the subepithelial space, and eventually the glomerulus is totally destroyed. Patients with glomerular amyloid may present with heavy proteinuria or NS. The end result of glomerular destruction is renal failure and death in uremia.

Hereditary Nephritis

Hereditary nephritis is an assemblage of heterogeneous hereditary–familial renal diseases associated primarily with glomerular injury. Alport's syndrome, the best known of the group, is characterized by nephritis accompanied by nerve deafness and various disorders of the eye, including lens dislocation, posterior cataracts, and corneal dystrophy. The mode of inheritance is heterogeneous, either X-linked or autosomal dominant. Males are more frequently and severely affected, and are more likely to progress to renal failure.

Defective GBM synthesis underlies the renal lesions. The initial histologic changes involve the glomeruli with segmental proliferation or sclerosis, or both. As the disease progresses, there is increasing glomerulosclerosis, vascular narrowing, tubular atrophy, and interstitial fibrosis. With electron microscopy, the basement membrane shows irregular foci of thickening or attenuation, with pronounced splitting and lamination of the lamina densa. The tubular basement membranes are similarly altered.

Hematuria is the most common presenting sign, together with RBC casts. Proteinuria may be observed but rarely NS. Symptoms in boys and young men appear at 5 to 20 years of age, with the onset of overt renal failure between the ages of 20 to 50 years. Women who inherit the allele are usually asymptomatic and have little functional impairment. For an example of Alport's syndrome, refer to Case Study 10-8.

DISEASES AFFECTING TUBULES AND INTERSTITIUM

Acute Tubular Necrosis

Acute tubular necrosis (ATN) is characterized morphologically by destruction of tubular epithelial cells and clinically by acute suppression of renal function. ATN is the most common cause of ARF.[9] ATN is a reversible condition with a variety of causes ranging from severe trauma to acute pancreatitis. A common factor in the etiology is a period of inadequate blood flow to the peripheral organs, usually accompanied by marked hypotension and shock.

There are two distinct types of ATN, ischemic and toxic. Tubular epithelial cells are particularly sensitive to anoxia and ischemia, which result in a variety of structural and functional changes. Because the medulla receives a small proportion of renal blood flow, it is particularly susceptible to ischemia, so that the cortical and medullary tubules (including the functionally important thick ascending limb of Henle) are affected. The main causes of ischemic ATN are sepsis (bacterial infections), shock (severe burns), and trauma (crushing injuries, surgical procedures).

Several characteristics predispose the tubules to toxic injury, including their large, electrically charged surface (needed for tubular reabsorption), active transport systems for ions and organic acids, and capacity to concentrate solutes. Many agents are nephrotoxic, including drugs such as gentamicin and other antibiotics; radiographic contrast agents; and toxins, including heavy metals (mercury), organic solvents (carbon tetrachloride), and other poisons (mushrooms, pesticides).

ATN occurs quite frequently because of the multitude of etiologies. Its reversibility adds to its clinical importance because proper management means the difference between full recovery and death.

With ischemic ATN, tubular necrosis is patchy, with relatively short lengths being affected throughout the nephron—from the medullary segments of the proximal tubules and ascending loops of Henle to the collecting ducts. The tubular basement membrane is often disrupted because of the complete necrosis of the tubular cells, so that the tubular lumen is exposed to the renal interstitium. Renal cell fragments, consisting of three or more tubular cells, shed intact and, primarily originating in the collecting duct, are sloughed into the urine.

In contrast, with toxic ATN, extensive necrosis is present along proximal tubule segments (usually not involving the basement membranes), together with necrosis of the distal tubule, particularly the ascending loop of Henle. Finding the large, distinctive proximal convoluted tubule cells in the urine sediment is strong evidence for toxic ATN.[9] Cast formation in the distal convoluted tubules and collecting ducts is observed in both types of ATN, but an increased number and variety of casts (granular, renal tubular cell, waxy, and broad) in the urine sediment is associated with ischemic ATN.

Clinically, ATN may be divided into three phases: initiating, maintenance, and recovery. In the ischemic form of ATN, the initiating phase may be abrupt, lasting for about 36 hours, and involving only a slight decline in urine output with a rise in BUN. During the maintenance phase, oliguria (a sustained decrease in urine output to between 40 to 400 mL/day) occurs with salt and water overload, rising BUN, hyperkalemia, metabolic acidosis, and other manifestations of renal failure and uremia.

The recovery phase begins with a steady increase in urine output and may reach up to 3 L/day. Because the tubules are still damaged, large amounts of water, sodium, and potassium are lost in the "urinary flood."[9] Rather than hyperkalemia, hypokalemia may become a clinical problem. Eventually, concentrating ability improves, renal tubular function is restored, BUN and creatinine levels begin to return to normal, and most patients who reach the recovery phase eventually return to normal.

Urinary Tract Infections and Tubulointerstitial Nephritis

A lower UTI may involve the urethra (urethritis), the bladder (cystitis), or both. Similarly , an upper UTI may involve the renal pelvis alone (pyelitis) or the interstitium together with the renal pelvis (PN). UTIs are very common disorders and may be asymptomatic (e.g., asymptomatic bacteriuria) or may remain localized in the bladder (cystitis) without leading to renal infection.

Although any bacterial or fungal agent can potentially cause a UTI, gram-negative bacteria that are normal inhabitants of the intestinal tract are the etiologic agents for more than 85% of the cases. Originating in fecal matter, these organisms gain entrance to the urinary tract because of various factors, and there they proliferate and cause an infection. The most common organism is *Escherichia coli* followed by *Proteus*, *Klebsiella*, and *Enterobacter* species.

Pain or a burning sensation on urination (dysuria) are characteristic signs of cystitis and sometimes are accompanied by lower abdominal pain. Urinalysis reveals leukocyturia and bacteriuria but no casts (differentiating a lower UTI from an upper UTI, in which casts are observed). Some hematuria and proteinuria may be observed, as well as increased numbers of transitional epithelial cells in the sediment. A quantitative bacterial culture of the urine yielding ≥100,000 colony-forming units (CFU)/mL is usually considered diagnostic for an infection.

Included in tubulointerstitial nephritis (TIN) is a group of renal diseases characterized by histologic and functional alterations mainly involving the tubules and interstitium. TIN can be acute or chronic, and the causes and different pathogenic mechanisms are listed in Table 10-6.

Histologically, acute TIN is characterized by interstitial edema, frequently with leukocytic infiltration and focal tubular necrosis. With the chronic form, there is an infiltration of mononuclear cells, prominent interstitial fibrosis, and widespread tubular atrophy. The absence of signs pointing to glomerular injury (such as nephritic or NS) together with positive signs of defects in tubular function separate TIN from the glomerular diseases.

TABLE 10-6
Tubulointerstitial Diseases

Infections
Acute bacterial pyelonephritis
Chronic pyelonephritis (including reflux nephropathy)
Other infections (e.g., viruses, parasites)

Toxins
Drugs
    Acute hypersensitivity interstitial nephritis
    Analgesic abuse nephritis
Heavy metals
    Lead, cadmium

Metabolic Diseases
Urate nephropathy
Nephrocalcinosis (hypercalcemic nephropathy)
Hypokalemic nephropathy
Oxalate nephropathy

Physical Factors
Chronic urinary tract obstruction
Radiation nephritis

Neoplasms
Multiple myeloma

Immunologic Reactions
Transplant rejection
Tubulointerstitial disease associated with glomerulonephritis
Sjögren's syndrome

Vascular Diseases

Miscellaneous
Balkan nephropathy
Nephronophthsis–medullary cystic disease complex
Other rare causes (sarcoidosis)
Idiopathic interstitial nephritis

(From Cotran RS, Kuman V, Robbins SL. *Robbins pathologic basis of disease.* 5th ed. Philadelphia: WB Saunders, 1994.)

PYELONEPHRITIS Pyelonephritis, one of the most common diseases of the kidney, is a renal disorder that affects the tubules, the interstitium, and the renal pelvis. There are two forms, acute and chronic.

As illustrated in Figure 10-7, there are two routes by which bacteria can reach the kidneys. One pathway is through the bloodstream (hematogenous infection). The other is from the lower urinary tract (ascending infection)—the most common cause of clinical PN.

Colonization of the urethra occurs first; the organisms then gain entrance into the bladder. Organisms that enter the bladder are usually cleared by the flushing action of urination as well as by antibacterial mechanisms. With stasis related to obstruction or bladder dysfunction, the bladder is not completely emptied and bacteria may multiply, as seen frequently in patients with benign prostatic hypertrophy, tumors, or calculi.

Although obstruction is an important antecedent for ascending infection, bacteria may ascend the ureter into the pelvis because of incompetence of the vesicoureteral orifice, thus allowing urine to reflux from the bladder into the ureters (vesicoureteral reflux). For examples of PN and UTIs, refer to Case Studies 10-3, 10-4, 10-9, 10-13, and 10-15. In addition, Chapter 9 has several examples of UTIs.

ACUTE PYELONEPHRITIS This is an acute bacterial infection of the kidney (hematogenous or ascending) involving the renal tubules, interstitium, and renal pelvis. It is characterized by patchy, interstitial, suppurative inflammation and tubular necrosis. Suppuration may manifest as discrete focal abscesses or as large, wedge-shaped areas of coalescent suppuration.

Initially, the neutrophilic infiltration is limited to the interstitial tissue, although eventually the reaction involves the tubules and produces a characteristic abscess with destruction of the engulfed tubules. The glomeruli appear to be resistant to the infection and rarely become involved.

Clinically, the onset of acute PN is usually sudden, with pain at the costovertebral angle (flank) together with systemic evidence of infection (i.e., fever and malaise). Signs of bladder and urethral irritation such as dysuria, a burning sensation, frequency, and urgency are usually evident.

Urinalysis reveals bacteria and large numbers of leukocytes (pyuria) and other inflammatory cells (macrophages) derived from the inflammatory infiltrate in the kidney. Pyuria does not differentiate upper from lower UTI, but the finding of leukocyte casts indicates renal involvement because casts are formed only in tubules. Other types of casts may also be observed (e.g., granular, renal tubular epithelial cell [RTE], broad). Uncomplicated acute PN usually follows a benign course, and with appropriate antibiotic therapy,

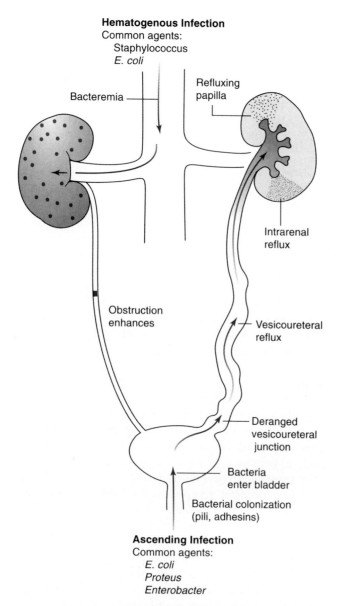

Hematogenous Infection
Common agents:
Staphylococcus
E. coli

Bacteremia

Refluxing
papilla

Intrarenal
reflux

Obstruction
enhances

Vesicoureteral
reflux

Deranged
vesicoureteral
junction

Bacteria
enter bladder

Bacterial colonization
(pili, adhesins)

Ascending Infection
Common agents:
E. coli
Proteus
Enterobacter

FIGURE 10-7 Schematic representation of pathways of renal infection. *Hematogenous* infection results from bacteremic spread. More common is *ascending* infection, which results from a combination of urinary bladder infection, vesicoureteral reflux, and intrarenal reflux. (From Cotran RS, Kuman V, Robbins SL. *Robbins pathologic basis of disease.* 5th ed. Philadelphia: WB Saunders, 1994.)

symptoms disappear within a few days. Permanent renal damage may develop if predisposing conditions are not resolved so that repeated infections occur.

CHRONIC PYELONEPHRITIS Chronic PN (CPN) is characterized by chronic tubulointerstitial inflammation and renal scarring associated with pathologic involvement of the calyces and pelvis. Nearly all of the diseases listed in Table 10-6 produce chronic tubulointerstitial

changes, but only CPN and analgesic abuse nephropathy affect the calyces. The chronic interstitial inflammation associated with CPN results in fibrosis and irregular scarring. CPN is characterized by the coarse, discrete, corticomedullary scar overlying a dilated, blunted, or deformed calyx.[9]

There are two forms of CPN, chronic obstructive and chronic reflux associated. In chronic obstructive PN, recurrent infections superimposed on diffuse or localized obstructive lesions lead to recurrent episodes of renal inflammation and scarring.

Reflux nephropathy is the most common form of CPN and may be vesicoureteral or intrarenal. Vesicoureteral reflux is most often due to a congenital, inherited anatomic abnormality of the vesicoureteric junction that allows the backward flow (reflux) of urine up the ureters to the kidneys. Intrarenal reflux occurs in the renal pelvis, resulting in the movement of urine back up the collecting ducts into the renal cortex because of anatomic variations in the renal papillae.

The course of chronic obstructive PN may be insidious at the beginning or it may involve clinical manifestations of acute recurrent PN with back pain, fever, frequent pyuria, and bacteriuria. Patients with reflux CPN may come to medical attention relatively late in the course of the disease because of the gradual onset of renal insufficiency and HTN, or because of the finding of pyuria or bacteriuria on routine urinalysis. As tubular function is lost (especially concentrating ability), polyuria and nocturia develop, and as the disease progresses with the development of HTN, renal blood flow and GFR are affected. CRF develops in approximately 11% to 20% of CPN patients, requiring dialysis or renal transplantation.

Tubulointerstitial Nephritis Induced by Drugs and Toxins

In TIN, renal injury may be produced in at least three ways: 1) an immediate allergic response in the interstitium (e.g., methicillin); 2) ARF from direct and acute damage to the tubules (e.g., heavy metals); or 3) subtle, cumulative tubular injury requiring years to become evident (e.g., analgesic abuse nephropathy).

ACUTE DRUG-INDUCED INTERSTITIAL NEPHRITIS A constantly increasing number of drugs potentiate this well-recognized adverse reaction, which was first reported after the use of sulfonamides.[9] Acute TIN occurs most frequently with the synthetic penicillins (methicillin, ampicillin), other synthetic antibiotics (rifampin), diuretics (thiazides), nonsteroidal antiinflammatory agents (phenylbutazone), and miscellaneous drugs (phenindione, cimetidine).

Onset begins about 15 days after exposure to the drug and is manifested by fever, eosinophilia (possibly transient), a skin rash (about 25% of patients), and renal abnormalities, including hematuria, mild proteinuria, and leukocyturia (including eosinophils). In approximately 50% of cases, the serum creatinine level is increased or ARF with oliguria develops, particularly in older patients. Histologically, the interstitium shows pronounced edema and infiltration by mononuclear cells (particularly lymphocytes), eosinophils, and neutrophils. Occasionally, a few plasma cells and basophils are observed.

It is thought that the drugs act as haptens that bind to some cytoplasmic or extracellular component of tubular cells (during secretion by the tubules) and become immunogenic.[9] Injury results from IgE- and cell-mediated immune reactions against the tubular cells or their basement membranes. Routine urinalysis demonstrates hematuria, mild proteinuria, and leukocyturia without bacteria. Eosinophiluria is also found, and leukocyte or eosinophil casts may also be observed. Withdrawal of the offending drug can result in full recovery of renal function (although it may take several months), but irreversible damage may occur occasionally in elderly individuals.

ANALGESIC ABUSE NEPHROPATHY This form of chronic renal disease is caused by excessive intake of analgesic mixtures, leading to chronic TIN with renal papillary necrosis.[9] The incidence of analgesic nephropathy is distributed worldwide and corresponds with the consumption of analgesics in various populations.

The renal damage was first related to phenacetin. Most patients consume phenacetin-containing preparations, although a few cases are related to ingestion of aspirin, phenacetin, or acetaminophen alone. The disease usually develops in those who ingest large quantities of analgesic mixtures, more than 2 kg of aspirin or phenacetin over a 3-year period.

Events leading to renal damage start with papillary necrosis, then cortical TIN as a secondary manifestation. Acetaminophen, the metabolite of phenacetin, injures cells by covalent binding as well as oxidative damage.[9] Aspirin apparently predisposes the papilla to ischemia so that papillary damage results from a combination of the direct toxic effect of phenacetin metabolites coupled with ischemic injury to both tubular cells and vessels.

Analgesic nephropathy is more common in women than in men and is observed especially in individuals afflicted with recurrent headaches and muscular pain, in psychoneurotic patients, and in factory workers. As would be expected with lesions in the papilla, early renal findings include inability to concentrate the urine. Renal stones may develop because of acquired distal renal tubular acidosis (RTA). Other symptoms include

headache, anemia, gastrointestinal problems, and HTN together with UTIs for about 50% of patients. Although progressive impairment of renal function may lead to CRF, drug withdrawal and proper therapy for infection as needed may either stabilize or actually improve renal function. A serious complication that sometimes occurs is the development of transitional papillary carcinoma of the renal pelvis.

Other Tubulointerstitial Diseases

URATE NEPHROPATHY Three types of nephropathy may develop in patients with hyperuricemic disorders. Acute uric acid nephropathy results from the precipitation of uric acid crystals in the renal tubules, mainly in the collecting ducts, resulting in nephron obstruction and the development of ARF. This type is seen particularly in patients with leukemias and lymphomas as a result of chemotherapy, which brings about the destruction of neoplastic cells (and their nuclei) and the elaboration of uric acid. The acidic pH in collecting ducts favors the precipitation of uric acid.

Chronic urate nephropathy, also known as gouty nephropathy, occurs in patients manifesting more protracted forms of hyperuricemia. Monosodium urate crystals are deposited in the distal tubules, collecting ducts, and the interstitium. The deposits of birefringent, needle-like crystals often have a distinct histologic appearance (a tophus), surrounded by foreign body giant cells, other mononuclear cells, and a fibrotic reaction. Cortical atrophy and scarring result from tubular obstruction by the urates.

Because of the rather high frequency of HTN in patients with gout, arterial and arteriolar thickening is often observed. Many patients with gout in whom a chronic nephropathy actually develops show signs of increased exposure to lead, primarily through drinking "moonshine" whiskey contaminated with lead.

Nephrolithiasis is the third renal syndrome in hyperuricemia. Uric acid stones are manifested in 22% of patients with gout and in 42% of patients with secondary hyperuricemia associated with rapid cell turnover (e.g., leukemias).

HYPERCALCEMIA AND NEPHROCALCINOSIS In disorders associated with hypercalcemia, such as hyperparathyroidism, multiple myeloma, vitamin D intoxication, metastatic bone disease, or excess calcium intake (milk-alkali syndrome), calcium stones may form in the kdney, and calcium may be deposited as well (nephrocalcinosis). Extensive calcinosis may induce a form of chronic tubulointerstitial disease and renal insufficiency.

Observations include mitochondrial distortion, evidence of cell injury, and calcium deposits in the mitochondria, cytoplasm, and basement membrane. Calcified cellular debris plug the tubular lumina and lead to obstructive atrophy of nephrons with interstitial fibrosis and nonspecific chronic inflammation. Entire areas of the cortex drained by calcified tubules may atrophy, producing alternating areas of normal and of scarred parenchyma in such kidneys.

The first sign of the disorder is the inability to produce a concentrated urine. Other tubular defects such as tubular acidosis and salt-losing nephritis may be seen also. If damage continues, a slowly progressive renal insufficiency develops, usually as a result of nephrocalcinosis, although many patients also have calcium stones and secondary PN.

MULTIPLE MYELOMA Multiple myeloma (plasma cell myeloma) is a progressive and ultimately fatal neoplastic disease characterized by marrow plasma cell tumors that either produce excessive amounts of an intact monoclonal immunoglobulin (IgG, IgA, IgD, or IgE) together with free monoclonal kappa or lambda light chains (Bence Jones proteins), or produce only the Bence Jones proteins and not the immunoglobulin. Overt renal insufficiency occurs in half of the patients with this disease. The kidneys may be affected by nonrenal malignant tumors in several ways. The two most common are related to complications caused by the tumor (hypercalcemia, hyperuricemia) or to effects of therapy (irradiation, chemotherapy).

Up to 80% of myeloma patients produce Bence Jones proteins (immunoglobulin light chains), which are freely filtered by the glomeruli, excreted in the urine, and are the main cause of the renal dysfunction. Bence Jones proteins appear to cause renal toxicity by two mechanisms: 1) direct toxicity, especially in the proximal tubule, after absorption of the proteins by the tubular cells, which interferes with lysosomal function[26]; and 2) by combining with the urinary Tamm-Horsfall glycoprotein to form large, histologically distinct tubular casts that obstruct the tubular lumina and also induce a peritubular inflammatory reaction.

Clinically the most common renal manifestation is the subtle and slowly progressive development of CRF extending over several months to years. Conversely, ARF with oliguria may occur suddenly, related to such factors such as dehydration, hypercalcemia, acute infection, and treatment with nephrotoxic antibiotics.

Tubular Dysfunction

Primary renal disease or secondary influences may result in renal tubular dysfunction. The effects may involve either depressed tubule secretion or reabsorption; or impairment of urine concentration or dilution. Isolated portions of the tubule (e.g., proximal tubule) may be affected while other portions retain normal function. The GFR is usually normal because the disorders do not affect the glomeruli.

CYSTINOSIS AND CYSTINURIA Cystinosis is inherited as an autosomal recessive trait. It is a metabolic defect associated with abnormal accumulations of cystine in cells of various body tissues caused by defective transport across lysosomal membranes. Cystine crystals are deposited in the cornea, conjunctiva, bone marrow, lymph nodes, spleen, liver, kidneys, fibroblasts, and leukocytes. Genetic heterogeneity is suggested because there are three forms of the disorder.

The most severe form of cystinosis is the nephropathic manifestation, which appears in infancy. In the kidney, cystine crystals accumulate in the glomerular epithelial cells, the proximal tubular cells, and the interstitial cells. The deposits cause generalized proximal tubular dysfunction and development of Fanconi's syndrome. Actually, the multiple proximal tubular defects associated with Fanconi's syndrome were first recognized in children with cystinosis.[14] As discussed later under the heading of Fanconi's Syndrome, bicarbonate wasting results in an alkaline urine. Because cystine becomes soluble at an alkaline pH, cystine crystals are almost never seen in the urine of these patients. In fact, cystine calculus formation has been reported in only one individual with cystinosis.[27]

With severe cystinosis, children often contract more generalized renal disease, resulting in glomerular dysfunction and renal failure. Without renal dialysis or a kidney transplant, these children usually die before puberty as a result of the extensive renal damage.

The juvenile and adult forms of cystinosis are extremely rare. The juvenile form appears in the second decade of life, is intermediate in its severity, and is associated with the development of progressive azotemia in the second or third decades. In the adult form, the cystine concentration in many cells is elevated but is lower than in the first two forms; the kidney is spared, and the condition is considered benign. Although ocular deposits of cystine are common, retinopathy is rare. Indeed, some patients with nonnephropathic cystinosis are discovered later in life when a routine ophthalmologic evaluation reveals cystine deposits in their eyes.

Although low-sulfur diets, ascorbic acid supplements, and various drugs have generally failed to prevent the development of CRF in cystinosis patients, the cystine-depleting agent cysteamine bitartrate (Cystagon) has yielded some success. Although renal stones are not a major problem with cystinosis patients, progressive renal failure requires supportive care, including dialysis. Renal transplantation has also proved successful for some patients.[12]

Cystinuria, inherited as an autosomal recessive trait, is a defect of the renal tubules characterized by the urinary excretion of large amounts of the amino acid cystine together with the dibasic amino acids arginine, lysine, and ornithine. In an acid urine, cystine is the least soluble of the group, so that with increased concentration, precipitation in the urinary tract results in the formation of cystine crystals and stones. The radiopaque cystine stones form in the renal pelvis (staghorn calculi are common) or in the bladder. Because of obstruction, UTIs and renal failure may develop.

Treatment involves sufficient water intake to increase urine volume in order to decrease the concentration of cystine, and alkalinization of the urine to a pH greater than 7.5 to increase the solubility of the cystine. Oral administration of D-penicillamine may be part of the therapy. This drug converts cystine to a more soluble form, penicillamine-cysteine disulfide. Disadvantages of the drug include its cost and several undesirable side effects, including fever, rash, arthralgias, proteinuria, NS, pancytopenia, or an SLE-like reaction. For an example of cystinuria with renal stones, refer to Case Study 10-12.

RENAL TUBULAR ACIDOSIS RTA represents a group of disorders, either primary or secondary, that are characterized by impaired ability to secrete hydrogen ions in the distal tubule or to reabsorb bicarbonate ions in the proximal tubule, leading to chronic metabolic acidosis. Although several forms of RTA have been identified based on their renal tubular defects, there are only two major forms: distal RTA (type I) and proximal RTA (type II).

Distal RTA is mostly a sporadic disorder, although familial cases occur either in association with another inherited disease or rarely as an isolated autosomal dominant disease. The sporadic cases may develop as a primary (idiopathic) disease, most common in women, or as a secondary disease associated with a predisposing cause such as an autoimmune disorder with hypergammaglobulinemia, therapy with amphotericin B or lithium, renal transplantation, nephrocalcinosis, or renal medullary cystic disease. The tubular defect is the inability to secrete hydrogen ions against a concentration gradient, so that urine pH does not fall below approximately 6.

The chronic metabolic acidosis induces potassium wasting and depletion, leading to muscle weakness, hyporeflexia, and paralysis. The accumulation of acid exhausts the serum buffers and eventually the body uses bone calcium (as the carbonate) to buffer the serum. The continued loss of bone calcium results in rickets and osteomalacia, as well as nephrocalcinosis and stones. Eventually, renal parenchymal damage and CRF may develop.

Proximal RTA is characterized by a diminished capacity of the proximal tubules to reabsorb bicarbonate ion from the filtrate so that at normal levels of plasma bicarbonate, increased amounts are lost and excreted in the urine (the threshold for the appearance of bicarbonate in the urine is lowered). The proximal form of RTA may accompany several inherited diseases, including Fanconi's syndrome and Wilson's disease, or it may be associated with multiple myeloma, renal transplantation, certain toxins (lead, cadmium, mercury) or treatment with certain drugs (sulfonamides, outdated tetracycline, acetazolamide). Although severe bone disease and hypercalciuria are observed in proximal RTA, nephrocalcinosis and ureteral stones are not common.

For both types of RTA, oral administration of bicarbonate relieves the symptoms and prevents or stabilizes renal failure and bone disease. The dosage regimen for bicarbonate differs for the two types of RTA: moderate amounts for the distal form and massive dosages for the proximal form. Potassium supplements may be required in selected cases after alkalinization.

FANCONI'S SYNDROME This is a generalized disorder of proximal renal tubule transport (acquired or inherited) resulting in impaired reabsorption of glucose, phosphate, amino acids, bicarbonate, uric acid, water, potassium, and sodium. For a given individual, any one or all of these defects may be observed.

As an inherited trait, Fanconi's syndrome is usually seen together with another genetic disorder, particularly cystinosis (the most common association in children), in which case it is expressed as an autosomal recessive disease. Acquired Fanconi's syndrome may be caused by outdated tetracycline, renal transplantation, multiple myeloma, and toxins (heavy metals) or other chemical agents.

The chief clinical features, which usually appear in infancy with the hereditary form of the syndrome, include growth failure, chronic proximal tubular acidosis, hypophosphatemic rickets, hypokalemia, polyuria, and polydipsia.

HYPOPHOSPHATEMIC RICKETS (VITAMIN D–RESISTANT RICKETS) This disorder, which is usually familial, is characterized by impaired reabsorption of phosphate in the proximal renal tubules (with resultant hypophosphatemia), defective intestinal absorption of calcium, and rickets or osteomalacia that is unresponsive to vitamin D. The familial form is inherited as an X-linked dominant trait. Acquired cases are rare and are sometimes associated with benign tumors.

A spectrum of abnormalities is manifested with the disease, from hypophosphatemia alone, to severe rickets or osteomalacia with bowing of the legs and other bone deformities, pseudofractures, bone pain, and short stature. Although blood calcium levels are normal, blood phosphate levels are decreased and serum alkaline phosphatase (ALP) is often elevated. Spinal and pelvic rickets seen in vitamin D deficiency are rarely found with hypophosphatemic rickets. Onset is usually at less than 1 year of age. Treatment consists of oral phosphate together with vitamin D (to initiate bone healing). A few cases of adult onset have been improved dramatically after removal of a benign fibrosing hemangiosarcoma.

RENAL GLUCOSURIA (RENAL GLYCOSURIA) This disease is characterized by the excretion of glucose in the urine when the blood glucose levels are normal or low, and may be associated with many renal tubular defects involving aminoaciduria and renal tubular acidosis.[5] When it is manifested as an isolated finding with otherwise normal renal function, it is usually inherited as an autosomal dominant trait, although occasionally it may be inherited as a recessive trait.

The maximum rate for the active transport of substances by the renal tubules is termed the transport maximum (T_m). The T_m for glucose is normally 320 mg/minute. In type A renal glucosuria, the T_m for glucose is reduced and sugar escapes into the urine. In type B, the T_m is normal but the renal threshold for glucose reabsorption is reduced so that glucose appears in the urine at a lower-than-normal plasma concentration. Renal glucosuria is asymptomatic, without serious sequelae, and does not require treatment.[5]

NEPHROGENIC DIABETES INSIPIDUS In this disease, renal function is normal except the renal tubules do not respond to antidiuretic hormone (ADH). In the neurogenic form of diabetes insipidus (DI), insufficient ADH is released by the posterior pituitary.

Nephrogenic DI occurs as an X-linked (probably recessive) disease. Boys affected with the defect are completely unresponsive to ADH, whereas heterozygous girls show normal or slightly impaired responsiveness to ADH. The consequences of nephrogenic DI are polydipsia, polyuria, and hypotonic urine, the same features as are seen in neurogenic DI (from which nephrogenic DI must be distinguished). Nephrogenic DI usually appears soon after birth. Because the infant cannot communicate its thirst, severe water depletion may result in hypernatremia, fever, vomiting, and convulsions. Brain damage with permanent mental retardation may occur if the diagnosis is not made promptly. Urine osmolality is usually 50 to 100 mOsm/kg (normal range, 275–300 mOsm/kg). The GFR is normal, and there are no symptoms of any other defect of tubular function.

Nephrogenic DI is treated by ensuring that the patient has an adequate free water intake. Although polyuria and polydipsia may be nuisances, serious problems seldom occur as long as the patient can increase his water intake in response to thirst. Thiazide diuretics may be helpful in treating the disease.[5]

HARTNUP'S DISEASE This rare genetic disorder, in which consanguinity is common, is transmitted as an autosomal recessive trait. It is characterized by a pellagra-like skin rash, cerebellar ataxia, psychiatric illness, mental retardation, short stature, headaches, collapsing or fainting, and aminoaciduria. Because of a transport defect, the intestinal absorption of the entire group of neutral amino acids (including the crucial amino acid tryptophan) is impaired, as well as the renal tubule reabsorption of the same group of amino acids.

Pellagra is a deficiency disorder due to an insufficient dietary supply of niacin (vitamin B_3 or nicotinic acid) or the amino acid tryptophan, which the body converts to niacin. Many diets causing pellagra are low in good-quality protein as well as in vitamins, so that pellagra is usually due to a combined deficiency of tryptophan and niacin.

The coenzyme nicotinamide adenine dinucleotide is derived in part from niacin. Because about half of the requirement for niacin is satisfied through synthesis from dietary tryptophan, a deficiency in the supply of tryptophan may lead to a deficiency of niacin and the symptoms of pellagra.

Loss of tryptophan in the urine of patients with Hartnup's disease, although quantitatively of less importance than the intestinal absorption defect, would contribute to the reduced production of niacin. Both the pellagra-like rash and neurologic symptoms of Hartnup's disease respond to the administration of niacin or nicotinamide.

Diagnosis is made by demonstrating the characteristic amino acid excretion pattern in the urine, together with the presence of indoles and other tryptophan degradation products in the urine. The eventual prognosis of Hartnup's disease is good, and the frequency of attacks usually diminishes with age. Treatment includes maintaining good nutritional status and supplementing the diet with niacin (or niacinamide).

DISEASES OF BLOOD VESSELS

The renal blood vessels are secondarily involved in nearly all diseases of the kidney.[9] Systemic vascular disease (such as various forms of vasculitis) may also involve renal blood vessels but are not considered in the following discussion.

Benign Nephrosclerosis

Benign nephrosclerosis (BNS), or benign HTN, is the term associated with a lesion of arterioles described as hyaline arteriolosclerosis, a condition frequently observed in elderly patients. The vascular lesion consists of a homogeneous, pink-staining, hyaline thickening of the walls of arterioles with loss of underlying structural detail and with narrowing of the lumen. The effect in the kidney is the formation of focal ischemia in the renal parenchyma supplied by the thickened, narrowed arteriole. Some degree of BNS is found at autopsy in many individuals older than 60 years of age. HTN increases the incidence and severity of the lesions.

Although there is usually a moderate reduction in renal plasma flow with BNS, the GFR is normal or only slightly reduced, and uncomplicated BNS alone rarely causes renal insufficiency or uremia. There may be mild proteinuria occasionally. Although renal failure may eventually develop in 5% of patients with prolonged benign HTN, in most cases it results from the development of the accelerated or malignant phase of HTN (malignant nephrosclerosis).

Malignant Nephrosclerosis (Malignant Hypertension)

Malignant nephrosclerosis may occasionally develop in previously normotensive individuals but often is superimposed on preexisting essential benign HTN, secondary forms of HTN, or an underlying chronic renal disease, especially GN or reflux nephropathy. Malignant nephrosclerosis is relatively uncommon, occurring in 1% to 5% of all patients with HTN. Uncomplicated malignant nephrosclerosis usually affects younger individuals, especially men and blacks.

The most striking histologic alteration is fibrinoid necrosis in the arterioles and the capillary tuft. Proliferation of intraglomerular cells as well as epithelial crescents may be observed. Interlobular arteries usually show considerable intimal thickening. The glomeruli may become necrotic and infiltrated with neutrophils, and the glomerular capillaries may thrombose (necrotizing glomerulitis) so that the vascular lumen is virtually destroyed.

Malignant HTN is usually associated with very high levels of renin, angiotensin, and aldosterone. Although the initial stimulus for hyperreninemia is not clear, studies suggest that vasoconstriction and severe increases in blood pressure accentuate the vascular necrosis occurring in renal arterioles and arterioles in other organs. The increase in blood pressure causes endothelial injury, platelet thrombosis, fibroid necrosis, and intravascular coagulation. By inducing ischemia, these changes maintain the destructive pattern of HTN and elevated blood levels of renin, angiotensin, and aldosterone.

Malignant HTN is characterized by diastolic pressures greater than 130 mm Hg, retinopathy, cardiovascular abnormalities, and varying degrees of renal insufficiency. Early symptoms are most often related to increased intracranial pressure, including headaches, nausea, vomiting, and visual impairments (blurring of vision or "spots before the eyes"). A hypertensive crisis may occur, with loss of consciousness or even convulsions.

Urinary findings depend on the stage of the disease and include proteinuria, microscopic hematuria, an occasional RBC cast, granular casts (commonly), and eventually broad casts and waxy casts. The newer antihypertensive drugs have improved the prognosis for these patients so that about 75% survive 5 years and 50% survive with precrisis renal function.[9]

Renal Artery Stenosis

Even though unilateral renal artery stenosis is a relatively uncommon cause of HTN (2–5% of cases), it is important because it is the most common curable form of HTN. Surgery (renal revascularization) is successful in 70% to 80% of carefully selected cases. The hypertensive effect, at least initially, is due to stimulation of renin secretion by the juxtaglomerular apparatus with production of the potent vasoconstrictor angiotensin II.

Occlusion at the origin of the renal artery due to an atheromatous plaque is the leading cause (70% of cases) of renal artery stenosis. It is usually unilateral but may occur bilaterally. This cause occurs more commonly in men, especially with advancing age and with DM.

Another type of lesion, fibromuscular dysplasia of the renal artery, also leads to stenosis. This is characterized by a fibrous or fibromuscular thickening involving the intima, the media, or the adventitia of the artery. These stenoses are more common in women and tend to occur in the third and fourth decades of life. These lesions usually occur in the middle or distal portion of the renal artery and consist of a single, well-defined constriction or a series of narrowings.

With either type of stenosis, the kidney shows signs of diffuse ischemic atrophy, with crowded glomeruli, atrophic tubules, interstitial fibrosis, and focal inflammatory infiltrate. Clinically, these patients resemble those presenting with essential HTN. Diagnosis may be aided by observing elevated plasma or renal vein renin, a response to captopril (inhibitor of angiotensin-converting enzyme), renal scans, and intravenous pyelography (IVP). Arteriography is required to localize the stenotic lesion.

Thrombotic Microangiopathies

These diseases have overlapping clinical manifestations and are characterized morphologically by thrombosis in the interlobular arteries, the afferent arterioles, and the glomeruli, as well as necrosis and thickening of the vessel walls. The morphologic changes are similar to those seen in malignant HTN, but with the thrombotic microangiopathies, they precede the appearance of HTN or may even be seen in its absence. Clinically, microangiopathic hemolytic anemia, thrombocytopenia, and renal failure are observed.

Included here are childhood hemolytic–uremic syndrome, various forms of adult hemolytic–uremic syndrome, and thrombotic thrombocytopenic purpura.[9] Even though the disorders may have diverse causes, all appear to be triggered by endothelial injury and intravascular thrombosis. Etiologies include bacterial endotoxins and cytotoxins, cytokines, viruses, or possibly antiendothelial antibodies.

CLASSIC (CHILDHOOD) HEMOLYTIC–UREMIC SYNDROME Classic (childhood) hemolytic–uremic syndrome is the best characterized of the microangiopathic syndromes because 75% of cases occur in children with an intestinal infection involving verocytotoxin-producing *E. coli*. These toxins, which are similar to shiga toxins produced by *Shigella* species, cause damage to vero cells in culture, hence the name "verocytotoxins." Epidemics have been traced to infected ground meat (hamburgers), and the disease is one of the main causes of ARF in children.

Usually following a gastrointestinal or flulike illness, the syndrome is manifested by a sudden onset of bleeding (especially hematemesis and melena), severe oliguria, hematuria, a microangiopathic hemolytic anemia, and in some cases, prominent neurologic changes. About half of the patients experience HTN.

The shiga-like toxin has a variety of effects on endothelium, causing increased adhesion of leukocytes, production of factors that favor vasoconstriction, and lysis of endothelium. Thrombosis and vasoconstriction are enhanced, resulting in the characteristic microangiopathy. Proper management of the renal failure with dialysis enables most patients to recover in a matter of weeks, although the long-term prognosis (15–25 years) is not uniformly favorable.

ADULT HEMOLYTIC–UREMIC SYNDROME Adult hemolytic–uremic syndrome is similar to the childhood syndrome and occurs under a variety of settings: in association with infection (e.g., *E. coli* septicemia, shigellosis); in women in relation to complications of pregnancy or the postpartum period; in association with vascular diseases such as SLE or malignant HTN; from the effects of chemotherapeutic agents; and hereditary hemolytic–uremic syndrome (also occurring in children).

THROMBOTIC THROMBOCYTOPENIC PURPURA Thrombotic thrombocytopenic purpura is characterized by fever, neurologic symptoms, hemolytic anemia, thrombocytopenic purpura, and thrombi in the glomerular capillaries and afferent arterioles. Most patients are younger than 40 years of age and female. Because of the overlap of this condition with the hemolytic–uremic syndrome, some workers consider both diseases to be part of the spectrum of the same entity. However, with thrombotic thrombocytopenic purpura, central nervous system involvement is a dominant feature, whereas only about 50% of patients experience renal involvement.

Histologic features include eosinophilic granular thrombi in the terminal part of the interlobular arteries, afferent arterioles, and glomerular capillaries. These thrombi are composed of both platelets and fibrin and are found in the arterioles of other organs throughout the body. The disease has a high fatality rate, but exchange transfusions and corticosteroid therapy have reduced mortality to less than 50%.

Sickle Cell Disease Nephropathy

A variety of alterations in renal morphology and function that produce clinically significant abnormalities may be associated with sickle cell disease in both the homozygous and the heterozygous forms. "Sickle cell nephropathy" is the term given to the various manifestations.

Hematuria and diminished concentrating ability are the most common clinical and functional abnormalities. It is thought that these effects are largely due to the accelerated sickling in the hypertonic, hypoxic conditions in the renal medulla. The sickling increases the viscosity of the blood during its passage through the vasa recta, leading to plugging of the vessels and decreased flow. Cortical scarring associated with patchy papillary necrosis may be found in both homozygotes and heterozygotes. Approximately 30% of patients experience proteinuria, which is usually mild to moderate. However, overt NS may develop associated with an MPGN lesion.

Urinary Tract Obstruction (Obstructive Uropathy)

It is important to recognize UO since it increases susceptibility to infection and to stone formation. If obstruction is not corrected, it almost always leads to permanent renal atrophy (termed hydronephrosis or obstructive atrophy). Many causes of obstruction can be corrected surgically or treated medically. Figure 10-

8 summarizes the interrelationships of the obstructive lesions of the urinary tract.

Common causes of UO include congenital anomalies, urinary calculi, benign prostatic hypertrophy, tumors, inflammation, sloughed papillae or blood clots, normal pregnancy, uterine prolapse and cystocele, and functional disorders.[9] Progressive atrophy of the kidney due to obstruction to the outflow of urine is termed "hydronephrosis," a condition characterized by dilatation of the renal pelvis and calyces.

Glomerular filtration persists for some time even with complete obstruction because the filtrate diffuses back into the renal interstitium and perirenal spaces, then to the lymphatic and finally the venous systems. Because of this continuous filtration, the calyces and pelvis become dilated. Because the pressure in the pelvis is transmitted back through the collecting ducts into the cortex, renal atrophy occurs. The pressure also compresses the renal vasculature of the medulla, resulting in diminished inner medullary blood flow. These effects are reversible but, if prolonged, lead to functional alterations in the medulla. Initially the alterations are largely tubular, seen primarily as impaired concentrating ability. Later on, the GFR begins to be affected.

Clinically, acute obstruction may present with pain associated with the distention of the collecting system or the renal capsule; calculi lodged in the ureters may produce renal colic. Unilateral hydronephrosis may go undetected for long periods of time because the unaffected kidney is able to maintain adequate renal function. With bilateral partial obstruction, the earliest sign is the inability to concentrate the urine, as reflected by polyuria and nocturia. In some patients, a picture of TIN will have developed with scarring and atrophy of the papilla and medulla. Such patients commonly have HTN. Complete bilateral obstruction produces oliguria or anuria and requires immediate attention.

For examples of UO, refer to Case Studies 10-9 and 10-14.

Urolithiasis (Renal Calculi, Stones)

Although most calculi form in the kidney, they may develop at any level in the urinary tract. As a frequent clinical problem, urolithiasis affects 5% to 10% of Americans during their lifetime. Stones develop in men more frequently than in women. The peak age at onset is from 20 to 30 years of age.

It has been known for a long time that there are familial and hereditary tendencies for stone formation. Many of the inborn errors of metabolism (e.g., gout, cystinuria) are examples of hereditary diseases associated with excessive production and excretion of stone-forming substances.

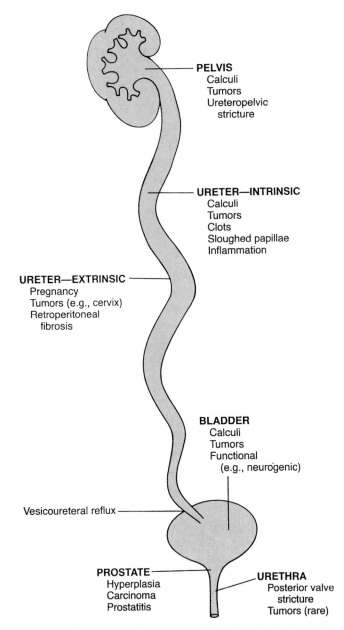

FIGURE 10-8 Obstructive lesions of the urinary tract. (From Cotran RS, Kumar V, Robbins SL. *Robbins pathologic basis of disease.* 5th ed. Philadelphia: WB Saunders Company, 1994.)

Most stones (about 75%) contain calcium, mostly calcium oxalate or calcium oxalate mixed with calcium phosphate. So-called "triple stones" or "struvite stones," which are composed of magnesium ammonium phosphate (the triple phosphate crystals of urinalysis), make up another 15% of the calculi encountered. Uric acid calculi account for 6% of the stones formed, whereas the rest (1–2%) are composed of cystine.

All calculi contain an organic matrix of mucoprotein that comprises 1% to 5% of the stone by weight. Although many factors are involved in the initiation and formation of calculi, the most important determinant is an increased urinary concentration of the constituents making up the stone to the point of supersaturation. For some metabolically normal patients, a low urine volume favors supersaturation.

Stone formation may not necessarily be associated with a concomitant increase of the constituents in the blood. About 25% of patients in whom calcium stones develop do not have hypercalcemia or hypercalciuria, and about 50% of individuals with uric acid stones do not have hyperuricemia or hyperuricosuria. On the other hand, individuals manifesting hypercalciuria, hyperoxaluria, and hyperuricemia are at risk for development of renal stones. Sometimes renal tubular reabsorption mechanisms may be dysfunctional, resulting in increased excretion of the constituent in the urine. Another possibility is increased intestinal absorption of the constituent resulting from dietary increases or from hereditary tendencies.

Magnesium ammonium phosphate stones are most often formed after infections by urea-splitting bacteria (e.g., *Proteus* species), which convert urea to ammonia so that the pH of the urine shifts to the alkaline side and causes the precipitation of the magnesium ammonium phosphate salts. Besides an increased concentration of stone constituents, changes in urinary pH, decreased urine volume, and the presence of bacteria, a factor enhancing stone formation is a deficiency in inhibitors of crystal formation in the urine (e.g., pyrophosphate, diphosphonate, citrate, glycosaminoglycans, and a glycoprotein called nephrocalcin).[9]

One final factor that is important in the formation of calculi is the presence of a foreign body "seed," which provides a nucleus that fosters crystallization. The seed or nucleus for the formation and growth of a crystal (the beginning of stone formation) can be an object like another crystal, a bit of debris, a clump of bacteria, a fibrin clot, or an epithelial cell.

Although calculi may be present without producing any symptoms or significant renal damage, they are most often discovered when the urinary tract becomes obstructed or the stones produce ulceration and bleeding. Smaller stones usually are the most hazardous because they may pass into the ureters and produce an excruciating pain (known as renal colic) as well as ureteral obstruction. The pain starts in the kidney region and radiates downward and forward to include the abdomen, genitalia, and legs. The pain is often accompanied by nausea, vomiting, sweating, and a frequent urge to urinate. The larger stones, which cannot enter the ureters, remain in the renal pelvis and first manifest themselves by producing hematuria. As they gradually enlarge they create a "cast" of the pelvic and calyceal spaces of the kidney.

By increasing fluid intake to produce a dilute urine

and by modifying the diet to eliminate excesses of certain constituents, patients are able to help prevent calculus formation. The pH of the urine can be manipulated to maintain an acid or alkaline reaction as needed to ensure the solubility of the solute causing the problem. Drugs may be used to convert a solute to a more soluble form, as with the administration of D-penicillamine to convert cystine to a more soluble compound. Controlling infections with antibiotics to eliminate urea-splitting bacteria helps minimize calculus formation.

After a stone has formed, there are several methods available for its destruction or removal. Cystoscopy can be used to crush and remove the stone if it is located in the lower third of the ureter or is in the bladder. More recently, lithotripsy (the use of sound waves to disintegrate the stone in situ) has been successfully used instead of surgery. If an obstruction is present or the patient is at risk for progressive deterioration, surgical removal may be the best option. For examples of urolithiasis, refer to Case Studies 10-10 and 10-12.

Acute and Chronic Renal Failure

ACUTE RENAL FAILURE

One definition of ARF[3] is any condition, regardless of cause or pathogenesis, resulting in sudden suppression of kidney function: decreased GFR; oliguria (urine output <400 mL/day) or anuria; and rapid, steadily increasing azotemia. The traditional pathophysiologic–anatomic classification takes into account the fact that the kidneys function sequentially by creating an ultrafiltrate of arterial blood, processing this ultrafiltrate by tubular epithelial reabsorption and secretion, and eliminating the elaborated urine through ureteral, vesicular, and urethral channels. From this, the three major categories of ARF can be defined: prerenal ARF (reduction in renal perfusion), intrinsic renal ARF (acute, severe parenchymal renal damage), and postrenal ARF (obstruction to the excretion of normally elaborated urine).

Prerenal ARF may be associated with depletion of fluid and electrolytes, hemorrhage, septicemia, cardiac failure, liver failure, burns, surgical procedures, and acute diarrhea as well as vomiting. The urine sediment in prerenal ARF is unremarkable, but urine volume and sodium concentration are reduced, whereas urinary osmolality and urine-to-plasma ratios for osmolality, creatinine, and urea are increased. Approximately 25% of ARF presentations are prerenal.

Renal ARF accounts for approximately 65% of ARF cases. Renal damage characterizes this category and can result from any number of glomerular, tubular, interstitial, or vascular disease processes. The clinical presentation for nearly all of the cases of renal ARF is ATN. With progression of the condition, destruction of the renal tubules results in a loss of water and electrolytes. With primary renal injury, the sediment characteristically contains tubular cells, tubular cell casts, and many brown granular casts.[5] Eosinophiluria suggests allergic TIN, and RBC casts reflect vasculitis or GN.

Postrenal ARF results from obstructions in urine flow and accounts for about 10% of ARF cases. The increase in hydrostatic pressure within the tubules and Bowman's space disrupts the normal filtration pressure across the glomerular filtration barrier so that the GFR is decreased. With continued back-pressure, the tubules eventually become damaged and renal function declines. The urine sediment in postrenal ARF may not be particularly distinctive, although WBCs and RBCs may be found, together with granular and renal tubular cell casts.[5]

CHRONIC RENAL FAILURE

CRF is a clinical condition resulting from a multitude of pathologic processes leading to the progressive loss of renal function caused by an irreversible and intrinsic renal disease. A variety of clinical manifestations may exist among the various diseases causing CRF. The feature common to all is a diminished GFR. The GFR slowly but continuously decreases, which becomes clinically recognizable only after 80% to 85% of normal renal function as been lost. This corresponds to a GFR of about 15 to 20 mL/minute.[7]

Functionally, CRF can be grouped into three stages: diminished renal reserve, renal insufficiency (failure), and uremia.[6] With diminished renal reserve, patients are asymptomatic and homeostasis is preserved even though there is measurable loss of renal function. With renal insufficiency, a patient may have only vague symptoms despite a slight azotemia, although nocturia is noted at this stage because of failure to concentrate the urine. As renal dysfunction develops further, disturbances in fluid and electrolyte balance are observed, azotemia increases, and systemic manifestations (uremia) occur.

In the uremic state, the GFR is less than 6 mL/minute/m^2. The first manifestations of uremia are often lassitude, fatigue, and decreased mental acuity. Neuromuscular features include coarse muscular twitches, peripheral neuropathies with sensory and motor phenomena, muscle cramps, and convulsions. Other clinical features include anorexia, nausea, vomiting, weight loss, HTN, stomatitis, and an unpleasant taste in the mouth.

CRF eventually progresses to end-stage renal disease (end-stage kidneys). The patient requires dialysis or renal transplantation to survive. Urinalysis findings for end-stage renal disease include isosthenuria (fixed specific gravity at 1.010), proteinuria, hematuria, and several types of casts, especially waxy and broad casts, which are characteristic for end-stage renal failure. The many different types of kidney diseases that may result in CRF, together with their frequency of occurrence, include DM (34%), HTN (nephrosclerosis, 29%), GN (14%), interstitial nephritis (3%), cystic kidney disease (3%), and other or unknown (15%).[30]

For examples of CRF, refer to Case Studies 10-5, 10-6, and 10-11.

Metabolic Diseases and Screening Tests

Urinalysis plays an important role in providing initial diagnostic information concerning metabolic dysfunctions of both renal and nonrenal origin. Screening tests performed in the urinalysis laboratory may detect a substance or suggest its presence in a patient's urine and alert the physician to the need for more sensitive, quantitative clinical procedures to identify the specific substance.

The Porphyrias

This is a heterogeneous group of hereditary (primary) or acquired (secondary) disorders in which certain enzyme activities of the heme biosynthetic pathway are partially or almost completely deficient. In general, each porphyria is caused by a single enzyme deficiency. Increased amounts of porphyrins or their precursors (e.g., delta-aminolevulinic acid [ALA] and porphobilinogen [PBG]) are produced, accumulate in tissues, or are excreted in urine and feces.

Historically, various systems have been used to classify the porphyrias. Before the biosynthetic pathway for the porphyrins had been worked out, names were given that reflected the typical age of presentation, such as "congenital erythropoietic porphyria." Later, the tissue of origin was used. This system defines four categories: erythropoietic porphyria (EP), hepatic porphyria, erythropoietic/hepatic (mixed) porphyria, and toxic porphyria. These categories are outlined in Table 10-7.

Another approach divides the disorders into three groups according to clinical symptoms: 1) neurologic only (acute intermittent porphyria [AIP]), 2) cutaneous only (porphyria cutanea tarda, EP, erythropoietic protoporphyria), and 3) both neurologic and cutaneous (variegate porphyria, hereditary coproporphyria).

As shown in Figure 10-9, the first intermediate formed in the pathway to heme is ALA. The next compound in the sequence is PBG, which is a single pyrrole ring. As the biosynthesis proceeds, various tetrapyrrole precursors ("porphyrinogens") are produced.

The porphyrin precursors ALA, PBG, and the porphyrinogens (uroporphyrinogen, coproporphyrinogen, and protoporphyringen) are colorless and nonfluorescent compounds. Conversely, the oxidized form of PBG (porphobilin), and the porphyrins (oxidation products of the porphyrinogens—uroporphyrin, coproporphyrin, and protoporphyrin) are dark red or purple, and are intensely fluorescent. In the normal case, the biosynthesis of heme is closely regulated in the body so that only trace amounts of porphyrins are formed. However, with enzyme deficiencies as manifested in the porphyrias, various precursors accumulate as well as their oxidized products, so that increased amounts may be found in blood, urine, and feces. The clinical and laboratory findings for the porphyrias are summarized in Table 10-8.

The two cardinal symptoms of the porphyrias are photosensitivity and neurologic manifestations. For some porphyrias, only neurologic symptoms are observed; for others, only photosensitivity; and for some, a combination of the two. Photosensitivity occurs because of the absorption of light by the porphyrins at about 400 nm with subsequent formation of oxy-

gen free radicals, which cause substantial damage to tissues, cells, subcellular elements, and various biomolecules. The photosensitivity may be expressed as cutaneous lesions (extensive blistering or bullae), a burning sensation, inflammatory skin reactions (edema, erythema, itching), and scarring.

The neurologic disturbances are thought to involve either the accumulation of ALA and PBG, deficient heme synthesis, or increased tryptophan in the central nervous system due to decreased hepatic tryptophan pyrrolase (oxygenase) activity.[6] The neurologic manifestations may include hysteria, psychosis, dysesthesia, seizures, abdominal pain, diarrhea, constipation, muscular paralysis, and respiratory failure.

Noting the color of the specimen during the physical examination of a urine can yield information concerning a possible case of porphyria or a porphyric attack. Urine containing large amounts of porphobilin, the oxidation product of PBG, may appear dark red, often described as a "port wine" color, as may occur during an acute attack of AIP (Swedish porphyria).[6] Also, different urine specimens that initially had a normal color may change to shades of red after standing at room temperature for several hours because of the photooxidation of PBG. Another example of the occurrence of a red-pigmented urine is with congenital EP. As shown in Figure 10-9, this is due to the excessive excretion of coproporphyrin I and uroporphyrin I.[36]

TABLE 10-7
Classification of the Porphyrias

	Heredity	Photosensitivity or Skin Involvement	Onset	Acute Symptoms: Abdominal Pain or Psychological Symptoms
Erythropoietic				
Erythropoietic porphyria	Recessive	Yes	Infancy	No
Erythropoietic protoporphyria	Dominant	Yes	Infancy	No
Hepatic				
Acute intermittent porphyria	Dominant	No	Adolescence	Yes
Variegate porphyria	Dominant	Variable	Young adult	Variable
Hereditary coproporphyria	Dominant	Variable	Young adult	Yes
Porphyria cutanea tarda	Familial = dominant	Yes		No
	Sporadic = renal dialysis		All ages (peak in middle age)	
Erythropoietic and hepatic				
Hepatoerythropoietic porphyria	Recessive	Yes	Childhood	No
Acquired (toxic)				
Drug-induced	NA*	Yes	Variable	No
Lead	NA	No	Variable	Yes

* NA, not applicable.

(Ravel R. *Clinical laboratory medicine*. St. Louis: Mosby, 1995.)

Ehrlich's reaction (discussed in Chapter 7) can be used to screen for PBG. The Watson-Schwartz test (see Chapter 7) may be used to differentiate between the presence of urobilinogen (the normal urine constituent, which is also Ehrlich positive) and PBG. A more rapid method to screen for the presence of PBG is the Hoesch test (see Chapter 7). Ehrlich's reagent can also be used to screen for increased ALA; first, ALA is condensed with ethyl acetoacetate to form a pyrrole, and this derivative is purified by extraction into ethyl acetate.[20] This pyrrole derivative in ethyl acetate can now be reacted with Ehrlich's reagent to give a cherry-red compound that can be measured spectrophotometrically at 555 nm.

When porphyrins dissolved in organic solvents are illuminated by ultraviolet light they emit a strong red fluorescence. This color is so characteristic that it is frequently used to detect small amounts of free porphyrins. One method to screen for porphyrins involves their extraction into a mixture of glacial acetic acid and ethyl acetate.[33] With a Wood's lamp, negative reactions have a faint blue fluorescence. Positive specimens fluoresce as pink, violet, or red, depending on the concentration of porphyrins. To rule out interfering substances, the organic layer can be removed to a separate tube, acidified with 0.5 mL of hydrochloric acid (3 N), and the mixture shaken well. Only porphyrins are extracted into the acid layer, which fluoresces a bright orange-red.[17]

Aminoacidopathies

Among other signs, inborn errors of amino acid metabolism may be manifested by aminoaciduria—i.e, by increased amino acids in the urine. Broadly defined, aminoacidurias may be either "renal" or "overflow."

The renal aminoacidurias are characterized by normal levels of the amino acids in the blood but increased levels in the urine resulting from defective renal tubular reabsorption. Cystinuria is an example of the renal type. The renal tubular disorders are considered as a group earlier in this chapter.

The overflow type is identified by increased concentrations of one or more amino acids in the blood but a normal renal clearance. Some of these overflow aminoacidurias are considered in the following section.

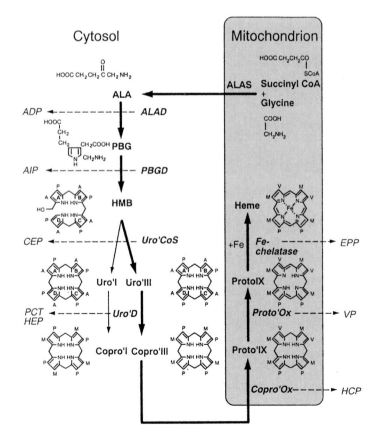

FIGURE 10-9 Enzymes and intermediates in the heme biosynthetic pathway. Pyrrole ring designation is shown in the structures of hydroxymethylbilane, uroporphyrinogen I and III. In uroporphyrinogen III, β-substituent groups in ring D have undergone "flipping", i.e., the ring is reversed. ADP = α-aminolevulinic acid dehydratase porphyria; AIP = acute intermittent porphyria; ALA = δ-aminolevulinic acid; ALAD = δ-aminolevulinic acid dehydratase; ALAS = δ-aminolevulinic acid synthase; CEP = congenital erythropoietic porphyria; Copro' = coproporphyrinogen; Copro'Ox = Copro' oxidase; EPP = erythropoietic protoporphyria; HCP = hereditary coproporphyria; HEP = hepatoerythropoietic porphyria; HMB = hydroxymethylbilane; PBG = porphobilinogen; PBGD = porphobilinogen deaminase; PCT = porphyria cutanea tarda; Proto' = protoporphyrinogen; Proto'Ox = Proto' oxidase; Uro' = uroporphyrinogen; Uro'Cos = Uro'III cosynthase; VP = variegate porphyria. A: $-CH_2COOH$; M: $-CH_3$; P: $-CH_2CH_2COOH$; V:$-CH = CH_2$. (From Berkow R. ed. *The Merck manual of diagnosis and therapy*. 16th ed. Rahway, NJ: Merck and Co. Publications, 1992.)

TABLE 10-8
Clinical and Laboratory Findings of the Porphyrias

Porphyria	Clinical Symptoms	Laboratory Findings*			
		Red Cells	Plasma	Urine	Stool
AIP	Neurologic Nausea, vomiting, abdominal pain, diarrhea, constipation, ileus, dysuria, muscle hypotonia, respiratory insufficiency, sensory neuropathy, seizures	—	—	ALA, PBG	—
ADP	Neurologic (same as AIP)	Zn-PP	—	ALA	—
CEP	Photosensitivity Bullae, crusts, scar formation, sclerodermoid, hyperpigmentation and hypopigmentation, hypertrichosis, erythrodontia, hemoltyic anemia, splenomegaly	Uro I, Copro I	Uro I, Copro I	Uro I, Copro I	—
PCT	Photosensitivity Skin fragility, bullae, crusts, sclerodermoid, hyper and hypopigmentation, hypertrichosis	—	Uro, 7-carboxyl	Uro, 7-carboxyl	Uro, 7-carboxyl, Isocopro
HEP	Photosensitivity (same as CEP)	Zn-PP	Uro, 7-carboxyl	Uro, 7-carboxyl	Uro, 7-carboxyl, Isocopro
HCP	Neurologic and photosensitivity (same as AIP and PCT)	—	Copro	ALA, PBG, Copro	Copro
VP	Neurologic and photosensitivity (same as AIP and PCT)	—	Proto	ALA, PBG	Proto
EP	Photosensitivity Burning sensation, edema, erythema, itching, scarring, vesicles	Proto	Proto	—	Proto

ADP, delta-aminolevulinic acid dehydratase porphyria; AIP, acute intermittent porphyria; ALA, delta-aminolevulinic acid; CEP, congenital erythropoietic porphyria; Copro, coproporphyrin; EP, erythropoietic porphyria; HCP, hereditary coproporphyria; HEP, hepatoerythropoietic porphyria; PCT, porphyria cutanea tarda; PBG, porphobilinogen; Proto, protoporphyrin; Uro, uroporphyrin; VP, variegate porphyria; Zn-PP, Zn-protoporphyrin.

* Laboratory findings show increased levels, which are abnormal. It is difficult to provide approximate values because normal values vary depending on laboratory.

(From Berkow R ed. *The Merck manual of diagnosis and therapy.* 16th ed. Rahway, NJ: Merck and Co. Publications, 1992.)

PHENYLKETONURIA

Among several variants of this inborn error of metabolism, the most frequently encountered form is "classic phenylketonuria" (PKU). This disorder is quite common in persons of Scandinavian descent and is distinctly uncommon in African Americans and Jews.[29]

Phenylketonuria is inherited as an autosomal recessive trait. It is characterized by a severe lack of the hepatic enzyme phenylalanine hydroxylase, so that phenylalanine is not converted into tyrosine. Consequently,

phenylalanine accumulates, together with its metabolites phenylpyruvic acid, phenyllactic acid, and phenylacetic acid. As these compounds build up in the blood, they eventually are excreted in large amounts in the urine ("overflow").

Phenylpyruvic acid accounts for the name of the disorder, PKU. Some of the metabolites are excreted in the sweat, so that an infant with this disorder, as well as the infant's urine, have a characteristic musty or mousy odor, mainly due, perhaps, to the phenylacetic acid. It is thought that excess phenylalanine or its metabolites contribute to the brain damage in patients with PKU.

At birth, babies with PKU appear unaffected, but on a normal diet (milk), they soon manifest a rising level of phenylalanine in the blood and progressive mental retardation. Early signs include feeding difficulties, vomiting, and failure to thrive. Fewer than 4% of untreated PKU children have IQ values greater than 50 or 60.[29] Approximately one third of the untreated children never learn to walk, and about two thirds cannot talk.

Seizures and other neurologic abnormalities are often manifested, as well as decreased pigmentation of hair and skin and mental retardation in untreated children. The hyperphenylalaninemia and mental retardation can be avoided by restricting dietary intake of phenylalanine early in life.

A number of screening procedures for hyperphenylalaninemia are available. All states have mandated that infants be tested for PKU in the immediate postnatal period.

Although screening tests for urine are available (nonspecific ferric chloride or Phenistix), initial screening for PKU is not done in the urinalysis laboratory because too much time may elapse before urinary excretion of phenylalanine and its metabolites is observed. Meanwhile, the neurologic damage may be occurring. For this reason, the specimen of choice is blood.

The best known screening procedure for PKU is the bacterial inhibition test developed by Guthrie. In this time-honored bioassay, blood obtained from the infant by means of a heel stick is allowed to soak into circles marked on an absorbent paper card. The blood is allowed to dry. Standardized discs from these circles are punched out and placed on culture media streaked with *Bacillus subtilis*. Increased phenylalanine in the infant's blood counteracts the effect of beta-2-thienylalanine, an inhibitor of *B. subtilis* that is present in the media, and the bacteria grow in a halo around the filter paper disk containing the blood.

Phenylketonuria variants have been found in about 10% of patients with apparent PKU. The metabolic system for converting phenylalanine to tyrosine is actually a group of at least four enzymes and coenzymes.[24] Classic PKU is produced by a deficiency in the hydroxylase enzyme; a deficiency in one of the other components of the system produces variant PKU. An important variant is caused by a deficiency of the hydroxylase cofactor tetrahydrobiopterin. In this case, a phenylalanine-deficient diet is not enough to control the disease and additional therapy is required. On the other hand, some patients with different variants of PKU do not require a phenylalanine-free diet.

ALKAPTONURIA (OCHRONOSIS)

More than 600 cases of this autosomal recessive trait have been reported, with an estimated incidence of 2 to 5 cases per million live births.[25] The metabolic defect is a lack of the hepatic enzyme homogentisic acid oxidase, as shown in Figure 10-10.

Homogentisic acid (HGA, dihydroxyphenylacetic acid) accumulates in cells and body fluids and is excreted in the urine. The most striking clinical laboratory manifestation of the disorder is the darkening of urine after standing in air or after the addition of alkali. HGA is oxidized by the oxygen in the air to a brownish black pigment. Late in the disease, patients manifest a dark blue to black pigmentation in cartilage and connective tissues (ochronosis) and a form of degenerative arthritis due to the oxidation of HGA to benzoquinone acetate, which polymerizes and binds to cartilage and other connective tissues. The ochronosis is especially noticed in the ears.

Alkaptonuria is usually not diagnosed until ochronosis and arthritis occur in middle age. However, if the dark stain in a diaper is noticed and investigated, the disorder may be diagnosed in neonates. Although there is no satisfactory treatment for alkaptonuria, if the diagnosis is made early, it may be beneficial to restrict dietary tyrosine or its precursor, phenylalanine.[31]

Urinary screening tests rely on the reducing ability of the HGA. These tests include the ferric chloride test (transient, very dark blue color), and copper reduction methods such as Benedict's test and the Clinitest (manifested as false-positive results for glucose). Adding alkali to freshly voided urine causes a dark color to develop, hence the term "alkali lover" or alkaptonuria.[33] Adding silver nitrate and ammonium hydroxide to the urine produces a black color. Confirmatory tests can be carried out with thin-layer chromatography or high-performance liquid chromatography.

TYROSINOSIS, TYROSINEMIA, AND RELATED DISORDERS

Tyrosinosis (hereditary tyrosinemia type I, hepatorenal tyrosinemia) is a rare disorder caused by a deficiency of the enzyme fumarylacetoacetate hydrolase, as shown in Figure 10-10. The enzyme deficiency results in elevated levels of tyrosine in the blood and urine, elevated levels of methionine in the blood, and increased serum levels of alpha-fetoprotein.

The primary effects of the disease are related to the liver and kidneys. Liver damage varies from acute failure and death in infancy to a more chronic state that leads to cirrhosis later in life. The kidney damage leads

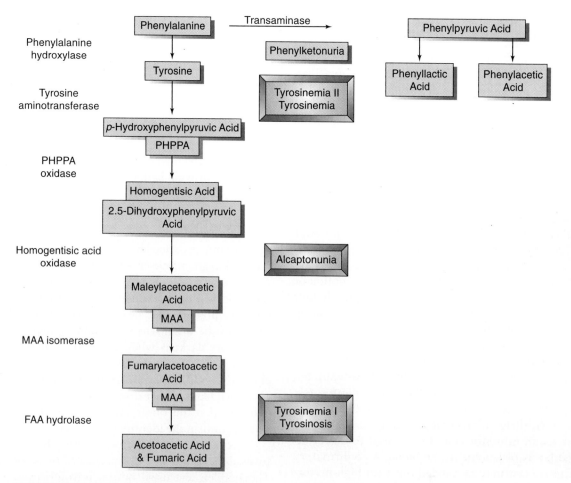

FIGURE 10-10 Metabolic pathway of phenylalanine. (From Anderson SD, Cockayne S. *Clinical chemistry*. Philadelphia: WB Saunders Company, 1993.)

to Fanconi's syndrome with vitamin D–resistant rickets, hyperphosphaturia, glucosuria, and aminoaciduria.

Infants with acute tyrosinosis manifest diarrhea, vomiting, and a cabbage-like odor, as well as failure to thrive. Chronic tyrosinosis is associated with milder symptoms, but death ensues by the age of 10 years. Therapy consists of a diet low in tyrosine and phenylalanine, and in some cases, low in methionine also.

Most cases of type I tyrosinemia have been found in an isolated French-Canadian population in Quebec.[32] Elsewhere, the disease has an incidence of about 1 in 100,000. Although dietary restriction corrects the biochemical change, it does not halt the progressive liver damage.

The inherited metabolic defect in tyrosinemia type II is a deficiency in the hepatic enzyme tyrosine aminotransferase, illustrated in Figure 10-10. Inflammation and lesions of the eye and skin may occur from the intracellular deposition of tyrosine crystals. Some cases may manifest mental retardation. Blood and urine lev-

els of tyrosine are elevated. In contrast to tyrosinemia type I, blood levels of methionine are not elevated.

Neonatal tyrosinemia is a manifestation of hepatic immaturity and the inability to synthesize adequate enzymes. Serum tyrosine levels are elevated in asymptomatic premature infants and in full-term infants of low birth weight. The condition is benign, and there is no liver or renal disease. Within 4 to 8 weeks, as the liver matures, serum levels of tyrosine decrease to adult levels and the tyrosinemia resolves.

For all of the disorders of tyrosinemia, tyrosinuria is observed, and the characteristic fine, silky, needle-like crystals of tyrosine may form in acid urine. Leucine crystals may accompany the tyrosine crystals. A nonspecific screening method for tyrosine in urine uses the reagent nitrosonaphthol, which forms soluble red complexes with tyrosine as well as with tyramine (the product of tyrosine decarboxylation). Confirmatory tests might use chromatography or one of the quantitative serum assays.

MAPLE SYRUP URINE DISEASE (BRANCHED-CHAIN KETONURIA)

Maple syrup urine disease is an autosomal recessive disorder involving the absence (or greatly reduced activity) of the alpha-keto acid decarboxylase required to metabolize leucine, valine, and isoleucine. Plasma, cerebrospinal fluid, and urinary levels of leucine, isoleucine, and valine, together with their alpha-keto acids, are elevated. The urine has the odor of maple syrup or burnt sugar because of the high concentration of the aliphatic keto acids.[32]

Several variants of maple syrup urine disease have been identified clinically and biochemically. In the classic case, the infant displays symptoms soon after birth (during the first week) that include feeding difficulties, vomiting, seizures, and lethargy. If not diagnosed and treated appropriately, mental retardation or death can occur. Therapy involves replacing dietary protein with a mixture of amino acids excluding leucine, isoleucine, and valine.

Dinitrophenylhydrazine can be used in a nonspecific screening test to detect increased levels of keto acids in the urine (forming insoluble yellow-white hydrazones with the acids), and the ferric chloride test (nonspecific) gives a gray-blue color with the keto acids. A Guthrie microbiologic assay using 4-aza-leucine as an inhibitor can also be used to detect increased levels of leucine in the blood. A confirmatory quantitative test may be carried out with high-performance liquid chromatography.

HOMOCYSTINURIA

A group of disorders, the homocystinurias are characterized by increased levels of homocysteine in body tissues. Classic homocystinuria is due to a deficiency or absence of the enzyme cystathionine synthase, which converts homocysteine to cystathionine. This enzymatic defect results in the accumulation of methionine (the precursor for homocysteine), homocysteine, and homocystine in blood and urine. A diet low in methionine and high in cystine prevents pathologic changes if initiated early in life.[25]

Symptoms of the disorder are not observed at birth but develop with time. One of the most common observations is dislocation of the ocular lens, which occurs in the first few years, often followed by myopia, glaucoma, and retinal detachment. Other abnormalities include osteoporosis, genu valgum (knock-knee), frequent chest, vertebral, and foot deformities, and, occasionally, mental retardation. If death occurs it is usually related to cardiovascular problems. Afflicted individuals manifest arterial or venous thromboemboli (probably related to enhanced platelet stickiness) that may cause mental retardation or death.

The cyanide–nitroprusside test produces a reddish color with homocystinuria that must be differentiated from the possibility of a positive test due to cystine. The silver–nitroprusside test, which uses silver (as silver nitrate) as the reductant in place of cyanide, is positive for homocystine but not for cystine. There is a Guthrie microbiologic assay designed to detect increased levels of plasma methionine using the growth inhibitor, methionine sulfoximine. The screening tests for homocystine have been converted to spectrophotometric procedures that provide better detection at low levels.[33]

MELANURIA

Melanin, produced by melanocytes from tyrosine, is the dark pigment observed in the hair, skin, and eyes. Melanomas of the skin or retina (tumors consisting of melanocytes) may produce enough of the pigments or colorless precursors to be excreted (melanuria) and detected in the urine. Urine containing melanin and its precursors darkens when exposed to air or sunlight. The amount of darkening depends on the melanin concentration and the exposure time, and the urine may even turn black. Other disorders result in darkening of urine, so that this observation needs further investigation to confirm the identity of the darkening substance.

Screening tests[32] include ferric chloride, which turns dark brown in the presence of melanogens. The Thormählen test uses sodium nitroferricyanide solution and produces a color with melanogens (when glacial acetic acid is added to the reaction mixture) that varies from greenish blue to bluish black.[32] Ammoniacal silver nitrate may be used and slowly darkens as a result of the formation of both melanin and colloidal silver.

Disorders of Carbohydrate Metabolism

DIABETES MELLITUS

DM, the most important disease that results in hyperglycemia, is not a single, well-defined disorder but rather a heterogeneous group of disorders. In one classification, the three types of DM are type I or insulin-dependent DM (IDDM); type II or non–insulin-dependent DM (NIDDM); and "other types" of diabetes that are secondary to conditions such as pancreatic or endocrine disease; administration of particular hormones, drugs, or chemicals; and some genetic syndromes or certain environmental conditions.

DM type I is characterized by an absolute deficiency of insulin resulting from the destruction or degeneration of the beta cells of the pancreatic islets of Langerhans. It is the most severe form of DM and is characterized by an abrupt onset of symptoms and the development of ketoacidosis. These patients require insulin and the disease most frequently occurs in juveniles.

DM type II is a milder form of diabetes characterized by a relative deficiency of insulin activity because of insulin resistance. Insulin levels may be normal, but there is an insufficient peripheral response to the insulin. Type II patients are not prone to ketosis and usually do not require insulin. NIDDM usually occurs in adults after age 40 years and progresses slowly.

In both types of DM, hyperglycemia develops because glucose is not used or is underused, and glucosuria occurs when the plasma level of glucose exceeds the renal threshold, between 180 to 200 mg/dL. Glucosuria leads to polyuria and polydipsia. Although the urine appears dilute, the specific gravity is considerably increased because of the increased concentration of urinary glucose. In those patients prone to ketosis, the ketone bodies acetoacetate, acetone, and beta-hydroxybutyric acid are formed and excreted in the urine (ketonuria).

The effects of DM are often observed during a routine urinalysis. The reagent test strip is positive for glucose, and if the patient is experiencing diabetic ketoacidosis, the test strip is also positive for ketones. For an example of diabetic ketoacidosis, refer to Chapter 9, Case Study 9-6.

Testing for microalbuminuria as a means to provide an early warning of impending diabetic nephropathy (and the need for tighter glycemic control) is discussed in Chapter 7.

GALACTOSEMIA

This is an autosomal recessive disorder of galactose metabolism. Lactose, which is the major carbohydrate in mammalian milk, is a disaccharide composed of glu-

cose and galactose. Lactose is split into its component sugars by the enzyme lactase in the intestinal microvilli. In normal metabolism, galactose is converted to glucose in three steps, as shown in Figure 10-11.

Of the two variants of galactosemia, the more common one is a total lack of galactose-1-phosphate uridyl transferase (the enzyme responsible for reaction 2, Fig. 10-11). This enzyme defect leads to an accumulation of galactose-1-phosphate in many areas of the body, including the liver, spleen, lens of the eye, kidneys, heart muscle, cerebral cortex, and erythrocytes. Galactitol also accumulates in the tissues because alternative metabolic pathways are activated. Soon after birth, signs of the disorder become evident, with failure to thrive, vomiting, and diarrhea appearing within a few days after starting the ingestion of milk. During the first week of life, jaundice and hepatomegaly are usually observed and cataracts develop within a few weeks. Within the first 6 to 12 months of life, mental retardation becomes evident.

Treatment consists of early removal of galactose from the diet, and, if started soon after birth, this prevents the cataracts and liver damage and permits almost normal mental development. A positive urinalysis screening test for a reducing sugar other than glucose suggests the possibility of galactosuria, and the diagnosis could be confirmed by measuring the level of the transferase enzyme in leukocytes or erythrocytes. Cultured fibroblasts from amniotic fluid may be tested for the enzyme to provide antenatal diagnosis.

The less common variant of galactosemia involves a deficiency of the enzyme galactokinase (responsible for reaction 1, Fig. 10-11). As with the more common variant, blood and urinary galactose levels are elevated, but with galactokinase deficiency, no liver or brain impairment occurs. However, unless galactose is eliminated from the diet, cataracts develop rapidly. Tests for the transferase enzyme are normal, but assays for galactokinase activity reveal its absence.

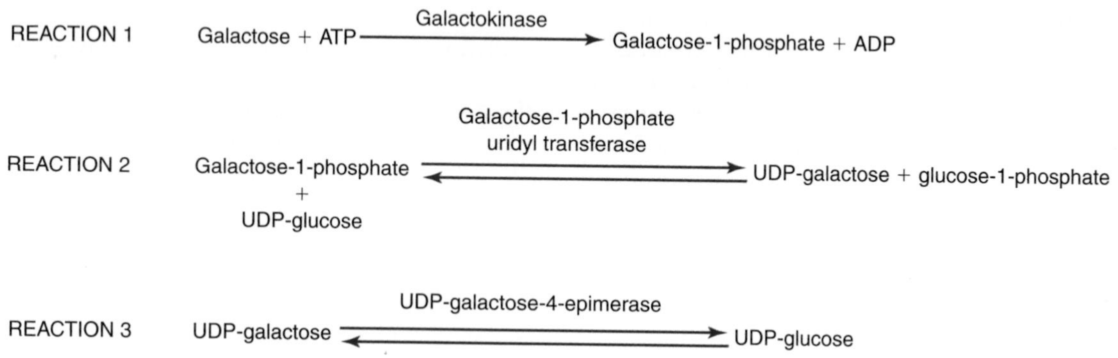

REACTION 1   Galactose + ATP —— Galactokinase ——→ Galactose-1-phosphate + ADP

REACTION 2   Galactose-1-phosphate + UDP-glucose ⇄ Galactose-1-phosphate uridyl transferase ⇄ UDP-galactose + glucose-1-phosphate

REACTION 3   UDP-galactose ⇄ UDP-galactose-4-epimerase ⇄ UDP-glucose

FIGURE 10-11 Pathway of galactose metabolism (From Cotran RS, Kumar V, Robbins SL. *Robbins pathologic basis of disease*. 5th ed. Philadelphia; WB Saunders Company, 1994.)

MUCOPOLYSACCHARIDOSES

The mucopolysaccharidoses (MPS) are one of a group of lysosomal storage diseases resulting from genetically determined deficiencies of specific lysosomal enzymes. The acid mucopolysaccharides (glycosaminoglycans) are structural components of cartilage, bone, skin, and connective tissues, and consist of a protein core with numerous polysaccharide branches containing hexosamine sulfates and hexuronic acids. They are normally degraded by lysosomal enzymes. In the MPS these enzymes are deficient.

Fragments of incompletely metabolized polysaccharide, including dermatan sulfate, heparan (not heparin) sulfate, keratan sulfate, and chondroitin sulfate, accumulate in the lysosomes of connective tissue cells. Various tissues and organs of the body are involved. Manifestations include severe somatic and neurologic changes.

There are several clinical variants of the disorders, numbered MPS I to VII. One variant, Hunter's syndrome, is inherited as an X-linked recessive trait, but all the other MPS are inherited as autosomal recessive traits.

In general, the MPS are progressive disorders involving multiple organs of the body, including the liver, spleen, heart, and blood vessels. Most are characterized by coarse facial features, clouding of the cornea, joint stiffness, and mental retardation.[9] Characteristic facial features include thick lips, an open mouth, and a flattened nasal bridge. Accumulated mucopolysaccharides are often excreted in the urine.

Hurler's syndrome (MPS I H) occurs because of a deficiency of alpha-L-iduronidase (a lysosomal exoglycosidase that removes iduronic acid from the nonreducing terminus of polysaccharide chains) and is one of the most severe forms of MPS. Affected children appear normal at birth, but growth is retarded, hepatosplenomegaly is observed by 6 to 24 months of age, and, as observed with other forms of MPS, coarse facial features and skeletal deformities develop. Death, often due to cardiovascular complications, occurs by 6 to 10 years of age. The single MPS inherited as an X-linked recessive, Hunter's syndrome or MPS II, has a milder clinical course and does not involve corneal clouding.

Three different urinary mucopolysaccharides are observed: dermatan sulfate, heparan sulfate, and keratan sulfate, and the excretion of a particular substance or substances depends on the specific metabolic disorder inherited. The most frequently used urinary screening tests[33] are the acid-albumin and cetyltrimethylammonium bromide turbidity tests. When these reagents are added to urine containing mucopolysaccharides, a thick, white turbidity forms.

MPS papers (Bayer Diagnostics, formerly Miles Diagnostics) containing "azure A" dye react with urine containing mucopolysaccharides to produce a blue color that cannot be washed away by a dilute, acidified methanol solution. Mucopolysaccharides in urine can be quantitated by measuring the hexuronic acid content, and electrophoresis can be used to identify the mucopolysaccharide excretion pattern. A direct assay of the particular enzyme in leukocytes or cultured skin fibroblasts provides the definitive diagnosis.

HEREDITARY FRUCTOSE INTOLERANCE

This disorder, inherited as an autosomal recessive trait, is caused by the absence of the enzyme fructose-1-phosphate aldolase (aldolase B). Fructose metabolism is illustrated in Figure 10-12.

This disorder is expressed as the metabolic inability to use fructose. If more than very small amounts of fructose (or sucrose, the disaccharide of glucose and fructose) are ingested, the individual experiences hypoglycemia, sweating, tremors, confusion, nausea, vomiting, and abdominal pain, as well as possible convulsions and coma. Cirrhosis of the liver and mental deterioration may develop. Proximal renal tubular acidosis may be manifested together with urinary loss of phosphate and glucose if ingestion of fructose is prolonged.

Infants with the disorder develop normally when fed only human or cow's milk, but show symptoms when fed formulas high in fructose or fruit juices. Diagnosis is suggested by the symptoms as well as by finding fructose (a reducing sugar) in the urine. Diagnosis is confirmed by demonstrating the absence of the enzyme by liver biopsy, or by demonstrating a fall in blood glucose 5 to 40 minutes after administering fructose (250 mg/kg, IV).[6]

Treatment involves excluding sources of fructose (e.g., sweet fruits, sucrose, sorbitol) from the diet. Fructose-induced hypoglycemic attacks may be treated by having the patient ingest glucose.

DEFICIENCY OF FRUCTOSE-1,6-DIPHOSPHATASE

Transmitted as an autosomal recessive trait, the deficiency of fructose-1,6-diphosphatase results in hypoglycemia because fructose-6-phosphate cannot be formed and thus glyconeogenesis cannot proceed. Acidosis is manifested because gluconeogenic precursors accumulate in the body (certain amino acids, lactic acid, and ketoacids). Individuals with this deficiency experience episodes of apnea, hyperventilation, hypoglycemia, ketosis, and lactic acidosis because of the severe impairment of gluconeogenesis.[28]

Diagnosis can be made by demonstrating the absence of the enzyme in liver biopsy specimens. Symp-

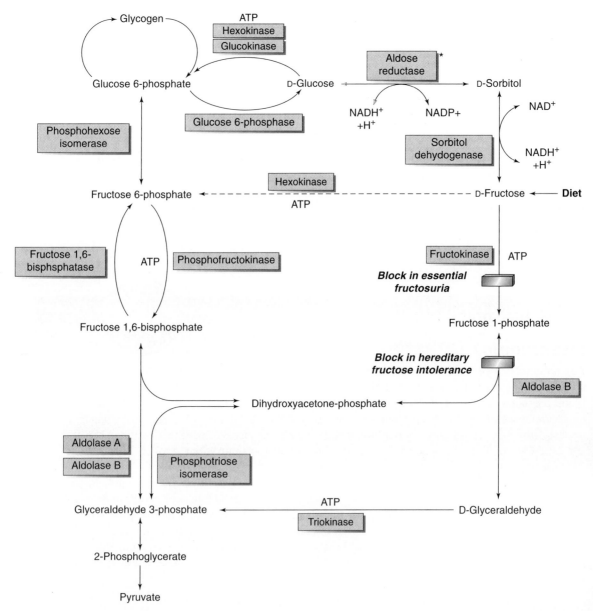

FIGURE 10-12 Metabolism of fructose. Aldolase A is found in all tissues except the liver, where only aldolase B is present. (*, not found in liver.) (From Murray RK, Granner DK, Mayes PA, Rodwell VW. *Harper's biochemistry*. 24th ed. Stamford, CT: Appleton and Lange, 1996.)

toms can be relieved by giving glucose orally (or IV if the hypoglycemia is severe), and management of the disorder includes frequent meals.

FRUCTOSURIA

Essential fructosuria is a benign condition resulting from a deficiency of the enzyme fructokinase. Serum fructose is elevated and fructose appears in the urine of affected individuals after the ingestion of sucrose or fructose. Although fructose does not react with the reagent strip method for glucose, it may give a false-positive test for glucose with copper reduction methods. The trait is transmitted as an autosomal recessive.

PENTOSURIA

An autosomal recessive trait, pentosuria is a benign condition characterized by the excretion of L-xylulose in the urine owing to the absence of the enzyme L-xylulose dehydrogenase. The trait occurs almost exclusively in the Jewish population, and, as observed with fructosuria, pentosuria may lead to false-positive results for glucose by copper reduction methods.

Diseases of Other Organ Systems

Hepatorenal Syndrome

In this syndrome, renal failure appears in patients with severe liver disease in the absence of any identifiable intrinsic morphologic or functional causes for the renal failure. It is characterized by progressively intense renal vasoconstriction.

Usually occurring in fulminant hepatitis or advanced cirrhosis with ascites, the hepatorenal syndrome begins suddenly with decreased urinary output (oliguria) and elevated BUN and creatinine levels. The kidneys are still able to form a concentrated urine that is hyperosmolar, has a very low sodium concentration (the result of hyperaldosteronism), and is devoid of proteins and abnormal sediment.

The most favored etiology is a reduction of renal blood flow, especially to the renal cortex, caused by vasoconstriction.[11] Some evidence suggests that an imbalance in the levels of vasodilator/vasoconstrictor hormones may be involved in the pathophysiology of the syndrome.[2] At autopsy, no permanent morphologic change is observed in the kidneys. If liver function can be restored in the patient, kidney function also markedly improves.

Illustrative Case Studies

CASE STUDY 10-1

This patient, a 29-year-old man, was referred to the hospital from the Immediate Care Center for influenza-like symptoms, headache, and HTN. Previous admissions had revolved around his blood pressure, uncontrolled HTN, increased cholesterol, increased creatinine and BUN, and hematuria. Assessment for this patient was hematuria with renal failure and HTN 2° to analgesic nephropathy, IgA nephropathy, or nephropathy 2° to collagen vascular disease. Creatinine clearance and total protein were determined on a 24-hour urine specimen with the following results: 3334 mg protein/24 hours (ref. range, <265 mg/24 hours) and a creatinine clearance of 43 mL/minute (ref. range, 85–125 mL/minute). A renal ultrasound examination showed small kidneys without any evidence of masses or cysts. A renal biopsy produced the following results: IgA nephropathy (Berger's disease, discussed earlier in this chapter) and arterial nephrosclerosis.

For the recent admission being considered here, the urinalysis was significant for blood moderate; WBCs 5–10/HPF; RBCs 50–100/HPF; and casts/LPF, 1–5 mixed, 0–1 waxy, rare WBC, TNTC granular. The significant elements observed in the urinary sediment for this patient are shown in Figures 10-13 to 10-19.

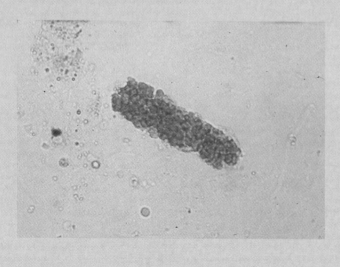

FIGURE 10-13 Hemoglobin/RBC cast. Urine sediment; SM stain; ×400.

continued

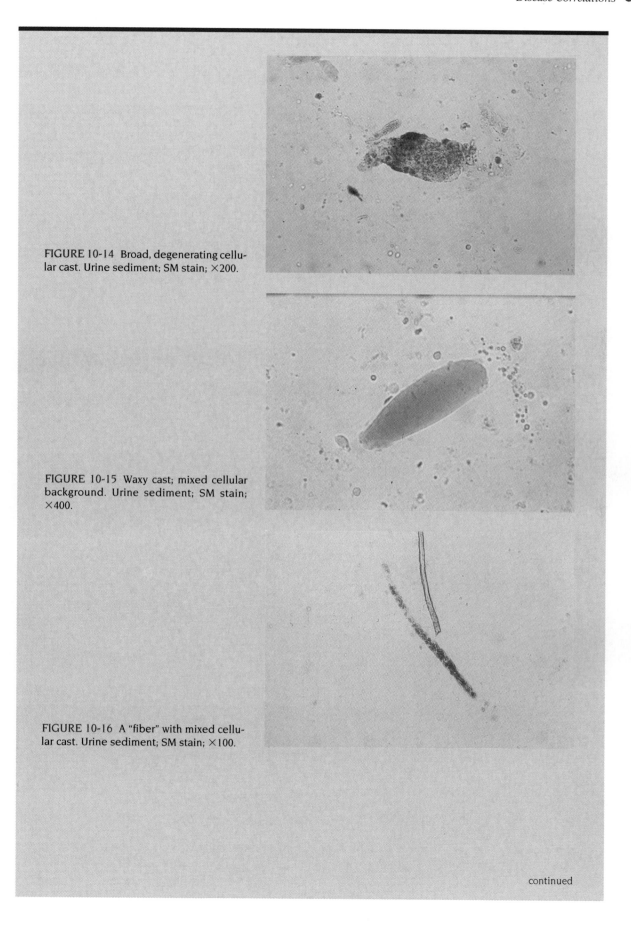

FIGURE 10-14 Broad, degenerating cellular cast. Urine sediment; SM stain; ×200.

FIGURE 10-15 Waxy cast; mixed cellular background. Urine sediment; SM stain; ×400.

FIGURE 10-16 A "fiber" with mixed cellular cast. Urine sediment; SM stain; ×100.

continued

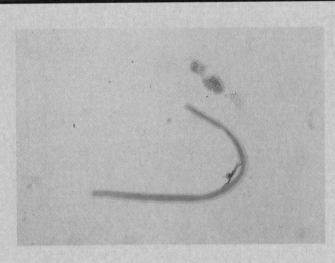

FIGURE 10-17 Waxy cast with granular cast fragments. Urine sediment; SM stain; ×100.

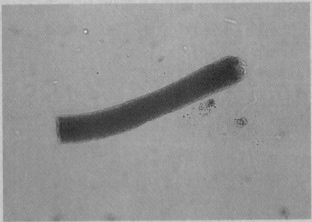

FIGURE 10-18 Granular/waxy cast. Urine sediment; SM stain; ×200.

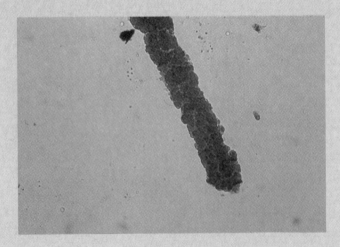

FIGURE 10-19 Cellular/granular cast. Urine sediment; SM stain; ×200.

continued

CASE STUDY 10-2

The patient, a 48-year-old man, had a history of alveolar proteinosis (chronic interstitial lung disease) that was diagnosed 2 years earlier. He had been recently discharged from the hospital after being treated for cryptococcal pneumonia. During his hospital stay, his treatment consisted of amphotericin B (IV), glucytosine, and prednisone. He was discharged after the fifth day in the hospital, but then he missed three doses of amphotericin B because of transportation problems.

He was subsequently seen in the ER complaining of severe shortness of breath (SOB). He was treated for SOB and sent home with supplies and instructions for breathing treatments. Four days later, his SOB had progressively worsened and he was subsequently admitted for SOB. His admission diagnosis was cryptococcal pneumonia, history of alveolar proteinosis, and renal insufficiency possibly 2° to amphotericin B therapy.

The admission urinalysis was significant for bilirubin small; blood small; protein 100 mg/dL; color orange; appearance hazy; WBCs 10—20/HPF; RBCs 0—2/HPF; bacteria few/HPF; casts TNTC RTE, TNTC hyaline/LPF; Ictotest positive. Medications at the time of admission included flucytosine, fluconazole, prednisone, and Pepcid.

After being admitted for SOB, the patient was transferred to the ICU. Overnight he started to desaturate, showing respiratory distress. He was intubated and placed on ventilator support. He began to show signs of septicemia, and blood cultures were positive for *Enterococcus fecalis*. He was placed on ampicillin and gentamicin, and continued on amphotericin B and fluconazole. His cardiovascular status continued to improve slowly, although it appeared that he was adrenally insufficient (polyuria and low blood pressure).

Three days after being placed in ICU, his urinalysis was significant for bilirubin small; WBCs 2–5/HPF; RBCs 0–2/HPF; epithelial cells few/HPF; bacteria 1+/HPF; casts 0–1 granular, 0–1 hyaline, rare WBC, rare waxy, rare mixed WBC and RBC/LPF; Ictotest positive; yeast rare. He was transferred from ICU to respiratory care and was started on prednisone, which was to be tapered gradually so as not to create adrenal problems.

The patient was discharged status postcryptococcal pneumonia, history of alveolar proteinosis, status postrespiratory failure, status postintubation and extubation, and status post–E. *fecalis* septicemia. The patient was to continue on fluconazole as well as prednisone (this to be gradually tapered). Examples of the formed elements observed in this patient's urine sediment during his hospitalization are provided in Figures 10-20 to 10-24 and are consistent with amphotericin B toxicity or renal ischemia/hypoxia. A photomicrograph of an India ink preparation of sputum from this patient showing *Cryptococcus* is also included in Figure 10-25.

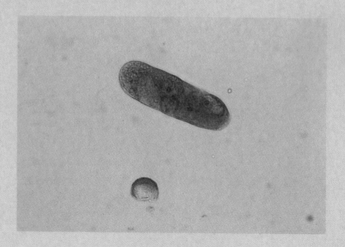

FIGURE 10-20 Multinucleated RTE cell; proximal tubule. Urine sediment; SM stain; ×400.

continued

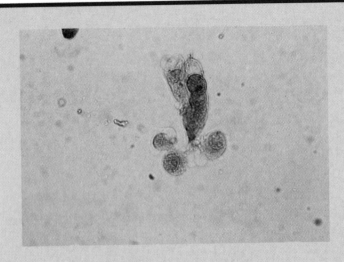

FIGURE 10-21 RTE cells (possibly regenerating); collecting duct. Urine sediment; SM stain; ×400.

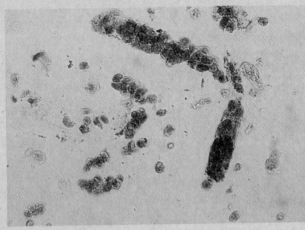

FIGURE 10-22 Mixed cellular casts (WBC/RTE). Urine sediment; SM stain; ×200.

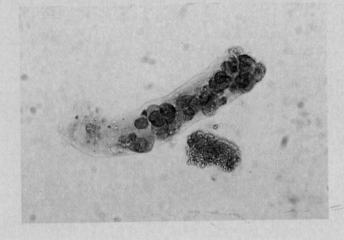

FIGURE 10-23 Small, coarsely granular cast; mixed cellular cast (WBC/RTE). Urine sediment; toluidine blue stain; ×400.

continued

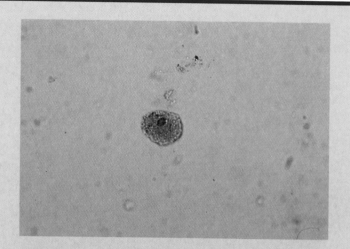

FIGURE 10-24 RTE cell; distal tubule. Urine sediment; toluidine blue stain; ×400.

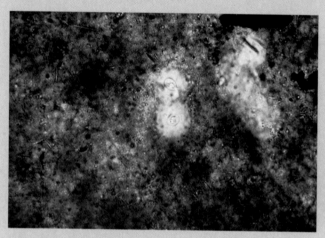

FIGURE 10-25 Sputum; India ink preparation; *Cryptococcus*. ×4000.

CASE STUDY 10-3

The Children's Protective Service brought this 18-year-old girl to the outpatient clinic for a routine OB check-up (IUP, 23 weeks) as a high-risk pregnancy. The patient also had a history of recurrent right-sided pyelonephritis (*Enterobacter aerogenes*), which the month before had been treated first with Cefotan (cefotetan) and then nitrofurantoin.

Her urinalysis was significant for: nitrite positive; leukocyte esterase small; appearance hazy; WBCs 50–100/HPF; RBCs 2–5/HPF; epithelial cells few squamous/HPF; bacteria 4+. The patient was evaluated and released with Bactrim for her UTI. The C&S result was colony count greater than 100,000 CFU/mL of E. *aerogenes*. Figures 10-26 and 10-27 show the appearance of the urinary sediment.

continued

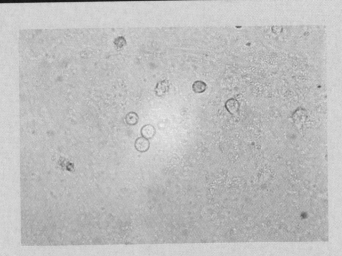

FIGURE 10-26 WBCs and bacteria. Urine sediment; SM stain; ×400.

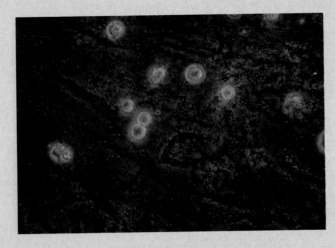

FIGURE 10-27 The same field of view as Figure 10-26, but with phase contrast showing WBCs and bacteria with mucus-like material in the background. Urine sediment; SM stain/phase contrast; ×400.

CASE STUDY 10-4

This patient, a 3-month-old girl, was brought to the ER by her mother because she had symptoms of fever and decreased appetite (not interested in her feedings). The baby had a history of UTIs as well as viral infections. The diagnosis of UTI was given and amoxicillin prescribed. The urinalysis (catheterized specimen) was significant for: WBCs 10–20/HPF; epithelial cells 1+/HPF; bacteria few/HPF. The urine C&S was colony count 50,000 to 100,000 CFU/mL of E. *coli*. The appearance of the urine sediment is presented in Figures 10-28 and 10-29.

continued

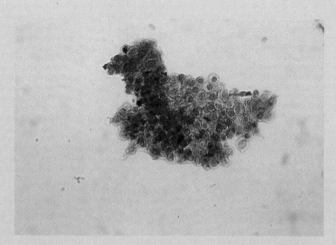

FIGURE 10-28 Cluster of small transitional epithelial cells, most likely dislodged by catheterization. Urine sediment; SM stain; ×200.

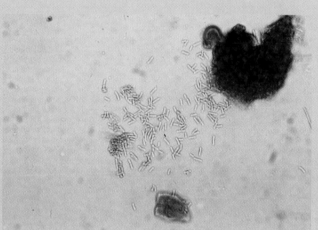

FIGURE 10-29 Cellular debris and bacteria. Urine sediment; SM stain; ×400.

CASE STUDY 10-5

A retired truck driver, this 74-year-old man was admitted through the ER complaining of dizziness and weakness after he fell trying to get out of bed. He was unable to get up out of a chair unaided and was weak and lethargic. He had a history of epileptic seizures from childhood, as well as CHF, HTN, IDDM, and CRF. He has had IDDM for more than 20 years. He had also been a heavy drinker until 3 years ago. On admission his medications were Dilantin, K-Dur (KCl), Lasix, and insulin.

On admission, a CT scan indicated a possible recent left frontal embolic event with some evidence for older embolic events and significant cerebral atrophy. His admission urinalysis was significant for protein 100 mg/dL; leukocyte esterase trace; appearance hazy; WBCs 5–10/HPF; RBCs negative; epithelial cells rare/HPF; bacteria rare/HPF; casts 1–5 WBC, 1–5 granular/LPF. The appearance of the urine sediment is shown in Figures 10-30 to 10-33 and is generally consistent with a picture of CRF.

continued

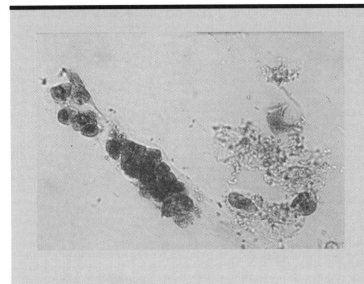

FIGURE 10-30 Mixed WBC/RTE cast. Urine sediment; SM stain; ×400.

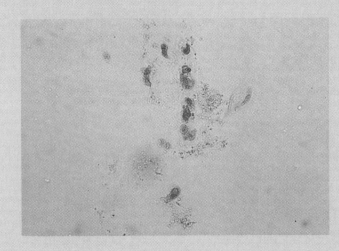

FIGURE 10-31 Mixed WBC/RTE cast. Urine sediment; SM stain; ×200.

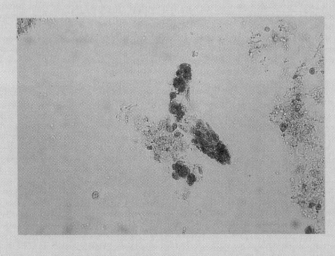

FIGURE 10-32 Mixed WBC/RTE casts. Urine sediment; SM stain; ×200.

continued

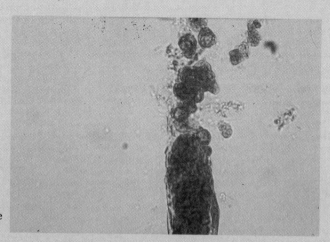

FIGURE 10-33 Mixed WBC/RTE cast. Urine sediment; SM stain; ×400.

CASE STUDY 10-6

A 71-year-old woman with a history of mild mental retardation was found at home confused, severely jaundiced, and very tired and agitated, a condition that had been progressing over the previous 2 to 3 days. She had been complaining of abdominal pain for the previous week. She had also been complaining of some diarrhea and constipation for the previous month and was scheduled to have a colonoscopy. She was admitted through the ER with the following assessment: severe anemia, possible gastrointestinal bleed; coagulopathy; liver failure; large breast mass; respiratory failure; renal insufficiency; altered mental status; and possible sepsis.

In the emergency room, the patient developed respiratory failure and finally metabolic acidosis. She was admitted to ICU, intubated, and placed on a ventilator to help her with breathing. She was found to have a lumpy mass on the right breast, crackles (moist rales) on auscultation, extreme pitting edema (3+) bilaterally on her legs, and a very icteric appearance.

Results of laboratory tests included a hemoglobin of 7 g/dL (ref. range, 12–16 g/dL); hematocrit of 21% (ref. range, 37–47%); WBC count 11,500/mm³ (4500–11,000/mm³); platelet count 102,000/mm³ (150,000–450,000/mm³); MCV 89 μm³ (80–96 μm³). Her ABGs were pH 7.30 (7.38–7.42); pCO₂ 30.5 mm Hg (35–45 mm Hg); pO₂ 67.7 mm Hg (75–85 mm Hg); bicarb 14.9 mEq/L (22–26 mEq/L); and an anion gap of 22 (1–11). She had a blood ammonia of 229 μg/dL (19–60 μg/dL); blood lactic acid of 9.5 mEq/L (0.9–1.7 mEq/L); total bilirubin of 8.2 mg/dL (0.2–1.5 mg/dL) with a conjugated bilirubin of 6.5 mg/dL (<0.3 mg/dL); ALP 1455 U/L (37–107 U/L); AST 1672 U/L (8–42 u/L); ALT 159 U/L (3–36 U/L); total protein of 4.4 g/dL (6.4–8.2 g/dL); albumin 1.6 g/dL (3.4–5.0 g/dL); LDH 3292 U/L (100–190 U/L); uric acid 13.3 mg/dL (2.4–5.1 mg/dL); BUN 110 mg/dL (5–25 mg/dL); creatinine 2.4 mg/dL (0.6–1.0 mg/dL); PT 19 seconds (11–15 seconds); PTT 34 seconds (<35 seconds).

Collectively, these tests provide a devastating picture of *anemia* (low hemoglobin and hematocrit); *respiratory failure and metabolic acidosis* (the ABG data and the blood lactic acid); *hepatic failure* (elevated bilirubin; elevated enzymes—ALT, AST, ALP, and LDH; low serum albumin and total protein; coagulopathy; elevated lactic acid; and elevated blood ammonia—giving rise to altered mental status); and *renal insufficiency* (elevated BUN, uric acid, and creatinine).

Once in the ICU, the patient underwent endoscopy and was found to have a large ulcer on her duodenum that was oozing blood, and this was cauterized. She received antibiotics for sepsis and was given fresh frozen plasma and vitamin K for coagulopathy. A biopsy of the breast was positive for adenocarcinoma with metastasis. A CT scan of the abdomen was then performed that showed widespread metastasis. Her grave condition was explained to the family and she was placed on dignity care. The patient died soon afterward, clinical cause being respiratory failure, hepatic failure, and renal failure 2° to metastatic breast cancer.

continued

Admission urinalysis was significant for bilirubin small; pH 5; color amber; appearance hazy; WBCs 0–2/HPF; RBCs rare; epithelials 1+ renal/HPF; casts 1–5 resembling RTE, rare resembling mixed WBC/RTE; Ictotest positive. The appearance of the urine sediment is shown in Figures 10-34 to 10-38, probably dominated by the respiratory failure (hypoxic damage), hepatic failure (spheroids resembling leucine), and renal failure 2° to metastatic breast cancer. In some instances, the formed elements appear to be slightly bile stained.

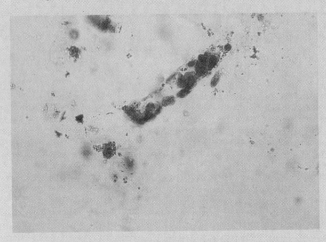

FIGURE 10-34 Mixed cellular cast (WBC/RTE). Urine sediment; SM stain; ×200.

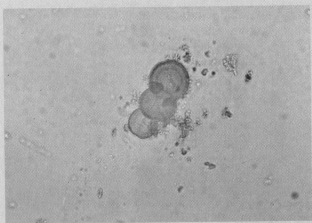

FIGURE 10-35 Spheroids resembling leucine, consistent with liver failure. Urine sediment; SM stain; ×400.

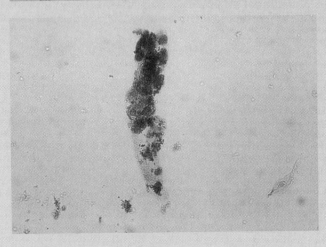

FIGURE 10-36 Granular/cellular (WBC) cast. Urine sediment; SM stain; ×200.

continued

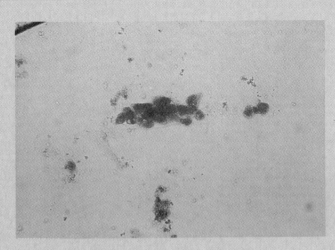

FIGURE 10-37 Mixed cellular cast (WBC/RTE). Urine sediment; SM stain; ×200.

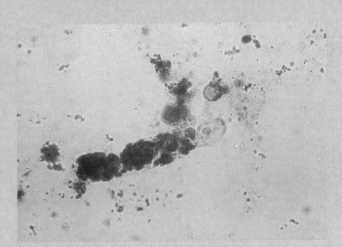

FIGURE 10-38 Two squamous epithelials; one transitional epithelial; and a mixed cellular cast (WBC/RTE). Urine sediment; SM stain; ×200.

CASE STUDY 10-7

A 60-year-old woman whose initial diagnosis by her private physician was SLE was admitted for exacerbation of her lupus: feeling tired and aching all over; swelling of the joints, hands and feet; a facial rash on the malar area and extending to the chest; dysphagia for 1 week; and HTN (155/95). Her admission Chem-10 was significant for BUN 95 mg/dL (ref. range, 5–25 mg/dL) and creatinine 2.3 (0.8–1.2 mg/dL), both renal markers and elevated. She was placed on prednisone for her SLE; an antibiotic (Keflex) for pharyngitis; Naprosyn (naproxen), an antiinflammatory/analgesic; Vasotec (enalapril maleate) for her HTN; Lasix (furosemide) for her edema; and a low-protein ("renal") diet.

While in the hospital she had a renal biopsy performed that demonstrated "arterial nephrosclerosis with mixed membranous and focal proliferative lupus GN." Immunofluorescence microscopy was also performed on frozen sections of the tissue and showed staining for multiple antibodies, complement (CI_q and C3), and kappa/lambda light chains.

Five days after admission, the results of a urinalysis were as follows: glucose, bilirubin, ketones, negative; specific gravity 1.020; blood moderate; pH 7; protein >300 mg/dL; urobilinogen 0.2 EU/dL; nitrite negative; leukocyte esterase moderate; WBCs 20–50/HPF; RBCs 10–20/HPF; epithelial cells 1+; occasional casts/LPF (waxy, granular, cellular); and bacteria few.

Figures 10-39 to 10-42 demonstrate the findings in the urine sediment for this case:

continued

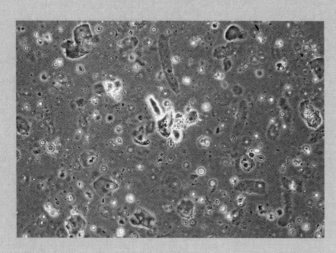

FIGURE 10-39 Low-power view of various cells and casts. Urine sediment; SM stain/phase contrast; ×100.

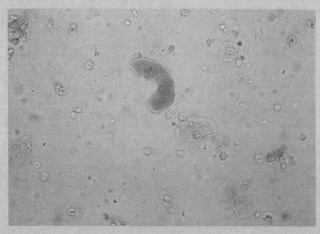

FIGURE 10-40 Waxy cast with mixed cellular background. Urine sediment; SM stain; ×200.

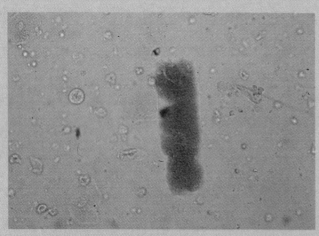

FIGURE 10-41 Broad granular cast with mixed cellular background. Urine sediment; SM stain; ×200.

continued

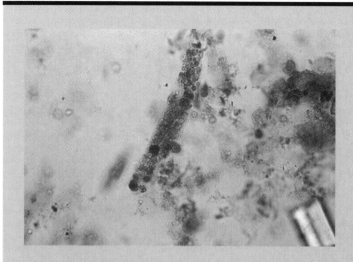

FIGURE 10-42 Mixed cellular cast with mixed cellular/debris background. Urine sediment; toluidine blue; ×200.

CASE STUDY 10-8

With a long history of chronic tonsillitis and adenoiditis, this 5-year-old boy was admitted for ton-sillectomy and adenoidectomy. There was also a family history of Alport's syndrome (hereditary nephritis) and the child had been diagnosed with this previously. Alport's syndrome is character-ized by intermittent hematuria, impairment of renal function, proteinuria, leukocyturia, and casts of various types.

The admission urinalysis was significant for blood large; protein trace mg/dL; color amber; ap-pearance hazy; WBCs 10–20/HPF; RBCs 50–100/HPF; and 1–5 RBC casts. Photomicrographs of the urinary sediment are not available, but the urinalysis in general is consistent with Alport's syn-drome.

CASE STUDY 10-9

This patient, a 62-year-old man, had been scheduled for surgery 7 months previously for a ure-thral stricture, but he had been putting it off and had a Foley catheter in place during that time because he was unable to void. He had a history of chronic UTIs.

The previous week, he presented to the ER complaining of bilateral flank pain and pain at the catheter site. During that visit he was treated for a UTI with Bactrim and discharged home. In the current instance, he was brought to the ER by ambulance complaining of inability to urinate owing to catheter blockage. The catheter was removed, and a large efflux of urine resulted, much to the relief of the patient. The Foley was replaced with an 18-French catheter and the patient was dis-charged home with Bactrim and instructions to drink plenty of fluids.

The urinalysis was significant for blood moderate; leukocyte esterase moderate; appearance hazy; WBCs/HPF TNTC; RBCs/HPF present; epithelial cells/HPF 2+; bacteria/HPF 1+; yeast pre-sent. A C&S on the urine indicated an infection with *Trichosporon beigelii* and *Candida parapsilosis*. The appearance of the urine sediment is illustrated in Figure 10-43.

continued

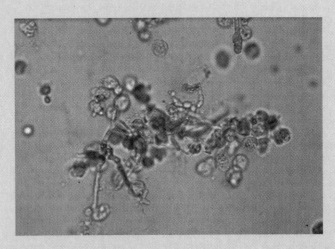

FIGURE 10-43 Yeast (including pseudo-hyphae); RBCs; WBCs. Urine sediment; SM stain; ×200.

CASE STUDY 10-10

This patient, a 31-year-old man, had a 3-year history of renal stones involving the left kidney. During a previous admission, an IVP revealed a large staghorn calculus in the left kidney and left renal hydronephrosis. The patient had undergone lithotripsy for obstructive uropathy on two previous occasions and had passed renal stones several times. The medical records included a photograph of some of the stones, which appeared to be rather smooth and yellow-brown. Crystallographic analysis indicated their composition was 5% calcium oxalate and 95% uric acid.

The admission described here was for cystoscopy and replacement of a stent in the left ureter. Urinalysis was significant for: blood large; protein 30 mg/dL; leukocyte esterase trace; color amber; appearance hazy; WBCs 5–10/HPF; RBCs TNTC/HPF; and epithelials few/HPF. The appearance of the sediment for this urine is illustrated in Figure 10-44.

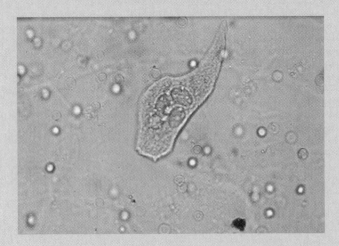

FIGURE 10-44 Mixed cellular background (RBCs; one reactive transitional epithelial). SM stain; ×400.

continued

CASE STUDY 10-11

The patient, a 58-year-old woman with a history of paroxysmal nocturnal dyspnea and orthopnea, CHF, COPD, HTN, and DM was admitted through the ER with worsening SOB. She had no complaints of chest pains, palpitations, fever, cough, nausea, or vomiting. The admitting diagnosis was CHF, R/O MI, exacerbated COPD, HTN, and DM. She was given breathing treatments (albuterol and Atrovent) and other supportive therapy. During her hospitalization, her CK went from 452 to 758 U/L (ref. range, 26–140 U/L), and at one point her CKMB was 7.6% (<5%). These results led to the diagnosis of subendocardial MI, which was thought to have triggered her CHF. Additional analyses during her hospitalization indicated a gradual decline in renal function, and on the day of discharge her BUN was 65 mg/dL (5–25 mg/dL) and serum creatinine was 3.8 mg/dL (0.8–1.2 mg/dL). Her discharge diagnosis was CHF, status postsubendocardial MI, HTN, DM, and renal failure. Her discharge medications were Vasotec, insulin, aspirin, Pepcid, and a Proventil (albuterol) inhaler.

Her admission urinalysis was significant for blood large; protein >300 mg/dL; leukocyte esterase small; appearance hazy; WBCs/HPF TNTC; RBCs/HPF TNTC; bacteria/HPF few; casts/LPF rare mixed WBC/RTE, 1–5 WBC, 10–20 granular; many glitter cells. C&S on the urine indicated 50,000–100,000 CFU/mL coag-positive *Staphylococcus*. The urine sediment for this case is illustrated in Figures 10-45 and 10-46.

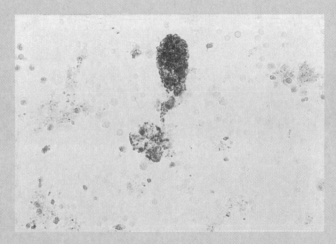

FIGURE 10-45 Granular cast with mixed cellular background. Urine sediment; SM stain; ×200.

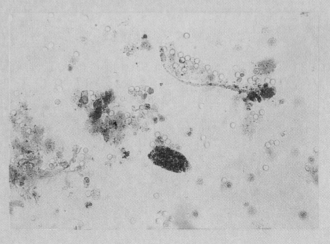

FIGURE 10-46 Granular cast with mixed cellular background. Urine sediment; SM stain; ×200.

continued

CASE STUDY 10-12

This patient, a 46-year-old woman, presented in the ER with severe left flank pain (lower quadrant). In her medical history, she indicated that she had been passing renal stones (both left and right) since the age of 14 years. Her previous medical history also included multiple ureterotomies (left and right) to remove renal stones. While in the ER facility, she passed a renal stone and this resolved the pain. After the stone passed, an IVP was carried out that revealed left hydronephrosis and obstruction, although no definite radiopaque calculus was observed.

The urinalysis was significant for blood large; protein 30 mg/dL; leukocyte esterase small; appearance cloudy; WBCs 0–2/HPF; RBCs 50–100/HPF; casts 5–10 granular/LPF; occasional crystals resembling cystine. The appearance of the sediment for this urine specimen, notable for the cystine crystals, is shown in Figures 10-47 to 10-50. The urine was tested with the cyanide-nitroprusside procedure resulting in a deep magenta color, a positive result for cystine.[17] No previous medical records on this patient were available to determine if any of the previous stones she had passed had ever been analyzed. However, the evidence strongly supported cystinuria.

Final diagnosis was NL with renal colic, left ureteral obstruction, and left hydronephrosis. At discharge she was advised to increase fluid intake, to return to the ER if she experienced worsening pain, or nausea, vomiting, or fever, and to keep her appointment with the urology clinic. The appearance of the urine sediment is illustrated in Figures 10-47 to 10-50.

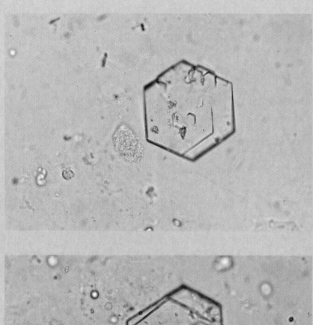

FIGURE 10-47 WBCs; squamous and transitional epithelials. Urine sediment; SM stain; ×400.

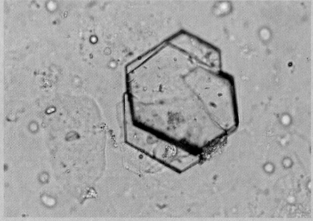

FIGURE 10-48 Cystine crystal. Urine sediment; ×200.

continued

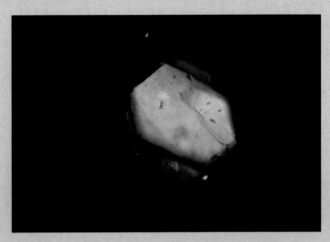

FIGURE 10-49 Cystine crystal; POL. Note that with polarized light only the thicker portion of the crystal is birefringent. Urine sediment; ×200.

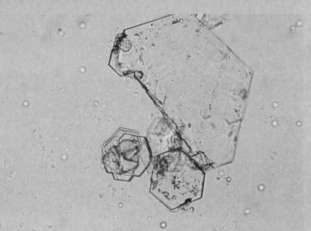

FIGURE 10-50 Cystine crystals. Urine sediment; ×100.

CASE STUDY 10-13

Presenting in the ER, this 38-year-old woman complained of right flank pain for the previous 3 days, together with a burning sensation on urination, and fever, chills, and nausea. She had been seen 6 days previously, diagnosed with UTI, and started on Bactrim. She returned to the ER because her symptoms were getting worse even though she had taken the medication. The assessment for this patient was pyelonephritis, renal lithiasis, hyperpyrexia, and dehydration.

Urinalysis was significant for: blood large; protein trace; leukocyte esterase trace; WBCs 5–10/HPF; RBCs TNTC/HPF; bacteria few; casts 0–1 granular/LPF. C&S on the urine resulted in several species, no significant growth. A sonogram of the right kidney indicated a small parenchymal calculus in the lower midzone; no stones were seen in the left kidney, and there was no evidence of either right or left hydronephrosis. Perhaps the Bactrim wiped out the bacteria, resulting in a negative C&S.

The appearance of the urine sediment is illustrated in Figures 10-51 to 10-54.

continued

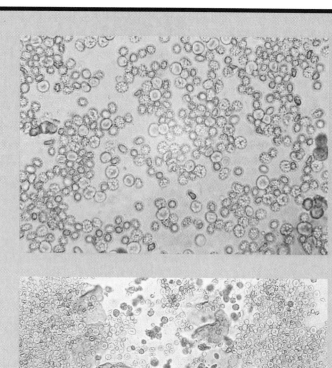

FIGURE 10-51 RBCs, some crenated. Urine sediment; SM stain; ×400.

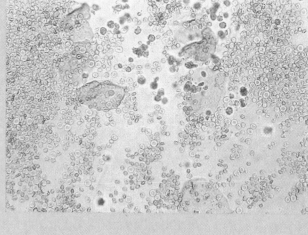

FIGURE 10-52 RBCs and mixed celular background. Urine sediment; SM stain; ×200.

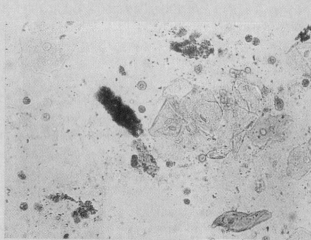

FIGURE 10-53 Granular cast with mixed cellular background. Urine sediment; toluidine blue stain; ×200.

continued

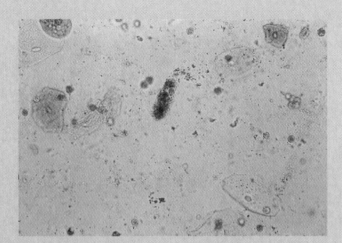

FIGURE 10-54 Mixed cellular/granular cast; mixed cellular background. Urine sediment; toluidine blue stain; ×200.

CASE STUDY 10-14

With a medical history of acute urinary retention, prostatic hypertrophy, urinary frequency, and frequent UTIs, this 73-year-old man was admitted because a previous examination had indicated a large mass in the prostate. The intent was to R/O prostate carcinoma versus bladder tumor. He complained of postvoid fullness and the feeling that he needed to urinate every 10 to 15 minutes.

A urine specimen was obtained by catheterization and the urinalysis was significant for blood moderate; leukocyte esterase trace; WBCs/HPF 2–5; RBCs/HPF 10–20; epithelials/HPF few squamous, rare renal. A C&S on the urine was negative. The urine sediment is illustrated in Figure 10-55 and shows transitional epithelial cells dislodged because of the catheterization.

A suprapubic total prostatectomy (for benign prostatic hypertrophy) was performed. He tolerated the procedure well and remained at bed rest for the postoperative period. He was afebrile at the time of discharge and was given Bactrim DS for any possible UTI and Tylenol with codeine for pain. He was fitted with a flushing Foley catheter and instructed how to drain his bladder and change the Foley bag until the entire unit was removed in the urology clinic during follow-up.

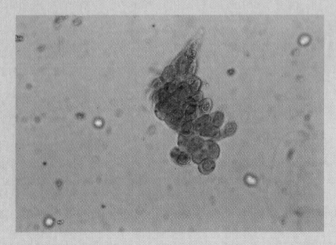

FIGURE 10-55 Group of transitional epithelial cells. Urine sediment; SM stain; ×400.

continued

CASE STUDY 10-15

After more than a week of fever and dysuria, this 22-year-old woman was seen in the ER because her condition had worsened to include extreme right flank pain and tenderness as well as bladder tenderness. She denied any nausea, vomiting, or diarrhea. She had also been coughing for about 5 days and had pain in her lower chest. Her admission diagnosis was right-sided pyelonephritis and possible septicemia.

After specimens for blood cultures were obtained, some morphine was administered for pain, and IV medications were started: Toradol (analgesic) and Rocephin (ceftriaxone sodium, broad-spectrum antibiotic).

Her admission urinalysis was significant for glucose 100 mg/dL; protein trace; nitrite negative; leukocyte esterase small; WBCs TNTC/HPF; RBCs rare/HPF; epithelial 4+/HPF; bacteria few/HPF. C&S on the urine demonstrated a colony count of greater than 100,000 CFU/ML of E. *coli*. Blood cultures were all negative. The appearance of the urinary sediment on admission is shown in Figure 10-56.

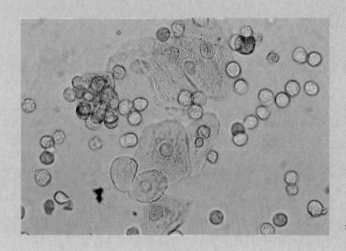

FIGURE 10-56 Cystine crystal. Urine sediment; ×200.

Case Histories and Study Questions

CASE HISTORY 10-1

A 20-year-old woman, having had no prenatal care, delivered a term baby at home 10 minutes before the arrival of an ambulance. She had a history of drug abuse, and on admission (with her newborn), her urine was positive for cocaine, although she denied using drugs during her pregnancy. C&S on the urine was negative. She was discharged home with her baby in due time and was warned about breast-feeding her baby while using drugs. She indicated she planned to bottle feed.

The results of the patient's urinalysis (catheter) on admission were glucose mg/dl negative; bilirubin negative; ketones 15 mg/dl; specific gravity 1.020; blood moderate;

continued

ph 6.0; protein 100 mg/dl; urobilinogen EU/dl 0.2; nitrite negative; leukocyte esterase small; color dark yellow; appearance slightly hazy; WBCs 20-50/HPF; RBCs 20-50/HPF; epithelial cells few squamous, rare RTE/HPF; bacteria few/HPF; and mucus moderate. The appearance of the urin sediment is shown in Figures 10-57 to 10-59

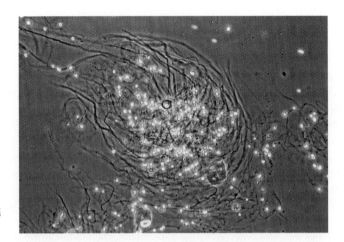

FIGURE 10-57 Urine sediment; SM stain/phase contrast; ×100.

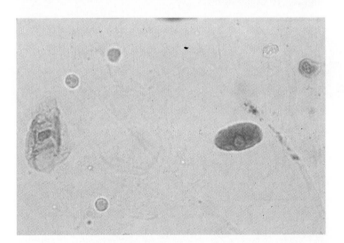

FIGURE 10-58 Urine sediment; SM stain; ×400.

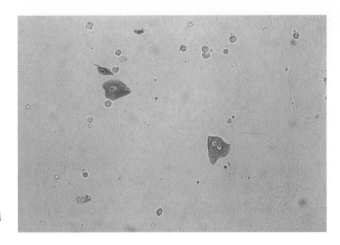

FIGURE 10-59 Urine sediment; SM stain; ×200.

continued

Study Questions for Case History 10-1

1. What aspects of the urinalysis do you find significant?
2. What pathophysiologic aspects of this case are illustrated in the urine sediment (Figs. 10-57 to 10-59)?

CASE HISTORY 10-2

As a referral from the family practice clinic, a 54-year-old woman was seen in the outpatient clinic for a routine urinalysis and to receive a routine Myochrysine (gold sodium thiomalate) injection for her RA. The patient's history was significant for thyroid CA 26 years ago, RA, COPD, and SLE 10 years ago. She also had fairly frequent panic attacks 2° to depression, for which she has been taking Zoloft (sertraline hydrochloride). The Myochrysine shots are maintenance therapy (indefinitely) for RA, given IM, 25 to 50 mg at 3- to 4-week intervals. Myochrysine side effects for the genitourinary tract include proteinuria (albuminuria), NS, nephritis, and ATN.

The results of the patient's urinalysis were glucose mg/dL negative; bilirubin small; ketones mg/dL trace; specific gravity 1.020; blood negative; pH 5.5; protein 30 mg/dL; urobilinogen EU/dL 0.2; nitrite negative; leukocyte esterase small; color amber; WBCs 10–20/HPF; RBCs 0–2/HPF; epithelials/HPF 1+ renal, few squamous, few transitional cells; bacteria 1+; casts/LPF, 3–10 hyaline, 0–1 granular, 0–1 resembling RTEs; Ictotest negative; mucus 2+. The types of formed elements seen in her urine sediment are illustrated in Figures 10-60 to 10-63.

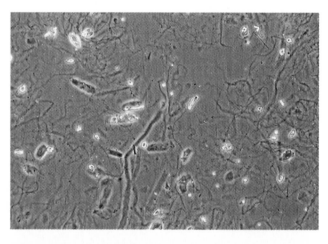

FIGURE 10-60 Urine sediment; SM stain/phase contrast; ×100.

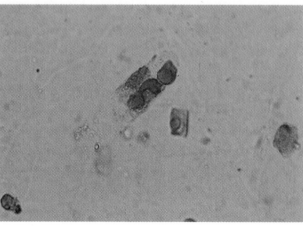

FIGURE 10-61 Urine sediment; SM stain; ×400.

continued

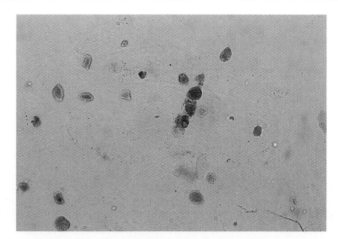

FIGURE 10-62 Urine sediment; SM stain; ×200.

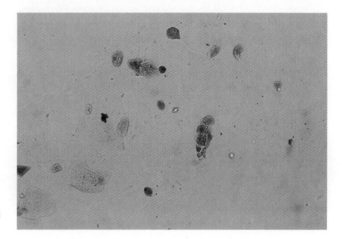

FIGURE 10-63 Urine sediment; SM stain; ×200.

Study Questions for Case History 10-2

1. What aspects of the urinalysis do you find significant?
2. What pathophysiologic aspects of this case are illustrated in the urine sediment (Figs. 10-60 to 10-63)?

CASE HISTORY 10-3

This 12-year-old girl, experiencing dysuria and right flank pain for the previous 3 days, was brought into the ER by her mother. The results of the patient's urinalysis were glucose mg/dL negative; bilirubin negative; ketones mg/dL negative; specific gravity 1.020; blood moderate; pH 6.0; protein mg/dL 30; urobilin 0.2; nitrite positive; leukocyte esterase small; color yellow; appearance hazy; WBCs TNTC/HPF; RBCs TNTC/HPF; epithelial cells/HPF 4+; bacteria 4+/HPF. A C&S was requested on the urine, and the report was *Klebsiella pneumoniae*, colony count greater than 100,000 CFU/mL. The appearance of the urinary sediment is shown in Figures 10-64 and 10-65.

Study Questions for Case History 10-2

1. What aspects of the urinalysis do you find significant?
2. What pathophysiologic aspects of the is case are illustrated by the urine sediment (Figs. 10-64 and 10-65)?
3. What diagnosis would you assign to this case?

continued

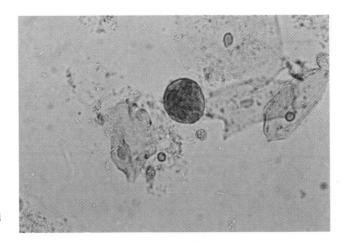

FIGURE 10-64 Urine sediment; SM stain; ×400.

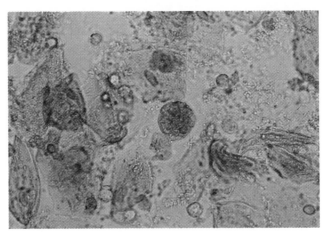

FIGURE 10-65 Urine sediment; SM stain; ×400.

CASE HISTORY 10-4

The patient, a 25-year-old woman, came to the ER for treatment after a 10-day period of lung congestion and coughing, intermittent fever (no nausea, vomiting, or chills), dysuria, hematuria, and urinary frequency and urgency, The urinalysis results were: glucose mg/dL negative; bilirubin negative; ketone mg/dL negative; specific gravity 1.005; blood negative; pH 5.0; protein mg/dL negative; urobilinogen EU/dL 0.2; nitrite negative; leukocyte esterase small; color yellow; WBCs/HPF 20–50 with a few clumps;

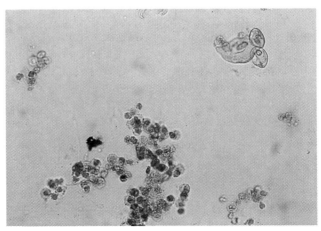

FIGURE 10-66 Urine sediment; SM stain; ×200.

continued

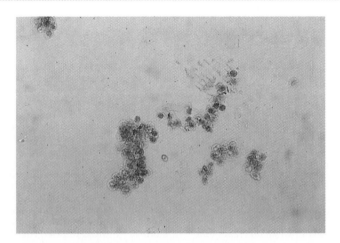

FIGURE 10-67 Urine sediment; SM stain; ×200.

RBCs/HPF negative; epithelial cells/HPF few; bacteria/HPF few. A C&S on the urine resulted in 50,000–100,000 CFU/mL of E. *coli.* The appearance of the urine sediment is shown in Figures 10-66 and 10-67.

Study Questions for Case History 10-4

1. What aspects of the urinalysis do you find significant?
2. What pathophysiologic aspects of this case are illustrated by the urine sediment (Figs. 10-66 and 10-67)?
3. What diagnosis would you assign to this case?

REFERENCES

1. Ballermann BJ, Levenson DJ, Brenner BM. Renin, angiotensin, kinins, prostaglandins, and leukotrienes. In: Brenner BM, Rector FC, eds. *The kidney.* 3rd ed. Philadelphia: WB Saunders (Ardmore Medical Books), 1986:281–340.
2. Bastl CP, Rudnick MR, Narins RG. Assessment of renal function: Characteristics of the functional and organic forms of acute renal failure. In: Seldin DW, Giebisch G, eds. *The kidney.* New York: Raven Press, 1985:1819–1836.
3. Berkow R, ed. *The Merck manual of diagnosis and therapy.* 14th ed. Rahway, NJ: Merck & Company Publications, 1982.
4. Berkow R, ed. *The Merck manual of diagnosis and therapy.* 16th ed. Rahway, NJ: Merck & Company Publications, 1992.
5. Brunzel NA. *Fundamentals of urine and body fluid analysis.* Philadelphia: WB Saunders, 1994.
6. Coe FL. Clinical and laboratory assessment of the patient with renal disease. In: Brenner BM, Rector FC, eds. *The kidney.* 3rd ed. Philadelphia: WB Saunders (Ardmore Medical Books), 1986:703–734.
7. Cotran RS, Kumar V, Robbins SL. *Robbins pathologic basis of disease.* 5th ed. Philadelphia: WB Saunders, 1994.
8. Crawford JM. The liver and the biliary tract. In: Cotran RS, Kumar V, Robbins SL, eds. *Robbins pathologic basis of disease.* 5th ed. Philadelphia: WB Saunders, 1994.
9. Cuppage FE, Chonko AM. Urate and uric acid nephropathy, cystinosis, and oxalosis. In: Tisher CC, Brenner BM, eds. *Renal pathology.* Philadelphia: JB Lippincott, 1989.
10. Emmett M, Seldin DW. Clinical syndromes of metabolic acidosis and metabolic alkalosis. In: Seldin DW, Giebisch G, eds. *The kidney.* New York: Raven Press, 1985:1567–1639.
11. Graff L. *A handbook of routine urinalysis,* Philadelphia: JB Lippincott, 1982.
12. Labbe RF. Porphyrins. In: Anderson SD, Cockayne S. *Clinical chemistry.* Philadelphia: WB Saunders, 1993:337–350.
13. Ravel R. *Clinical laboratory medicine.* St. Louis: Mosby, 1995.
14. Rodwell VW. Catabolism of proteins and of amino acid nitrogen. In: Murray RK, Granner DK, Mayes PA, Rodwell VW, eds. *Harper's biochemistry.* Norwalk, CT: Appleton & Lange, 1993.
15. Rose BD, Rennke HG. *Renal pathophysiology.* Baltimore: Williams & Wilkins, 1994.
16. Ross DL, Neely AE. *Textbook of urinalysis and body fluids.* Norwalk, CT: Appleton-Century-Crofts, 1983.
17. Sacks DB. Carbohydrates. In: Burtis CA, Ashwood ER, eds. *Tietz textbook of clinical chemistry.* 2nd ed. Philadelphia: WB Saunders, 1994.
18. Schofield D, Cotran RS. Diseases of infancy and childhood. In: Cotran RS, Kumar V, Robbins SL, eds. *Robbins pathologic basis of disease.* 5th ed. Philadelphia: WB Saunders, 1994.
19. Shayman JA, ed. *Renal pathophysiology.* Philadelphia: JB Lippincott, 1995.
20. Silverman LM, Christenson RH. Amino acids and proteins. In: Burtis CA, Ashwood ER, eds. *Tietz textbook of clinical chemistry.* 2nd ed. Philadelphia: WB Saunders, 1994.
21. Silverman LM, Christenson RH. Amino acids and proteins. In: Burtis CA, Ashwood ER, eds. *Tietz fundamentals of clinical chemistry.* 4th ed. Philadelphia: WB Saunders, 1996.
22. Strasinger SK. *Urinalysis and body fluids.* 3rd ed. Philadelphia: FA Davis, 1994.
23. Woo J, Henry JB. Metabolic intermediates and inorganic ions. In: Henry JB, ed. *Clinical diagnosis and management by laboratory methods.* 19th ed. Philadelphia: WB Saunders, 1996.

21. Silverman LM, Christenson RH. Amino acids and proteins. In: Burtis CA, Ashwood ER, eds. *Tietz fundamentals of clinical chemistry*. 4th ed. Philadelphia: WB Saunders, 1996.
22. Strasinger SK. *Urinalysis and body fluids*. 3rd ed. Philadelphia: FA Davis, 1994.
23. Woo J, Henry JB. Metabolic intermediates and inorganic ions. In: Henry JB, ed. *Clinical diagnosis and management by laboratory methods*. 19th ed. Philadelphia: WB Saunders, 1996.

BIBLIOGRAPHY

Anderson SC. Amino acid metabolism and related disorders. In: Anderson SD, Cockayne S, eds. *Clinical chemistry*. Philadelphia: WB Saunders, 1993:210–218.
Bennington JL, ed. *Saunders dictionary and encyclopedia of laboratory medicine and technology*. Philadelphia: WB Saunders, 1984.
Cotran RS, Rubin RH, Tolkoff-Rubin NE. Tubulointerstitial diseases. In: Brenner BM, Rector FC, eds. *The kidney*. 3rd ed. Philadelphia: WB Saunders (Ardmore Medical Books), 1986: 1143–1173.
DeFronzo RA, Thier SO. Inherited disorders of renal tubule function. In: Brenner BM, Rector FC, eds. *The kidney*. 3rd ed. Philadelphia: WB Saunders (Ardmore Medical Books), 1986: 1297–1339.
First MR. Renal function. In: Kaplan LA, Pesce AJ, eds. *Clinical chemistry*. 3rd ed. St. Louis: CV Mosby, 1996:484–504.
Geschickter CF, Antonovych TT. *The kidney in health and disease*. Philadelphia: JB Lippincott, 1971.
Henry JB, Lauzon RB, Schumann GB. Basic examination of urine. In: Henry JB, ed. *Clinical diagnosis and management by laboratory methods*. 19th ed. Philadelphia: WB Saunders, 1996: 411–456.
Jennette JC, Mandal AK. Kidney disorders in systemic diseases. In: Mandal AK, Jennette JC, eds. *Diagnosis and management of renal disease and hypertension*. Philadelphia: Lea & Febiger, 1988:295–335.
Mayes PA. The pentose phosphate pathway and other pathways of hexose metabolism. In: Murray RK, Granner DK, Mayes PA, Rodwell VW, eds. *Harper's biochemistry*. 24th ed. Stamford, CT: Appleton & Lange, 1996:205–215.
Morrison G, Geheb MA, Earley LE. Chronic renal failure. In: Seldin DW, Giebisch G, eds. *The kidney*. New York: Raven Press, 1985:1901–1943.
Nuttall KL. Porphyrins and disorders of porphyrin metabolism. In: Burtis CA, Ashwood ER, eds. *Tietz fundamentals of clinical chemistry*. 4th ed. Philadelphia: WB Saunders, 1996.
Threatte GA, Henry JB. Carbohydrates. In: Henry JB, ed. *Clinical diagnosis and management by laboratory methods*. 19th ed. Philadelphia: WB Saunders, 1996.
Vander AJ, Sherman JH, Luciano DS. *Human physiology*. New York: McGraw-Hill, 1994.

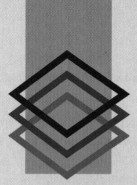

11

Cerebrospinal Fluid Analysis

ABBREVIATIONS USED IN THIS CHAPTER

ALL = acute lymphocytic leukemia

AZT = azidothymidine

CIE = counterimmunoelectrophoresis

CK = creatine kinase

CKBB = creatine kinase isoenzyme BB

CNS = central nervous system

C&S = culture and sensitivity

CSF = cerebrospinal fluid

CT = computed tomography

EEG = electroencephalogram

ER = emergency room

FTA-ABS = fluorescent treponemal antibody absorption test

HIV = human immunodeficiency virus

ICU = intensive care unit

IRIS = international remote imaging systems

LDH = lactate dehydrogenase

LP = lumbar puncture

MBP = myelin basic protein

R/O = rule out

RBC = red blood cell

SSA = sulfosalicylic acid

TCA = trichloroacetic acid

VDRL = Venereal Disease Research Laboratory

VP = ventriculoperitoneal

WBC = white blood cell

Introductory Case Study

This patient, a 3-year-old girl, had been taken to a rural clinic because of fever and vomiting during the previous 2 days. There were no signs of rhinorrhea, dysuria, or frequency, but there were indications of photophobia. Her temperature was 102°F, pulse 132, respirations 24, and blood pressure 110/70. She appeared lethargic and showed signs of malaise.

While in the clinic she had a tonic–clonic seizure that was treated with Ativan. She was then transported to the hospital by ambulance, and en route had another seizure that was treated with Diazepam. She was admitted with the diagnosis of acute hyperpyrexia R/O bacterial meningitis.

Results of CSF analysis (tube 3) were color white; appearance cloudy; supernatant colorless and clear; WBCs 3330/mm³; RBCs/mm³ 120; lymphocytes 3%; monocytes 3%; neutrophils 93%; mononuclear phagocytes 1%. The CSF Cytospin preparation (Figs. 11-1 and 11-2) demonstrates inflammatory cells and streptoccocal-like bacteria. The Gram stain preparation (Fig. 11-3) shows gram-positive cocci. The C&S on this specimen was positive for *Streptococcus pneumoniae* resistant to penicillin but sensitive to vancomycin. After appropriate treatment and recovery (Fig. 11-4), the child was discharged home in stable condition.

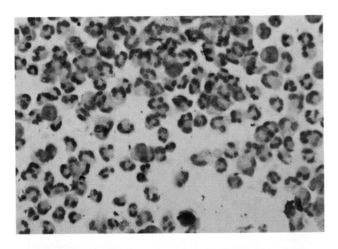

FIGURE 11-1 Cytospin preparation of CSF showing neutrophilic pleocytosis and bacteria resembling *Streptococcus*. Wright's stain: ×400.

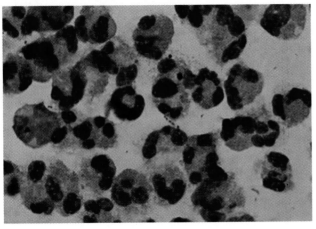

FIGURE 11-2 Same field of view as for Figure 11-1, but with higher magnification. Wright's stain: ×1000.

Continued

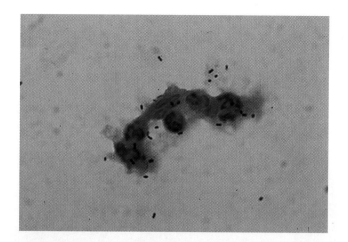

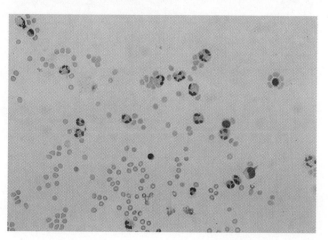

FIGURE 11-3 Direct Gram stain on CSF showing gram-positive cocci; ×1000.

FIGURE 11-4 Cytospin preparation of CSF after patient's recovery from streptococcal meningitis. Wright's stain; ×200.

Cerebrospinal Fluid Formation, Circulation, Composition

Three membranes (the meninges) envelop the brain and spinal cord. The outer membrane is the dura mater, the middle layer is the arachnoid mater, and the inner membrane is the pia mater, which adheres to the surface of the neural tissue. Cerebrospinal fluid (CSF) circulates in the space between the arachnoid and the pia mater and bathes the brain and spinal cord (Fig. 11-5). About 70% of the CSF is formed by the ventricular choroid plexuses (tufts of capillary blood vessels in the cerebral ventricles) by a combined process of active secretion and ultrafiltration from plasma.[5] The other 30% is formed at other sites, including the ependymal lining of the ventricles and the cerebral/subarachnoid space.

The total CSF volume is 90 to 150 mL in adults and 10 to 60 mL in neonates. The rate of formation in adults is about 500 mL/day or 20 mL/hour. The CSF acts as a protective, fluid cushion around the brain and helps prevent injury to the soft cerebral substance from forces of inertia and gravity. Variations in the amount of CSF permit the brain volume to remain undisturbed when the volume of the cerebral vessels changes, and thus the CSF also functions in volume regulation. Other functions of the CSF include the exchange of nutrients and metabolic wastes between the blood and the brain as well as the lubrication of the central nervous system (CNS).

The CSF exits from the ventricles through the foramina (see Fig. 11-5) and circulates over the cerebral hemispheres as well as downward over the spinal cord and nerve roots. Circulation of the CSF is very slow, allowing long contact with the CNS cells; this may account for the lower concentration of some substances in the CSF, such as glucose, compared with concentrations in plasma. The CSF is resorbed through the arachnoid villi in dural sinuses and also at dural reflections over cranial and spinal nerves. The arachnoid

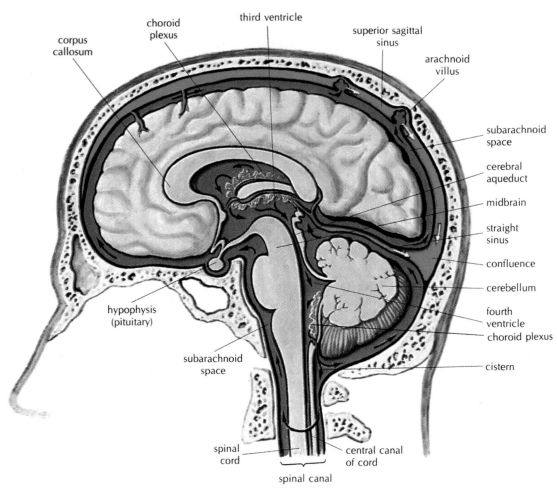

FIGURE 11-5 Flow of CSF from choroid plexuses back to the blood in dural sinuses is shown by the black arrows; flow of blood is shown by the white arrows. Flow of CSF from choroid plexuses back to blood in venous sinuses is shown by the black arrows; flow of blood is shown by the white arrows. (From Memmler RL, Cohen BJ, Wood KL. *The human body in health and disease*. 8th ed. Philadelphia: Lippincott-Raven Publishers, 1992.)

villi are herniations of arachnoid membrane into the lumen of the dural sinuses and represent an interface between blood and CSF.

The composition of the CSF is complex. Compared with their concentration in plasma, the concentration of some substances in the CSF is increased; for other substances, the concentration is decreased (Table 11-1). Even when cerebral metabolism is normal, alterations in the plasma are reflected in the CSF. Therefore, the concentration of substances in the CSF should always be compared with their concentration in the plasma.

Water, chloride, and CO_2 diffuse rapidly across the blood–CSF barrier, which is composed of the epithelium of the choroid plexuses and the endothelium of all capillaries in contact with the CSF. Lipid-soluble drugs (including anesthetics and alcohol) diffuse from plasma to the CSF in proportion to their lipid solubility. Glucose, urea, and creatinine diffuse freely but re-

quire several hours for equilibration. Substances such as penicillin and streptomycin that do not normally enter the CSF from the plasma may do so with membrane inflammation. Proteins diffuse slowly across the concentration gradient from plasma to CSF, and diffusion rates decrease with increasing molecular size.

Specimen Collection

The indications for performing a lumbar puncture can be divided into four major categories of disease: meningeal infection, subarachnoid hemorrhage, CNS malignancy, and demyelinating diseases. The absolute contraindication to performing a spinal puncture is infection at the puncture site, when a puncture may spread the infection into the meninges.[5] Bacteremia should not be considered a contraindication to lumbar

TABLE 11-1
Reference Values for Lumbar Cerebrospinal Fluid in Adults

	Conventional Units	SI Units
Protein	15–45 mg/dL	0.15–0.45 g/L
Prealbumin	2–7%	
Albumin	56–76%	
α_1-globulin	2–7%	
α_2-globulin	4–12%	
β-globulin	8–18%	
γ-globulin	3–12%	
Electrolytes		
Osmolality	280–300 mOsm/L	280–300 mmol/L
Sodium	135–150 mEq/L	135–150 mmol/L
Potassium	2.6–3.0 mEq/L	2.6–3.0 mmol/L
Chloride	115–130 mEq/L	115–130 mmol/L
Carbon dioxide content	20–25 mEq/L	20–25 mmol/L
Calcium	2.0–2.8 mEq/L	1.00–1.40 mmol/L
Magnesium	2.4–3.0 mEq/L	1.2–1.5 mmol/L
Lactate	10–22 mg/dL	1.1–2.4 mmol/L
pH		
Lumbar fluid	7.28–7.32	
Cisternal fluid	7.32–7.34	
pco_2		
Lumbar fluid	44–50 mm Hg	
Cisternal fluid	40–46 mm Hg	
po_2	40–44 mm Hg	
Other constituents		
Ammonia	10–35 μg/dL	5–20 μmol/L
Glutamine	5–20 mg/dL	0.3–1.4 mmol/L
Creatinine	0.6–1.2 mg/dL	50–110 μmol/L
Glucose	50–80 mg/dL	2.8–4.4 mmol/L
Iron	1–2 μg/dL	0.2–0.4 μmol/L
Phosphorus	1.2–2.0 mg/dL	0.4–0.6 mmol/L
Total lipid	1–2 mg/dL	0.01–0.02 g/L
Urea	6–16 mg/dL	3.0–6.5 mmol/L
Urate	0.5–3.0 mg/dL	30–180 μmol/L
Zinc	2–6 μg/dL	0.3–0.9 μmol/L

(From Krieg AF, Kjeldsberg CR. Cerebrospinal fluid and other body fluids. In: Henry JB, ed. P *Clinical diagnosis and management by laboratory methods.* 18th ed. Philadelphia: WB Saunders Company, 1991: 445–473.)

far down. For small children and infants, the interspace at L4–L5 is used because, for them, the cord may extend as low as L3–L4.

The procedure is performed aseptically after thorough cleansing of the patient's skin and application of a local anesthetic. After the needle has penetrated the dura mater and before collection of the specimens, the CSF pressure is measured by allowing the fluid to rise in a sterile, graduated manometer tube attached to the spinal needle. If opening pressure is normal, and if there is no marked fall in pressure when 1 to 2 mL of fluid is collected, then 10 to 20 mL of CSF may be slowly removed.

Usually, three specimens are collected in sequentially numbered, sterile tubes. Tests performed on the various tubes depend on laboratory protocol or the attending physician's request. One possible protocol would be chemistry/serology on tube 1; microbiology on tube 2; and cell count/differential on tube 3. A fourth tube may sometimes be collected to be stored in the refrigerator and observed for the formation of a "pellicle" when tubercular meningitis is suspected.

As with most laboratory procedures, examination of CSF is most useful when the results are correlated with the clinical findings, radiographic studies, and other laboratory studies (Table 11-2). Routinely, only a few tests need to be done; they should include the cell count, the differential count, the glucose level, and the protein level. Kjeldsberg and Knight further recom-

TABLE 11-2
Laboratory Tests on Cerebrospinal Fluid (CSF)

Routine
Opening CSF pressure
Cell count (total and differential)
Glucose (CSF/plasma ratio)
Protein

When Indicated
Cultures (bacteria, fungi, viruses, *Mycobacterium tuberculosis*)
Stains (Gram' stain, acid-fast stain)
Fungal and bacterial antigens
Cytology
Protein electrophoresis
VDRL test for syphilis
Myelin basic protein
Fibrin-derivative D-dimer

VDRL, Venereal Disease Research Laboratory.

(From Kjeldsberg CR, Knight JA. *Body fluids.* 3rd ed. Chicago: ASCP Press, 1993.)

puncture because an examination of the CSF can help rule out concurrent meningitis.

A relative contraindication is any sign of increased intracranial pressure from a suspected mass lesion. To reduce the risk of brain herniation in such instances, less invasive procedures such as a computed tomography (CT) scan or magnetic resonance imaging may be done before a decision is made to carry out lumbar puncture.

To avoid damage to the spinal cord in adults, the physician uses the interspace between L3 and L4 for a lumbar puncture because the cord does not extend that mend that if results for the opening pressure, CSF protein, cell count, and Cytospin differential are normal, no further studies need to be done in most instances.[5]

Examination

Physical Characteristics and Gross Examination

Table 11-3 summarizes the gross or physical examination of CSF. Normal CSF is crystal clear and colorless, with a viscosity about like water. Turbidity may be observed due to the presence of body cells, microorganisms, or flecks of protein. A traumatic tap introduces blood into the specimens that must be differentiated from blood resulting from a subarachnoid hemor-

rhage. In the case of a traumatic tap, there should be significant clearing of blood between the first and last tubes.

Subarachnoid bleeding results in the appearance of xanthochromia, which is a pink, orange, or yellowish discoloration of CSF supernatant after centrifugation. Within 1 to 4 hours after a subarachnoid hemorrhage, the CSF supernatant is pale pink—pale orange because of the appearance of oxyhemoglobin in the fluid. This peaks at about 24 to 36 hours and gradually disappears within 4 to 8 days.

About 12 hours after a subarachnoid hemorrhage, the CSF begins to show yellow xanthochromia because of the appearance of bilirubin. This peaks at about 2 to 4 days and gradually disappears during the next 2 to 4 weeks. Further, subarachnoid bleeding results in erythrophagocytosis, which is observed on

---

TABLE 11-3
Clinical Significance of Cerebrospinal Fluid Gross Appearance

Gross Appearance	Cause	Major Significance
Crystal clear		Normal
Smoky	RBCs	Hemorrhage (early, before RBC lysis)
		Traumatic tap
Cloudy, turbid	WBCs	Meningitis
	Microorganisms	Meningitis
	Protein	Disorders that affect blood–brain barrier
		Production of IgG within central nervous system
Fatty emulsion	Subdural fat	Aspirated during lumbar puncture
Clot and pedicle formation	Increased fibrinogen	Traumatic tap
		Subarachnoid block (Froin's syndrome)
		Suppurative meningitis
		Tuberculous meningitis
Bloody	RBCs	Hemorrhage
Xanthochromic	Hemoglobin	Old hemorrhage
		Lysed cells from traumatic tap
	Bilirubin	RBC breakdown
		Elevated serum bilirubin
	Merthiolate	Contamination
	Carotene	Increased serum levels (dietary)
	Protein	See above
	Melanin	Meningeal malignant melanoma
Oily	X-ray material	None
Greenish tinge	Myeloperoxidase	Purulent fluid
Viscous	Capsular polysaccharide	Cryptococcosis
	Mucus	Metastatic mucin-producing carcinomas
	Liquid nucleus pulposus	Needle injury to annulus fibrosus
Fat globules	Fat	Fat embolism

RBCs, red blood cells; WBCs, white blood cells.
(From Kjeldsberg CR, Knight JA. *Body fluids*. 3rd ed. Chicago: ASCP Press, 1993.)

microscopic examination. With some normal, premature infants (and even with some full-term infants), the CSF is xanthochromic because of immaturity of the blood–CSF barrier combined with increased bilirubin in the blood.

Clotting does not usually occur because the CSF contains so little fibrinogen. Clotting may be associated with a traumatic tap (and red clot), neurosyphilis, and tubercular meningitis (when a pellicle forms after refrigeration of the specimen).

Chemical Analyses

Krieg and Kjeldsberg[6] provide an excellent table of reference values for lumbar CSF in adults (see Table 11-1).

PROTEIN

Total Protein

Most serum proteins are present in the CSF (Table 11-4). Methods for determining total protein in CSF include turbidimetric methods (SSA or TCA), modified biuret methods, dye-binding methods, and immunochemical methods.

CSF total protein varies with age and with the site from which the specimen was obtained. For example, CSF obtained from the lumbar region has more total protein than a specimen obtained from the ventricles.

TABLE 11-4

Concentrations of Proteins in Plasma and Cerebrospinal Fluid (CSF)

Protein	CSF Concentration (mg/L)	Plasma/CSF Ratio
Prealbumin	17.3	14
Albumin	155.0	236
Transferrin	14.4	142
Ceruloplasmin	1.0	366
IgG	12.3	802
IgA	1.3	1346
α_2-macroglobulin	2.0	1111
Fibrinogen	0.6	4940
IgM	0.6	1167
β-lipoprotein	0.6	6213

Adapted from Felgenhauer K. *Klin Wochenschr* 1974; 52:1158.

(From Krieg AF, Kjeldsberg CR. Cerebrospinal fluid and other body fluids. In Henry JB, ed: *Clinical diagnosis and management by laboratory methods*. 18th ed. Philadelphia: WB Saunders Company, 1991.)

An example of the reference range for total protein in CSF is 15 to 45 mg/dL, and normal values change with age. Neonates have the highest values. Values decrease with age, owing to maturity of the blood–CSF barrier. After age 40 years, the values start increasing again. Conditions associated with increased total protein in CSF are shown in Table 11-5.

Increased protein in lumbar CSF (>65 mg/dL) is an important finding.[6] It is associated with a traumatic tap, which contaminates the CSF with plasma proteins; increased permeability of the blood–CSF barrier (e.g., as with infections, subarachnoid hemorrhage, toxic conditions); decreased reabsorption into the venous blood; and increased CNS synthesis of IgG (e.g., multiple sclerosis and neurosyphilis).

Decreased concentration of protein in lumbar CSF is associated with leakage from a dural tear; removal of a large volume of CSF as in pneumoencaphalography; increased cranial pressure causing increased filtration of CSF through arachnoid granulations of the dural sinuses; and hyperthyroidism.

Albumin and IgG

The CSF/serum albumin ratio may be used to evaluate the blood–CSF barrier:

$$\text{CSF/serum albumin ratio} = \frac{\text{Albumin}_{CSF}\ g/dL}{\text{Albumin}_{serum}\ g/dL}$$

The normal ratio is about 1/230.[6] This ratio is sometimes expressed as the CSF/serum albumin index, with Albumin$_{CSF}$ in milligrams per deciliter and the Albumin$_{serum}$ in grams per deciliter:

$$\text{CSF/serum albumin index} = \frac{\text{Albumin}_{CSF}\ mg/dL}{\text{Albumin}_{serum}\ g/dL}$$

The normal range for this index is about 4 to 8. Values of 9 to 14 are interpreted as slight impairment, values of 15 to 30 as moderate impairment, and values over 30 indicate severe impairment of the blood–CSF barrier. In newborns, the ratio is slightly elevated, falls to adult levels by age 6 months, and then gradually increases after 40 years of age. Increased ratios may be due to a traumatic tap as well as increased permeability of the blood–CSF barrier.[6]

Intrathecal production of IgG may be evaluated with the CSF/serum IgG ratio:

$$\text{CSF/serum IgG ratio} = \frac{\text{IgG}_{CSF}\ g/dL}{\text{IgG}_{serum}\ g/dL}$$

This ratio is normally 1/369. It may also be expressed as the CSF/serum IgG index:

TABLE 11-5
Conditions Associated with Increased Cerebrospinal Fluid (CSF) Total Protein

Condition	Comments
Traumatic tap	Normal pressure; CSF initially streaked with blood, with clearing
Increased permeability of blood–CSF barrier	
Infectious	
Bacterial meningitis	CSF protein 100–500 mg/dL; Gram' stain usually positive
Tuberculous meningitis	CSF protein 50–300 mg/dL; mixed cellular reaction typical
Fungal meningitis	CSF protein 50–300 mg/dL; special stains helpful
Viral meningoencephalitis	CSF protein usually under 100 mg/dL
Noninfectious	
Subarachnoid hemorrhage	Xanthochromia 2–4 hours after onset
Intracerebral hemorrhage	CSF protein 20–200 mg/dL; marked fall in pressure after removing small amount of CSF; xanthochromic fluid in 80%
Cerebral thrombosis	Slightly increased CSF protein in 40% of cases (usually under 100 mg/dL)
Endocrine conditions: diabetic neuropathy, myxedema, hyperadrenalism, hypoparathyroidism	CSF protein 50–150 mg/dL in about 50% in cases
Metabolic conditions; uremia, hypercalcemia, hypercapnia, dehydration	CSF protein slightly elevated (usually under 100 mg/dL)
Toxic conditions: ethanol, isopropanol, heavy metals, phenytoin, phenothiazines	CSF protein slightly elevated in about 40% of cases
Obstruction to circulation of CSF	
Mechanical obstruction (e.g., tumor, abscess)	Rapid fall in pressure on removal of CSF
Loculated effusion of CSF	Repeated taps may show progressive increase in CSF protein
Increased CNS synthesis of IgG and increased permeability of blood–CSF barrier	
Viral meningitis	About 20% of patients have increased CSF IgG
Guillain-Barré syndrome	CSF protein usually 100–400 mg/dL
Collagen diseases (e.g., periarteritis, lupus)	CSF protein usually under 400 mg/dL
Increased CNS synthesis of IgG	
Multiple sclerosis	CSF protein increased in about 40% (usually under 100 mg/dL)
Subacute sclerosing panencephalitis (SSPE)	CSF IgG almost invariably increased
Neurosyphilis	CSF protein usually under 100 mg/dL; about 20% have elevated IgG

(From Krieg AF, Kjeldsberg CR. Cerebrospinal fluid and other body fluids. In Henry JB, ed. *Clinical diagnosis and management by laboratory methods.* 18th ed. Philadelphia: WB Saunders Company, 1991.)

$$\text{CSF/serum IgG index} = \frac{\text{CSF}_{\text{CSF}}\text{ mg/dL}}{\text{IgG}_{\text{serum}}\text{ g/dL}}$$

The normal range for this index is about 3 to 8.

The CSF/serum IgG index may be divided by the CSF/serum albumin index to obtain the CSF IgG index:

$$\text{CSF IgG index} = \frac{\text{IgG}_{\text{CSF}}\text{ mg/dL}}{\text{IgG}_{\text{serum}}\text{ g/dL}} \times \frac{\text{Albumin}_{\text{serum}}\text{ g/dL}}{\text{Albumin}_{\text{CSF}}\text{ mg/dL}}$$

The normal range for this index varies but values exceeding 0.77 suggest increased IgG synthesis. About 90% of multiple sclerosis patients have a CSF IgG index over 0.77, although specificity is estimated to be in the range of 80% to 90% because increased CNS synthesis of IgG occurs in other inflammatory neurologic disorders.[6]

Electrophoresis

Before electrophoresis, the specimen is usually concentrated from 80- to 100-fold by dialysis. Normally there is a prealbumin and an albumin band; the gamma globulin area is decreased by about one half from the normal serum; and the beta area is increased by about twofold.

Oligoclonal banding (two or more discrete bands) in the gamma region of the CSF is observed in about 90% of multiple sclerosis patients. However, such banding has also been observed in other CNS disorders such as subacute sclerosing panencephalitis, neurosyphilis, cryptococcal meningitis, human immunodeficiency virus type I (HIV-I) infection, bacterial and viral meningitis, and Guillain-Barré syndrome. IgM is usually not found in the CSF, but it may be observed with changes in vascular permeability associated with meningitis, tumors, and multiple sclerosis.

Myelin Basic Protein

The presence of myelin basic protein (MBP) in CSF has been correlated with multiple sclerosis in about 90% of cases. Elevations occur during acute exacerbation and return to normal within about 2 weeks after the disease subsides. Levels under 4 ng/mL are usually considered normal, 4 to 8 ng/mL weakly positive, and over 8 ng/mL positive. However, other conditions besides multiple sclerosis are associated with elevated MBP (e.g., head trauma, hypoxia, myelopathy due to systemic lupus erythematosus, and intrathecal chemotherapy).

GLUCOSE

Glucose enters the CSF by both active transport and diffusion. CSF values need to be compared with corresponding values in plasma. Normally, adult CSF glucose is 60% to 70% of the plasma level. Three mechanisms are believed to cause decreased CSF glucose: impaired glucose transport, increased glycolytic activity in the CNS, and glucose utilization by leukocytes and microorganisms.

Using 40 mg/dL as the "normal" CSF glucose concentration, decreased CSF glucose is observed with about 50% to 80% sensitivity in acute or chronic meningitis, which may be bacterial, tuberculous, fungal, amebic, or parasitic. Decreased glucose is also observed in conditions such as systemic hypoglycemia, subarachnoid hemorrhage, neurosyphilis, and neoplasms involving the meninges. Increased CSF glucose does not suggest CNS disease, but is presumptive evidence of elevated plasma glucose.[6]

LACTATE

The primary source of lactate in the CSF is anaerobic metabolism in the CNS; thus, it is largely independent of blood lactate levels. In general, any condition associated with tissue hypoxia of the CNS may cause increased CSF lactate. Conditions associated with increased CSF lactate include cerebral infarct, traumatic brain injury, hypotension, meningitis, cerebral ischemia due to arteriosclerosis, low arterial pO_2, and hydrocephalus.

ENZYMES

Lactate dehydrogenase (LDH) is normally present in CSF, although establishing a reference range is difficult because of the variations in methods used to measure it. Many CNS diseases cause increased CSF LDH, such as ischemic necrosis, meningitis, leukemia, lymphoma, and metastatic carcinoma involving the CNS.[6] LDH isoenzymes may be clinically useful. LDH isoenzymes 4 and 5 predominate in granulocytes, 2 and 3 in lymphocytes, and 1 and 2 in brain tissue. Elevated isoenzymes 4 and 5 are seen in bacterial meningitis as a reflection of granulocyte interactions. Elevated isoenzymes 1, 2, and 3 are seen in viral meningitis, which reflects interaction of the CNS and lymphocytes.

Creatine kinase (CK) is also normally present in the CSF, primarily as the CKBB isoenzyme from brain tissue.

Cell Counts and Microscopic Examination

TOTAL CELL COUNT

The cell counts may be performed in a counting chamber with undiluted CSF. Crystal violet is used by some laboratories to stain the specimen before examination. As noted in Chapter 5, an instrument marketed by International Remote Imaging Systems (IRIS) performs the cell counts on CSF (and other body fluids) electronically. Cell counts on the CSF should be performed promptly because one study suggests that 40% of leukocytes may lyse after 2 hours at room temperature.[2] Specimens should be refrigerated if a delay of more than 1 hour is necessary.

Kjeldsberg and Knight give the values of 0 to 5/μL for normal leukocyte counts in adults.[5] Although no absolute agreement exists on the normal values for leukocyte counts for children, they suggest the following ranges: 0 to 30/μL in children younger than 1 year of age; 0 to 20/μL in children 1 to 4 years of age; and 0 to 10/μL in children 5 years of age to puberty.

Although RBC counts in CSF per se are of limited diagnostic value, they may be used to correct CSF leukocyte counts or the determination of CSF protein when a traumatic tap is suspected. Kjeldsberg and Knight give procedures for these corrections but point out that they are valid only if the cell count and the total protein concentration are determined for the same specimen of CSF.[5] Use of the corrections also assumes that all RBCs present are from the traumatic tap without any contribution from subarachnoid or intracerebral hemorrhage. The correction is limited because of the imprecision of the CSF RBC count.

Cells lining the ventricles (ependymal cells or choroid plexus cells) may occasionally be seen in both normal and abnormal CSF. These cells are more frequently found after a ventricular or cisternal tap, but they are also seen with a lumbar puncture procedure. Ependymal cells may be seen after traumatic brain injury, pneumoencephalography, surgery, myelography, ischemic infarction of the brain, and in children with hydrocephalus and ventricular shunts. These cells are rarely, if ever, seen in "normal" CSF obtained from lumbar puncture in adults. In children, however, they are occasionally seen in CSF when there are no apparent abnormalities.

From a cytologic point of view, it is difficult to differentiate between ependymal and choroid plexus cells in CSF. These cells may occur singly but occur more often in papillary clusters or sheets. The nuclei are round to oval and the size of small lymphocytes, whereas the cytoplasm is moderate to abundant and gray-blue. The nuclear chromatin is delicate and finely granular, with evenly distributed chromatin. Nucleoli are not present. The cytoplasmic borders may contain vacuoles, and occasionally cilia-like protrusions may be present. It is important to be able to recognize these cells because they may be mistaken for malignant cells.

DIFFERENTIAL COUNT

For many years there has been disagreement on whether neutrophils are present normally in CSF. Older literature suggests that even a single neutrophil is abnormal.

The use of a relatively new procedure, cytocentrifugation, has greatly improved the accuracy and preci-

---

TABLE 11-7
Causes for Increased Neutrophils in Cerebrospinal Fluid (CSF)

Meningitis
  Bacterial meningitis
  Early viral meningoencephalitis
  Early tuberculous meningitis
  Early mycotic meningitis
  Amebic encephalomyelitis
Other infections
  Cerebral abscess
  Subdural empyema
After seizures
After CNS* hemorrhage
  Subarachnoid hemorrhage
  Intracerebral hemorrhage
After CNS infarct
Reaction to repeated lumbar puncture
Injection of foreign materials into subarachnoid space (e.g., methotrexate, contrast media)
Metastatic tumor in contact with CSF

* CNS, central nervous system.
(From Krieg AF, Kjeldsberg CR. Cerebrospinal fluid and other body fluids. In Henry JB, ed. *Clinical diagnosis and management by laboratory methods.* 18th ed. Philadelphia: WB Saunders Company, 1991.)

---

sion of CSF differential counts. More recent studies indicate that a few neutrophils may occur in normal CSF (probably contamination from peripheral blood in a traumatic tap), and that up to 7% to 8% neutrophils is within normal limits, although there is no general agreement on an "upper limit of normal".[6] Table 11-6 shows suggested reference intervals for the differential cell count on CSF.

Increased numbers of neutrophils may occur in the conditions summarized in Table 11-7. The percentage of neutrophils often exceeds 60% in the early stages of acute bacterial meningitis, with a sensitivity at this cutoff level of about 90% to 95%. An initial neutrophilia may also be observed in early viral meningoencephalitis, but this usually changes to a lymphocytic response within 2 to 3 days. Other correlations for neutrophilic pleocytosis are indicated in Table 11-7.

Increased numbers of other cells have been reported for the conditions summarized in Table 11-8 (lymphocytes), Table 11-9 (plasma cells), and Table 11-10 (eosinophils). Increased numbers of basophils have little clinical significance. Increased numbers of monocytes are usually seen as part of a "mixed reaction" with neutrophils, lymphocytes, and plasma cells. This mixed reaction is characteristic of tuberculous meningitis, fungal meningitis, chronic bacterial meningitis, rup-

---

TABLE 11-6
Reference Intervals for Cerebrospinal Fluid Differential Counts by Cytocentrifuge

Cell Type	Adults (%)	Neonates (%)
Lymphocytes	62 ± 34	20 ± 18
Monocytes	36 ± 20	72 ± 22
Neutrophils	2 ± 5	3 ± 5
Histocytes	Rare	5 ± 4
Ependymal cells	Rare	Rare
Eosinophils	Rare	Rare

(From Krieg AF, Kjeldsberg CR. Cerebrospinal fluid and other body fluids. In Henry JB, ed. *Clinical diagnosis and management by laboratory methods.* 18th ed. Philadelphia: WB Saunders Company, 1991.)

TABLE 11-8
Causes for Increased Lymphocytes in Cerebrospinal Fluid

Meningitis
  Viral meningitis
  Tuberculous meningitis
  Fungal meningitis
  Syphilitic meningoencephalitis
  Leptospiral meningitis
  Bacterial meningitis due to unusual organisms (e.g.,
    Listeria monocytogenes)
  Parasitic infestations of the CNS (e.g., cysticercosis,
    trichinosis, toxoplasmosis)
  Aseptic meningitis due to septic focus adjacent to
    meninges
Degenerative disorders
  Subacute sclerosing panencephalitis
  Multiple sclerosis
  Encephalopathy due to drug abuse
  Guillan-Barré syndrome
  Acute disseminated encephalomyelitis
Other inflammatory conditions
  Sarcoidosis of meninges
  Polyneuritis
  Periarteritis involving the CNS

* CNS, central nervous system.

(From Krieg AF, Kjeldsberg CR. Cerebrospinal fluid and other body fluids. In Henry JB, ed. *Clinical diagnosis and management by laboratory methods.* 18th ed. Philadelphia: WB Saunders Company, 1991.)

TABLE 11-10
Causes for Eosinophilia in Cerebrospinal Fluid

Parasitic infestations
  Angiostrongylus cantonensis
  Taenia solium (cysticercosis)
  Gnathostoma spinigerum
  Schistosoma sp.
  Paragonimus westermani
  Fasciola hepatica
  Hypoderma bovis (larva migrans)
Fungal infections
  Coccidioides immitis
Rickettsial infections
  Rocky Mountain spotted fever
Other
  Foreign material (myelography)
  Sarcoidosis
  Intracranial shunt

(From Krieg AF, Kjeldsberg CR. Cerebrospinal fluid and other body fluids. In Henry JB, ed. *Clinical diagnosis and management by laboratory methods.* 18th ed. Philadelphia: WB Saunders Company, 1991.)

---

ture of brain abscess, leptospiral meningitis, *Toxoplasma* meningitis, and amebic encephalomyelitis.

With tuberculosis or mycotic meningitis, with foreign substances (e.g., ventricular drains), or CSF lipid derived from CNS injury (e.g., contusion), there may be increased numbers of macrophages observed, includ-

ing giant cells. Within 1 or 2 days after subarachnoid hemorrhage, macrophages containing phagocytized RBCs are seen. This may also occur after a traumatic tap. After another 2 to 4 days, dark brown granules of hemosiderin appear in the macrophages (termed "siderophages" because of the iron) and an iron stain (like Prussian blue) can be used to confirm its presence. The siderophages may persist for several months after the initial hemorrhage. Table 11-11 summarizes the predominant cells in the CSF and their clinical significance.

Immunology

TESTS FOR NEUROSYPHILIS

Since the early 1970s, the CSF fluorescent treponemal antibody test with absorption (CSF FTA-ABS) has been used to test for neurosyphilis with nearly 100% sensitivity and specificity. False-positive results in some cases may be related to traumatic tap and contamination by peripheral blood.

The CSF Venereal Disease Research Laboratory test (CSF VDRL) has poor sensitivity but its specificity is close to 100%, so that a reactive CSF VDRL test is considered diagnostic for neurosyphilis.

A nonreactive serum FTA-ABS essentially rules out syphilitic infection, including neurosyphilis. When neurosyphilis is not suggested by clinical findings, the

---

TABLE 11-9
Causes for Plasmacytosis in Cerebrospinal Fluid

Tuberculous meningitis

Syphilitic meningoencephalitis

Multiple sclerosis

Parasitic infestations of central nervous system

Subacute sclerosing panencephalitis

Guillain-Barré syndrome

Sarcoidosis

(From Krieg AF, Kjeldsberg CR. Cerebrospinal fluid and other body fluids. In Henry JB, ed. *Clinical diagnosis and management by laboratory methods.* 18th ed. Philadelphia: WB Saunders Company, 1991.)

TABLE 11-11
Predominant Cells in Cerebrospinal Fluid and Clinical Significance

Type of Cell	Clinical Significance
Lymphocyte	Viral, tubercular, and fungal meningitis, bacterial meningitis (occasionally), multiple sclerosis
Neutrophil	Bacterial meningitis, early viral, tubercular, and fungal meningitis, intracranial hemorrhage, intrathecal injections, meningeal malignancy
Mixed cellular reaction (lymphocyte, neutrophil, monocyte)	Partially treated bacterial meningitis, chronic bacterial meningitis, cerebral abscess, tubercular meningitis, fungal meningitis, amebic meningitis
Eosinophil	Parasitic infections, allergic reactions, intracranial shunts
Macrophage	Chronic meningitis, treated bacterial meningitis, intrathecal injections, intracranial hemorrhage
Erythrophage (containing red blood cells)	Hemorrhage (12 hr–1 wk)
Siderophage (containing hemosiderin)	Hemorrhage (2 days–2 mo)
Hematoidinophage (containing hematin crystals)	Hemorrhage (2–4 wk)
Lipophage (containing fat)	Brain necrosis, infarct, anoxia, or trauma
Plasma cells	Subacute and chronic inflammatory reactions, multiple sclerosis
Malignant lymphoid cells	Lymphoma, leukemia
Blasts	Leukemia, lymphoma
Other malignant cells	Primary brain tumor, metastatic tumor
Ependymal/choroid plexus cells	Trauma, surgery, ventricular shunts, neonate, intrathecal injections
Cartilage cells	Traumatic puncture
Bone marrow cells	Traumatic puncture
Primitive cell clusters (blastlike cells)	Intracranial hemorrhage in premature infant, neonate; possibly of germinal matrix origin

(From Kjeldsberg CR, Knight JA. *Body fluids*. 3rd ed. Chicago: ASCP Press, 1993.)

CSF VDRL is not indicated for patients with a negative serum FTA-ABS.

A negative CSF FTA-ABS in seropositive patients with neuropsychiatric signs makes the diagnosis of active neurosyphilis highly unlikely. If the CSF FTA-ABS is positive, a positive CSF VDRL is presumptive evidence of neurosyphilis (although a positive test may persist for many years after successful treatment).[6]

A patient with a positive CSF FTA-ABS and a negative CSF VDRL should have a neurologic evaluation for signs of neurosyphilis. Although not specific, an increased intrathecal synthesis of IgG, an elevated IgG index, or oligoclonal bands in the CSF are findings that may be observed with 75% to 80% of patients with active neurosyphilis.

OTHER IMMUNOLOGIC TESTS

Latex agglutination tests for cryptococcal antigens are of established value in the diagnosis of *Cryptococcus* meningitis, with a sensitivity which ranges from 60% to 99%. False-negative results occur in early stages of the disease as well as with patients infected with nonencapsulated variants of *Cryptococcus neoformans*. False-negative results due to prozone effect can be eliminated by diluting CSF specimens 1 : 10 before testing, whereas false-negative results due to immune complexes can be eliminated by enzymatic digestion (pronase), thus making bound antigen available for reaction. Specificity ranges from 80% to 99%. Rheumatoid factor and similar macroglobulins may give rise to false-positive results and may be eliminated by the use of pronase.

Coccidioides immitis antigens may be identified by serologic tests that have a sensitivity of approximately 70% to 80% and specificity in the range of 90% to 99%.

Mycobacterium tuberculosis antigens may be detected using enzyme-linked immunosorbent assay with a sensitivity of about 50% and specificity of approximately 96%. More experience is needed to evaluate the diagnostic performance of this procedure.[6]

Latex agglutination procedures may be used to detect antigens of *Hamophilus influenzae*, *Streptococcus pneumoniae*, *Neisseria meningitidis*, and group B streptococci in CSF. Sensitivity for *H. influenzae* is about 90%; for *S. pneumoniae*, about 60%; for *N. meningitidis*, about 50%; and for group B streptococci, about 90%. Specificity ranges from 90% to 97%. Although these tests are widely used, it has been suggested that they offer little advantage over Gram's stain for early diagnosis of bacterial meningitis.

Counterimmunoelectrophoresis (CIE) is a serologic procedure used by the microbiology laboratory for rapid detection and identification of bacterial antigens in the CSF. Because not all bacteria possess the chemical characteristics needed for the reaction to take place, CIE is limited to the detection and identification of *H. influenzae, S. pneumoniae, N. meningitidis, Escherichia coli*, and group B streptococci. Cross-over reactions, including one between *E. coli* and *H. influenzae*, may occur.

The usual support medium for CIE is a layer of agar prepared on a glass slide. Wells are punched at opposite ends of the slide. Antiserum is added to a well on one end, and the antigen (positive control or patient's CSF, presumably containing the antigen) is added to the well on the other end. The buffer and support medium are such that during electrophoresis the antibody migrates toward the cathode, and the antigen toward the anode—that is, antigen and antibody migrate toward each other. A precipitin line forms at the zone of equivalence just as with the usual simple double immunodiffusion system, but because the mobility of the reactants is enhanced by the electrophoresis, the results are visible in just a few minutes rather than in hours.

Microbiology

MICROSCOPIC EXAMINATION

Gram's stain with microscopic examination is the initial step in microbiologic evaluation of a CSF specimen. The sensitivity of Gram' stain is about 60% to 90% and may be increased by using Cytospin concentration rather than the regular centrifugation. For *M. tuberculosis*, the Ziehl-Neelsen stain is only about 40% sensitive, but when fluid from four serial spinal taps is examined, sensitivity may increase to approximately 80% to 90%. Somewhat better sensitivity may be possible using fluorescent rhodamine stain.

India ink preparations for *C. neoformans* have a sensitivity of about 25% to 50%, which is significantly less than the sensitivity of latex agglutination tests for cryptococcal antigens.[6] In some patients, mononuclear inflammatory cells may repel the carbon particles of India ink to produce "false-positive" results. It has been suggested that this problem may be prevented by the use of nigrosin in place of the India ink.

CULTURE

Common causes of meningitis include *H. influenzae, N. meningitidis*, and *S. pneumoniae*. Less frequent cases include staphylococci, streptococci, *Listeria monocytogenes*, coliform bacteria, *M. tuberculosis, C. neoformans* (and other fungi), leptospira, anaerobic bacteria, amebae, and parasites.

For common types of bacterial meningitis, aerobic culture methods provide a sensitivity in the range of 80% to 90%. However, if antibiotics are started before CSF is obtained for culture, bacteria may be difficult to isolate. For patients with tuberculous meningitis, the sensitivity of initial cultures is about 50%, increasing to approximately 80% on repeated cultures.

Clinical Correlations

Meningitis is the most important disease of the CNS to diagnose. Usually it can be treated if it is detected early enough, but if the diagnosis is overlooked, it is often rapidly fatal. The four main types of infectious agents are bacteria, fungi, mycobacteria, and viruses. In most instances, parasitic infections are rare.

Bacterial meningitis is characterized by elevated CSF protein, decreased CSF glucose, and pleocytosis with a predominance of polymorphonuclear leukocytes in the CSF. The pathogenic organisms are often seen on the Gram's stain; sometimes intracellular organisms are observed with Wright's stain preparations. Most commonly, the bacterial pathogens are *H. influenzae, S. pneumoniae, N. meningitidis*, and group B streptococci. Within 3 to 5 days after starting therapy, most signs and symptoms of meningitis have disappeared and the CSF shows a decrease in leukocyte count and a shift in the differential count to a predominance of mononuclear cells, as well as a gradual return of glucose and protein to normal levels.

Although neutrophils may predominate initially, viral meningitis is most often associated with a lymphocytosis in the CSF. Many different types of medium-sized and large, reactive lymphocytes are observed. The large, reactive lymphocytes need to be differentiated from the lymphoblasts seen in acute lymphoblastic leukemia (ALL). Many different types of lymphocytes are present in reactive lymphocytosis, whereas in ALL the lymphoblasts are generally uniform in size, shape, and appearance. In the later stages of viral meningitis, lymphocytes decrease in number, whereas monocytes and macrophages predominate.

A lymphocytic pleocytosis together with elevated CSF protein and low CSF glucose levels is a picture most commonly associated with meningitis caused by *M. tuberculosis*. However, a neutrophilic pleocytosis is not unusual in the early phase of the disease, and a persistent neutrophilia has been reported with *M. tuberculosis* meningitis.

For fungal meningitis, specific etiologic identification depends on the direct identification of the organisms in the CSF through microscopic examination, culture, or serologic detection of fungal antigens. Low or normal glucose levels and elevated protein levels are usually observed, along with a lymphocytic pleocytosis.

The effect of medical procedures should also be considered when making diagnoses based on laboratory examination of the CSF. For example, when a lumbar puncture has been repeated 8 to 12 hours after the initial puncture, the CSF may contain increased numbers of neutrophils, monocytes, and macrophages as well as occasional macrophages showing erythrophagocytosis. Pneumoencephalography and myelography may lead to pleocytosis with varying numbers of lymphocytes, neutrophils, monocytes, macrophages, and eosinophils. An increased number of monocytes and macrophages may be present for 2 to 3 weeks after the procedure.

Intracranial shunts for hydrocephalus may be associated with monocytosis and increased numbers of macrophages and eosinophils. The eosinophilic pleocytosis may represent an allergic reaction to the shunt.

Malignant cells from a variety of neoplasms may be seen in the CSF.[4] Examining the CSF is particularly valuable in the diagnosis of metastatic carcinoma, leukemic and lymphomatous involvement of the meninges, and certain primary CNS tumors. Of the primary CNS tumors, medulloblastoma is more likely to be associated with malignant cells in the CSF than gliomas and meningiomas.[4] When cells from metastatic tumors are detected in the CNS, melanoma and carcinoma of the lung, breast, and gastrointestinal tract are the most common. Malignant cells in the CSF may occur singly or more frequently in clumps. Occasionally, atypical lymphoid cells, macrophages, and clumps of ependymal or choroid plexus cells may be mistaken for tumor cells.

Quality Control

Commercial control materials are available for quality control of the chemical analyses on CSF, including chloride, glucose, IgG, lactic acid, LDH, sodium, and total protein.

Illustrative Case Studies

CASE STUDY 11-1

After reportedly being assaulted and struck repeatedly in the face during the previous evening, this patient, a 37-year-old man, was found by a family member the next morning at home on the floor (in the hallway), naked and unresponsive. There was no evidence of alcohol intoxication. He was brought into the ER in a semiconscious state, partially paralyzed but combative, making only incomprehensible sounds. He also showed some signs of meningitis. His admission diagnosis was closed head injury, contusions, bleeding edema, and meningitis.

The admission CT scan showed fluid in the left maxillary sinus and left ethmoid sinus, an or-

continued

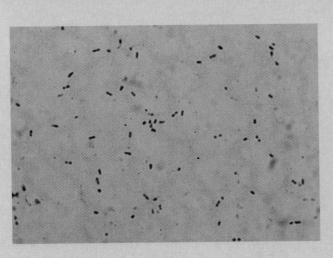

FIGURE 11-6 Direct Gram' stain of CSF showing gram-positive cocci; ×1000.

bital floor fracture on the left, mild bleeding edema, bifrontal medial contusion bleeding, and a right frontal contusion bleed. Results of the CSF analysis (tube 1) were color slightly xanthochromic; appearance slightly cloudy; supernatant slightly xanthochromic and hazy; WBCs/mm^3 7550; RBCs/mm^3 50; lymphocytes 1%; monocytes 1%; neutrophils 98%. Comment: bacteria present. The spinal fluid (Fig. 11-6) showed gram-positive cocci resembling *Streptococcus*, and the patient was started on penicillin. Later, gram-negative rods resembling enterics grew out of blood culture specimens, and he was placed on ciprofloxacin.

The patient did well in the hospital and was discharged to a rehabilitation center with the discharge diagnosis of bacterial meningitis, closed head injury, strokes due to sepsis, and evidence of mild short-term memory loss.

CASE STUDY 11-2

This patient, an infant girl, had been delivered by cesarean section from her 19-year-old mother at 31 weeks of pregnancy. The child showed respiratory distress and anemia as well as apnea and bradycardia of prematurity. She was placed on intermittent mandatory ventilation for the first 3 days of life, then extubated and kept on oxygen (nasal cannula).

Suggestions of sepsis developed and she was placed on vancomycin and cefotaxime. However, after 3 days, no sign of sepsis was seen in blood or urine, and the antibiotics were discontinued. On day 9 of life, the child experienced apnea and bradycardia again, and an infiltrate in her right lung was detected, so she was placed back on antibiotics. Four days later, all signs were negative for sepsis and the antibiotics were discontinued.

Also on the ninth day of life, an ultrasound of her head showed mildly enlarged ventricles as well as a right-sided grade 1 subependymal hemorrhage. Results of the CSF analysis (tube 1) were color xanthochromic; appearance hazy; supernatant xanthochromic and clear; WBCs/mm^3 28; RBCs/mm^3 490; lymphocytes 35%; monocytes 51%; neutrophils 7%; mononuclear phagocytes 7%. Comment: siderophages and erythrophagocytosis present. The CSF sediment is shown in Figures 11-7 and 11-8, which demonstrate erythrophagocytosis resulting from the hemorrhage. Supportive care was continued for several days, including blood (packed cells) for her apnea and anemia. Another ultrasound 4 weeks later showed the ventricles decreasing in size and no sign of a new hemorrhage. The infant was discharged home in stable condition with Similac with Iron.

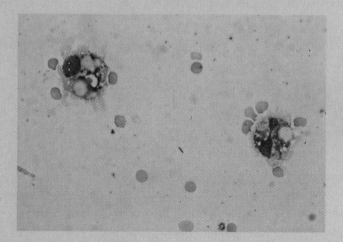

FIGURE 11-7 Cytospin preparation of CSF showing erythrophagocytosis. Wright's stain; ×400.

continued

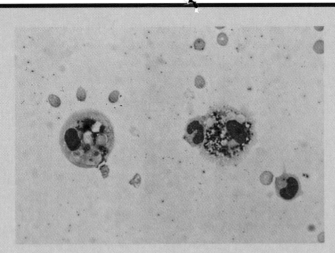

FIGURE 11-8 Cytospin preparation of CSF showing erythrophagocytosis. Wright's stain; ×400.

CASE STUDY 11-3

This 22-year-old woman had been diagnosed with *Coccidioides immitis* meningitis in 1991 and had been taking fluconazole for her infection. She was admitted through the urgent care clinic after experiencing nausea and vomiting with pains in her upper body (less when lying down) for the previous 2 weeks. A CSF serology was positive for C. *immitis*, and C. *immitis* was also cultured from this specimen. The patient was started on intrathecal injections of amphotericin B.

CSF analysis showed color colorless; appearance hazy; supernatant colorless and clear; WBCs/mm³ 320; RBCs/mm³ 203; lymphocytes 37%; plasma cells 2%; monocytes 3%; neutrophils 46%; mononuclear phagocytes 12%. The appearance of the CSF at admission is shown in Figure 11-9. As is common, no direct evidence of C. *immitis* was observed, even though the organism was cultured from this specimen.

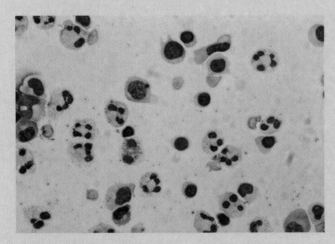

FIGURE 11-9 Cytospin preparation of CSF. Wright's stain; ×400.

CASE STUDY 11-4

This patient, a 25-year-old man, had been diagnosed 2 years earlier with *Coccidioides immitis* meningitis and was given fluconazole. However, he failed to keep his follow-up appointments. A year later he came back to the hospital, again with the chief complaint of persistent headaches and stiffness. This time he was placed on high-dose fluconazole and another attempt was made to follow him through the clinic, although with mixed success.

Eventually he came to the ER complaining of persistent and severe headaches, stiffness, malaise, and anorexia. He was admitted with the diagnosis of disseminated coccidioidomycosis

continued

and failure of fluconazole therapy requiring follow-up and intrathecal amphotericin B injections. Analysis of the admission lumbar puncture (LP) CSF (tube 1) showed appearance colorless and hazy; total vol. 6 mL; supernatant colorless and clear; WBCs 857/mm^3; RBCs/mm^3 0; lymphocytes 30%; plasma cells 6%; monocytes 12%; neutrophils 32%; eosinophils 11%; basophils 1%. The Cytospin preparation of this CSF specimen is illustrated in Figures 11-10 and 11-11, and the eosinophilia is evidence of the recrudescent *Coccidioides*.

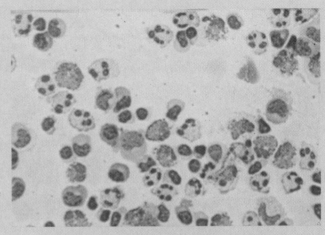

FIGURE 11-10 Cytospin preparation of CSF showing eosinophilia. Wright's stain; ×400.

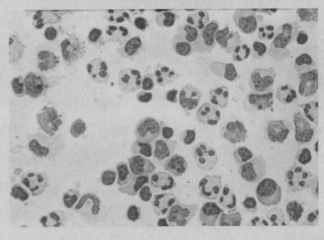

FIGURE 11-11 Cytospin preparation of CSF showing eosinophilia. Wright's stain; ×400.

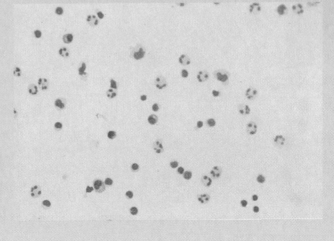

FIGURE 11-12 Cytospin preparation of CSF demonstrating the effect of amphotericin B injections on the patient's coccidioidomycosis: diminished white cell count and diminished eosinophilia. Wright's stain; ×200.

continued

After a month of treatments with amphotericin B, the patient was admitted again for evaluation and follow-up. The admission LP CSF (tube 1) showed color colorless; appearance very slightly hazy; supernatant colorless and clear; WBCs/mm^3 169; RBCs/mm^3 7; lymphocytes 68%; monocytes 5%; neutrophils 25%; eosinophils 2%. The Cytospin preparation of this specimen is illustrated in Figure 11-12, which shows some recovery compared with the previous month when amphotericin B injections were started.

CASE STUDY 11-5

After 2 weeks of neck and back pain together with fever, chills, and blackouts with some blurring of vision, this 27-year-old man (from the state prison) was admitted for evaluation. Results of CSF analysis were color colorless; appearance cloudy; supernatant colorless and clear; WBCs 9/mm^3; RBCs 18/mm^3; mononuclear phagocytes 100%. Many yeast forms were observed in the CSF (Figs. 11-13 and 11-14), and *Cryptococcus neoformans* was cultured from this specimen. A Gram stain on this specimen was positive for yeast forms, an India ink preparation demonstrated *Cryptococcus*-like cells, and blood cultures were also positive for *Cryptococcus*. The patient had a long history of IV drug abuse and was also at risk for acquired immunodeficiency syndrome.

The patient was treated aggressively with amphotericin B and flucytosine, but did not improve. He went into a coma while in the hospital and died with flat EEG tracings.

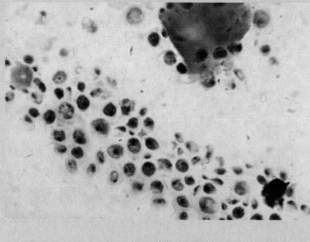

FIGURE 11-13 Cytospin preparation of CSF showing *Cryptococcus neoformans*. Wright's stain; ×1000.

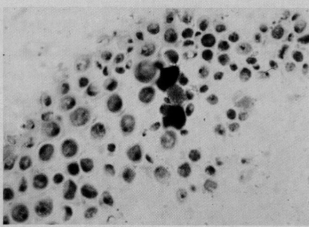

FIGURE 11-14 Cytospin preparation of CSF showing *Cryptococcus neoformans*. Wright's stain; ×1000.

continued

CASE STUDY 11-6

With a history of type II diabetes mellitus, seizure disorder, *Coccidioides* meningitis, and bilateral hydrocephalus, this 48-year-old man came into the ER complaining of extreme lethargy, decreased mental status, blackouts, memory loss, difficulty in speaking, and overall tremulousness. The hydrocephalus was being controlled by means of a VP (ventriculoperitoneal) shunt, and a CT scan indicated nondrainage of the left lateral ventricle. The Omaya reservoir area was shaved and a sterile 25-gauge needle was used to aspirate approximately 25 mL of clear CSF for studies. Admission diagnosis was altered mental status 2° to malfunction of VP shunt versus VP shunt infection (meningitis).

The Cytospin preparation of the CSF (Fig. 11-15) shows *Staphylococcus*-like bacteria. C&S for that specimen was positive for coag-negative *Staphylococcus* species, *Acinetobacter anitratus*, and *Pseudomonas aeruginosa*. The ventriculostomy sites had previously been changed several times because of infections. The infected VP shunt was removed, and a fresh shunt was fitted to a different site. The patient was treated with vancomycin, amikacin, and piperacillin, and eventually discharged in stable condition to a rehabilitation hospital.

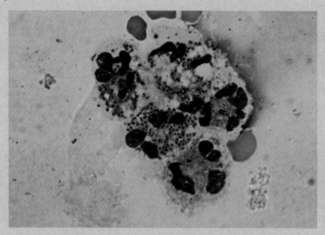

FIGURE 11-15 Cytospin preparation of CSF showing *Staphylococcus*-like bacteria. Wright's stain; ×1000.

CASE STUDY 11-7

Presenting to the ER with typical symptoms of meningitis, this 37-year-old man (state prison inmate) was admitted complaining of 3 to 4 months of severe headaches and some vomiting. He is HIV positive and also has been suffering from chronic diarrhea. CSF from lumbar puncture (tube 3) showed color colorless; appearance clear; WBC/mm³ 26; RBC/mm³ 31; lymphocytes 10%; monocytes 12%; neutrophils 72%; eosinophils 1%; basophils 5%; and the presence of budding yeast. The Cytospin preparation of this CSF is shown in Figures 11-16 and 11-17. The Gram stain on this spec-

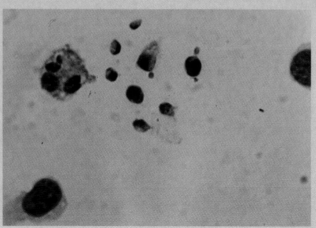

FIGURE 11-16 Cytospin preparation of CSF showing *Cryptococcus neoformans*. Wright's stain; ×1000.

continued

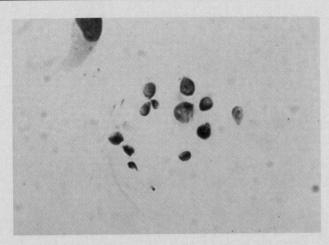

FIGURE 11-17 Cytospin preparation of CSF showing *Cryptococcus neoformans*. Wright's stain; ×1000.

imen showed moderate yeast forms, and the C&S was positive for *Cryptococcus neoformans*. He was given amphotericin B and flucytosine, but the treatment was complicated by renal insufficiency and bone marrow suppression. These problems were corrected by adjusting dosages so that subsequently he received amphotericin B three times a week and flucytosine daily. He was eventually discharged in stable condition.

CASE STUDY 11-8

This 6-month-old boy was brought into the ER unresponsive, mottled, and making little or no respiratory effort. His mother reported that he had been feverish and weak for the previous 2 days. The child was intubated and given mechanical ventilation. Intravenous lines were started in both legs, and he was successfully resuscitated. He was admitted to the ICU, placed on 100% oxygen, and started on rocephin and ampicillin. The admitting diagnosis was respiratory arrest, R/O sepsis, possibly meningitis.

The LP CSF (Fig. 11-18) showed gram-negative coccobacilli, and microbiology studies were initiated. Final diagnosis was *Haemophilus influenzae* meningitis, and the patient was discharged home with his parents to complete 6 days of therapy with intravenous vancomycin.

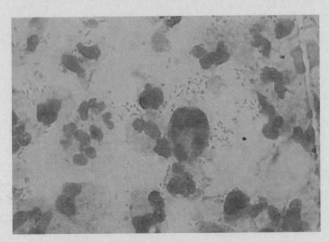

FIGURE 11-18 Gram's stain of CSF showing *Haemophilus influenzae*; ×1000.

Case Histories With Study Questions

CASE HISTORY 11-1

After several days of constant watery diarrhea, stomach pain, dysphagia, and weight loss, this 28-year-old man came to the ER. He appeared cachectic and was complaining of a severe frontal headache, but the CT scan was negative. He was found to have a severe immunodeficiency (CD4 count = 20) and was started on AZT. Analysis of the LP CSF showed color colorless; appearance hazy; supernatant clear and colorless; WBCs/mm³ 0; RBCs/mm³ 2; monocytes 0; neutrophils 0; and many (?) present. The spinal fluid appeared as shown in Figures 11-19 and 11-20. CSF C&S was positive for the (?), shown in Figures 11-19 and 11-20, and a Gram' stain on the specimen was confirmatory for (?). The patient was started on appropriate antibiotic therapy, was in and out of the hospital for a time, and finally expired in the hospital.

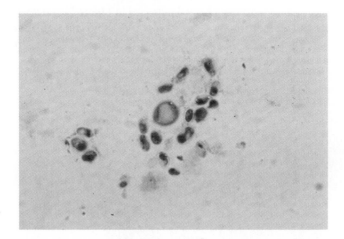

FIGURE 11-19 Cytospin preparation of CSF. Wright's stain; ×1000.

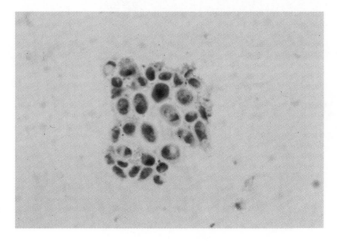

FIGURE 11-20 Cytospin preparation of CSF. Wright's stain; ×1000.

Study Questions for Case History 11-1

1. The cellular objects shown in Figures 11-19 and 11-20 are characteristic for:
   a. Amebic trophozoites
   b. Yeast forms of a fungus
   c. Fungal macroconidia
   d. Hydatid sand

continued

2. The most likely identification for the organism shown is:
   a. *Blastomyces dermatitidis*
   b. *Naegleria fowleri*
   c. *Cryptococcus neoformans*
   d. *Candida albicans*
3. Do you think the cell count and differential for this case are unusual? Explain.

CASE HISTORY 11-2

This patient, a 19-month-old boy, was brought into the ER by his mother after a 5-day history of restlessness, two to three vomiting episodes/day, and fever. The examination showed the child to be lethargic and sleepy with meningismus and stiff neck. The LP CSF showed color colorless; appearance cloudy; WBCs 2190/mm³; RBCs 250/mm³; lymphocytes 5%; monocytes 2%; neutrophils 94%; comment: many (?) seen. Other results included glucose 38 mg/dL (ref. range, 50–80 mg/dL), and protein 208 mg/dL (15–45 mg/dL)

The Cytospin preparation of the CSF is illustrated in Figures 11-21 and 11-22. The Gram' stain on the CSF demonstrated Gram-positive (?). The child responded well to antibiotics and had no seizures, weakness, or other abnormalities. After 10 days of treatment, he was discharged home in stable condition.

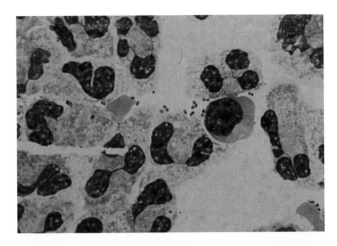

FIGURE 11-21 Cytospin preparation of CSF. Wright's stain; ×1000.

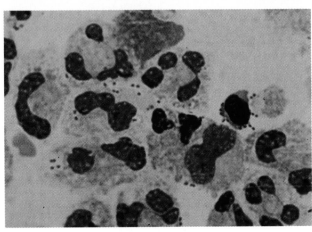

FIGURE 11-22 Cytospin preparation of CSF. Wright's stain; ×1000.

continued

Study Questions for Case History 11-2

1. What diagnosis seems most likely for this child ?
   a. Bacterial meningitis
   b. Viral meningitis
   c. Coccidioidomycosis
   d. Blastomycosis
2. In view of the Gram' stain result, of the following, what organism seems most likely from the morphology shown on the Cytospin preparation?
   a. *Haemophilus influenzae*
   b. *Neisseria meningitidis*
   c. *Blastomyces dermatitidis*
   d. *Streptococcus pneumoniae*

CASE HISTORY 11-3

This 40-year-old man was brought to the hospital by ambulance and was admitted through the ER complaining of headaches and increasing weakness on his right side. There was early evidence of hydrocephalus. The LP CSF showed (tube 1) color red; appearance bloody; supernatant xanthochromic and hazy; WBCs 667/mm^3; RBCs 116,000/mm^3; lymphocytes 25%; monocytes 10%; neutrophils 64%; eosinophils 1%. Figures 11-23 and 11-24 show the appearance of the Cytospin preparation of the CSF.

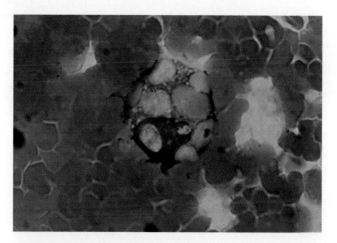

FIGURE 11-23 Cytospin preparation of CSF. Wright's stain; ×1000.

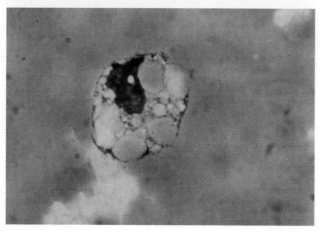

FIGURE 11-24 Cytospin preparation of CSF. Wright's stain; ×1000.

continued

Study Questions for Case History 11-3

1. The phenomenon illustrated here is termed:
    a. Lupus erythematosus cell formation
    b. Endospore formation
    c. Erythrophagocytosis
    d. Pinocytosis
2. The most likely cause for the phenomenon observed is:
    a. A traumatic tap
    b. Subarachnoid hemorrhage
    c. Multiple sclerosis
    d. Ankylosing spondylitis

REFERENCES

1. Chou G, Schmidley JW. Lysis of erythrocytes and leukocytes in traumatic lumbar puncture. *Arch Neurol* 1984;41:1084.
2. Kjeldsberg CR, Knight JA. *Body fluids*. Chicago: ASCP Press, 1983.
3. Kjeldsberg CR, Knight JA. *Body fluids*. 3rd ed. Chicago: ASCP Press, 1993.
4. Krieg AF, Kjeldsberg CR. Cerebrospinal fluid and other body fluids. In: Henry JB, ed. *Clinical diagnosis and management by laboratory methods*. 18th ed. Philadelphia: WB Saunders, 1991: 445–473.

BIBLIOGRAPHY

Brunzel NA. *Fundamentals of urine and body fluid analysis*. Philadelphia: WB Saunders, 1994.
International Remote Imaging Systems. *Technical literature*. Chatsworth, CA: IRIS, 1996.
Memmler RL, Cohen BJ, Wood DL. *The human body in health and disease*. 7th ed. Philadelphia: JB Lippincott, 1992.
Ringsrud KM, Linné JJ. *Urinalysis and body fluids: A color text and atlas*. St. Louis: Mosby–Year Book, 1995.
Strasinger SK. *Urinalysis and body fluids*. 3rd ed. Philadelphia: FA Davis, 1994.

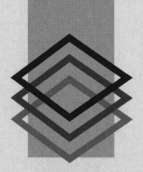

12 Seminal Fluid Analysis

Analysis of seminal fluid is usually carried out as part of a comprehensive investigation of infertility involving both partners of a childless marriage.[2]

Semen may also be studied to determine the effectiveness of a vasectomy; in forensic studies involving alleged or suspected rape; to evaluate semen quality for donation; and in paternity cases when sterility becomes an issue.

Physiology and Composition

Semen consists of a suspension of spermatozoa in the seminal plasma, which provides a nutritive medium of proper osmolality and volume and which also activates the spermatozoa to greater motility. Spermatozoa are produced in the testes, then matured and concentrated in the epididymides. It has been estimated that sperm may survive in the epididymides for up to 1 month.[2]

About 60% of the semen volume is derived from the seminal vesicles, which produce a viscid, neutral to slightly alkaline fluid. This fluid may be yellow or deeply pigmented depending on its flavin content. The substrate involved in the coagulation of semen after ejaculation is produced by the seminal vesicles. Fructose, the major nutrient for the spermatozoa, is also produced by the seminal vesicles. The prostate secretion (about 20% of the semen volume) is a slightly acidic, milky fluid that is rich in citric acid. The prostatic secretions also are rich in acid phosphatase and in proteolytic enzymes responsible for the coagulation and liquefaction of semen. The balance of the seminal fluid is produced by the epididymides, vasa deferentia, bulbourethral glands, and urethral glands.[2]

Ejaculation results in the mixing of three distinct fractions of semen that individually enter the urethra in rapid succession. The first fraction is a clear, viscid fluid probably produced by the urethral and bulbourethral glands. The second fraction is essentially prostatic secretion and contains most of the spermatozoa, plus relatively small amounts of secretions from the epididymides and vasa deferentia. The final fraction consists almost entirely of a mucoid secretion from the seminal vesicles.

Collection

Collection of a semen sample after a 3-day period of continence is usually the preferred procedure. The most satisfactory specimen is one collected by masturbation in a comfortable and private room near the physician's office or clinical laboratory. The patient should be provided with written and verbal instructions for the procedure. The entire ejaculate must be collected for analysis because the first portion may contain most of the spermatozoa. Containers can be wide-mouth, clean, glass jars or plastic containers such as those used for urine or sputum collection. However, if plastic is used, the specimen should be examined immediately on liquefaction or transferred to a glass container because storage in a plastic container reduces motility of the spermatozoa. Special Silastic condoms that are nontoxic to sperm may also be used.[2]

Specimens collected at a site distant from the laboratory should be brought in for analysis as soon as possible and no later than an hour after collection. The specimen should not be subjected to temperature extremes during transport to the laboratory. The container should be warmed to body temperature before collection, and it is best to keep the specimen at body temperature until liquefaction of the coagulum is complete (about 20 minutes). The container should be labeled with the patient's name, the period of sexual abstinence, and the date and time of specimen collection. Universal precautions must be followed by all personnel handling these specimens.

Physical Examination

Observed soon after ejaculation, semen is a highly viscid, opaque, white or gray-white coagulum with a distinct musty or acrid odor. Within about 20 minutes, the coagulum spontaneously liquefies to a translucent, turbid, viscous fluid. Liquefaction that is delayed beyond 60 minutes is abnormal and should be noted.

Increased turbidity may be associated with the presence of leukocytes, indicating an inflammatory process in some part of the reproductive tract. Viscosity may be observed while pouring the liquefied specimen from the collection container into the glass graduate for volume measurement. If viscosity is normal, a specimen can be poured drop by drop. Increased viscosity may be significant if it decreases sperm motility.

Normal semen volume averages from 1 to 5 mL. Volumes below or above this range have been associated with infertility.

Microscopic Examination

Although an automated instrument is available for counting spermatozoa (IRIS; see Chapter 5), the usual procedure is to use a hemacytometer once the speci-

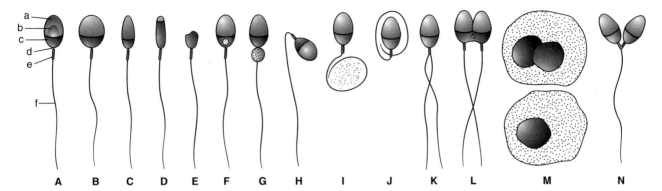

FIGURE 12-1 Semen analysis: sperm morphology. A, acrosome; B, nucleus (difficult to see); C, post-acrosomal cap; D, neckpiece; E, midpiece (short segment after neckpiece); F, tail. *a*, normal; *b*, normal (slightly different head shape); *c*, tapered head; *d*, tapered head with acrosome deficiency; *e*, acrosomal deficiency; *f*, head vacuole; G, cytoplasmic extrusion mass; H, bent head (bend of 45° or more); I, coiled tail; J, coiled tail; K, double tail; L, pairing phenomenon (sperm agglutination); M, sperm precursors (spermatids); N, bicephalic sperm. (From Ravel R. *Clinical laboratory medicine.* St. Louis, Mosby: 1995.)

men has liquefied. A 1:20 dilution is prepared with a micropipette by delivering an aliquot of the sample quantitatively into a premeasured amount of diluent, such as Isoton Plus.[1] After the hemacytometer is filled, 2 minutes are allowed for the sperm to settle before counting. The type of hemacytometer, the specimen dilution used, and the areas counted determine the conversion factor necessary to obtain the concentration of spermatozoa in millions per milliliter. Suggestions are provided for this procedure in Ringsrud and Linné.[7]

A normal sperm count is from 20 to 25 million/mL. Values above or below this range are usually considered abnormal and associated with infertility.[1] Yet, even men with sperm counts of 10 million/mL or less have been found to be fertile.[1,2]

Fertility is critically dependent on sperm motility because immotile sperm, even in high concentrations, are unable to reach an ovum and unite with it. To evaluate motility, a small drop of liquefied semen is mounted on a prewarmed (body temperature) slide with a coverslip ringed with coverslip. A total of at least 200 spermatozoa should be evaluated in several microscopic fields using the high dry objective, preferably with phase contrast. The percentage of spermatozoa showing actual progressive motion is determined.

One approach to evaluating the results assigns sperm to one of three categories: progressive motility, nonprogressive motility, and nonmotility. Spermatozoa showing progressive motility are graded according to the following scheme: grade I, minimal forward progression; grade II, poor to fair activity; grade III, good activity with tail movements visualized; grade IV, full activity with tail movements difficult to visualize.[2] If

normal semen is evaluated within an hour of collection, the sperm exhibit strong linear forward movement.[1]

Sperm morphology can be evaluated by making differential counts on smears prepared as for traditional blood smears and stained with Giemsa', Wright's, or Papanicolaou' stain. The morphology of normal and abnormal spermatozoa is illustrated in Figure 12-1. At least 200 spermatozoa should be examined under oil immersion and the percentage of abnormal forms recorded.[2] In general, more than 40% of the spermatozoa should have a normal appearance.[5] Other cells observed on the smear may include leukocytes, urethral epithelial cells, and immature spermatogenic cells.

The appearance of sperm in urine is illustrated in Figure 12-2.

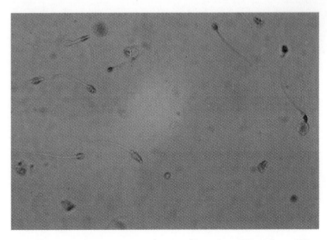

FIGURE 12-2 Spermatozoa observed in urine. SM stain; ×400.

REFERENCES

1. Brunzel NA. *Fundamentals of urine and body fluid analysis*. Philadelphia: WB Saunders, 1994.
2. Cannon DC, Henry JB. Seminal fluid. In: Henry JB, ed. *Clinical diagnosis and management by laboratory methods*. 18th ed. Philadelphia: WB Saunders, 1991:497–503

3. Kjeldsberg CR, Knight JA. *Body fluids*. Chicago: ASCP Press, 1983.
4. Ringsrud KM, Linné JJ. *Urinalysis and body fluids: A color text and atlas*. St. Louis: Mosby–Year Book, 1995.

BIBLIOGRAPHY

International Remote Imaging Systems. *Technical literature*. Chatsworth, CA: IRIS, 1996.
Kjeldsberg CR, Knight JA. *Body fluids*. 3rd ed. Chicago: ASCP Press, 1993

Ravel R. *Clinical laboratory medicine*. St. Louis: CV Mosby, 1995.
Strasinger SK. *Urinalysis and body fluids*. 3rd ed. Philadelphia: FA Davis, 1994.

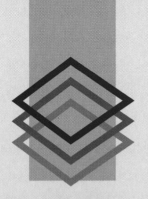

13 *Amniotic Fluid*

ABBREVIATIONS USED IN THIS CHAPTER

AChE = acetylcholinesterase

AF = amniotic fluid

AFP = alpha-fetoprotein

FSI = foam stability index

L = lecithin

L/S = lecithin/sphingomyelin
    ratio

NTD = neural tube defects

P = fluorescence polarization

PG = phosphatidylglycerol

PI = phosphatidylinositol

RBC = red blood cell

RDS = respiratory distress
    syndrome

S = sphingomyelin

TLC = thin-layer
    chromatography

Anatomy and Physiology

Of the two fetal membranes, the amnion is the innermost, lining the chorion and enclosing the amniotic fluid (AF) in which the fetus is suspended. The AF cushions and protects the fetus, enables it to move and grow, maintains an even temperature, and participates in fetal biochemical homeostasis. Various tissues contribute to this fluid, including the amniotic membrane, fetal cord, and the fetal gastrointestinal, respiratory, and renal systems.[11] Fetal urine is probably the major source of AF after the first trimester.

Early in gestation, the composition of the fluid is very much like a complex dialysate of the maternal serum.[5] With fetal growth, as pregnancy progresses, the fluid changes in many ways. The concentration of some analytes decreases (e.g., protein, sodium, glucose, chloride, bilirubin); that of others progressively increases (e.g., potassium, creatinine, urea, uric acid, amylase, alkaline phosphatase, and various phospholipids).

In addition to accurate measurement of the analytes and an estimation of the gestational age, an adequate interpretation of the parameters depends on whether the patient has a normal amount of AF. The volume of AF increases until about 34 weeks' gestation, decreases slightly through the 40th week, then decreases even more until the 42nd week. Fluid is added to the amniotic cavity by fetal urination and removed by fetal swallowing. Bidirectional water flux occurs between mother and fetus (placenta), fetus and AF (umbilical cord, skin), and AF and mother (amniotic membranes).[5]

Pathologic changes in AF volume may occur. Oligohydramnios refers to an abnormally low AF volume, such as with intrauterine growth retardation or abnormalities of the fetal urinary tract (bilateral renal agenesis and urethral obstruction). Polyhydramnios is an abnormally high AF volume observed with maternal diabetes mellitus, severe hemolytic disease of the newborn (isoimmune disease), fetal esophageal atresia, and anencephaly.

Specimen Collection and Handling

Amniotic fluid is obtained by amniocentesis, the aseptic aspiration of the fluid by hypodermic needle and syringe. It is generally accepted that the procedure can be performed safely by the 14th week of gestation. Before amniocentesis, an ultrasound examination is performed, although simultaneous ultrasonic examination may be combined with the amniocentesis. The ultrasound examination is used to confirm the fetal gestational age, detect gross fetal anomalies, verify fe-

tal cardiac activity, determine placental location, determine the volume of AF, determine the number of gestational sacks, and determine the optimal puncture site.

AF analyses in the second trimester are usually carried out to diagnose congenital disorders such as neural tube defects (NTD) and Down syndrome. Third trimester analyses provide information on the severity of isoimmune hemolytic disease and aid in assessing fetal maturity.

Transabdominal amniocentesis is the preferred method because vaginal amniocentesis is associated with an increased risk of infection and can also contaminate the specimen with vaginal bacteria, maternal vaginal cells, or both. The major risks of amniocentesis are trauma to the fetus, umbilical cord, and placenta; infection; spontaneous abortion; prematurely ruptured membranes; preterm labor; hemorrhage; and maternal isoimmunization.[7] Figure 13-1 shows the relationship of the amnion, fetus, and AF.

To preserve the cellular and biochemical constituents, the specimen should be processed as soon as possible after removal from the amniotic cavity. Specimen handling depends on the variety of tests intended. Protocols may include keeping the specimen on ice, protecting it from light, keeping it in the refrigerator or

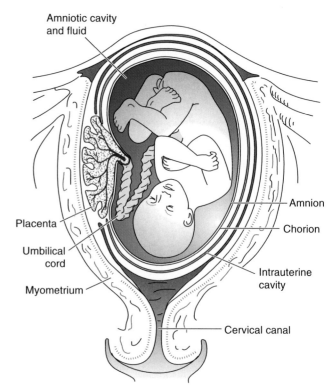

FIGURE 13-1 Schematic drawing of the anatomic relationships of the fetus and the amniotic fluid.(From Kjeldsberg CR, Knight JA. *Body fluids*. Chicago: ASCP Press, 1983.)

TABLE 13-1
Fluid Color and Associated Fetal Conditions

Color	Possible Associated Condition
Colorless to pale straw	Normal (appearance does not rule out erythroblastosis, however)
Yellow	Erythroblastosis
Green (meconium)	Fetal hypoxia (except during early pregnancy), meconium aspiration syndrome
Dark red-brown	Fetal death

(From Kjeldsberg CR, Knight JA. *Body fluids*. 3rd. Chicago: ASCP Press, 1993.)

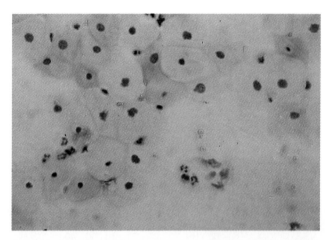

FIGURE 13-3 Numerous squamous epithelial cells and other cells observed in Cytospin preparation of amniotic fluid. Wright's stain. ×200.

at room temperature, or centrifuging it at various speeds according to specific test requirements.

Physical Examination

The color and turbidity of an AF specimen should be noted immediately after the sample is received in the laboratory. Table 13-1 provides several correlations of AF color and associated fetal conditions. Because oxyhemoglobin interferes with several tests (as noted later), it is important to remove any intact RBCs from the fluid by centrifugation before they hemolyze.

Early in pregnancy there is little or no particulate matter in the AF. By 16 weeks' gestation, large numbers of cells are present, having been shed from the surfaces of the amnion, skin, and tracheobronchial tree. As pregnancy continues, increased amounts of fetal cells

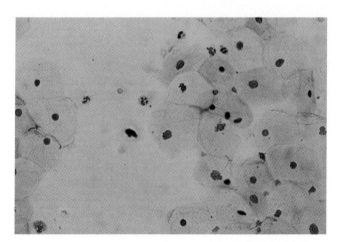

FIGURE 13-2 Numerous squamous epithelial cells and other cells observed in Cytospin preparation of amniotic fluid. Wright's stain; ×200.

and hair as well as vernix caseosa (caseous covering of fetal epidermis) appear in the fluid and contribute to its turbidity.

Microscopic Examination

For cytologic examination, smears may be made after centrifuging the specimen, although cytologic filters or cytocentrifuge procedures demonstrate morphologic characteristics more distinctly. The slides can be stained with the Papanicolaou, hematoxylin and eosin, Wright's, or Nile blue stains.

More than a dozen types of cells have been described in AF specimens. Figures 13-2 and 13-3 illustrate some of the cells observed in AF. Although the cytologic examination of AF may be of limited clinical value compared with other procedures used to analyze AF, microscopic examination of the specimen may provide additional information in the diagnosis of ruptured membranes and chorioamnionitis, the determination of fetal maturity, the determination of sex prenatally, and the detection of NTD.[7]

Clinical Disorders and Analysis of Amniotic Fluid
Neural Tube Defects

Alpha-fetoprotein (AFP) is an albumin-like protein that is initially produced in small quantities by the fetal yolk sac. Alpha-fetoprotein is produced in larger quantities

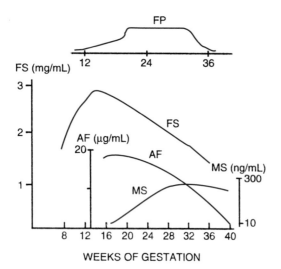

FIGURE 13-4 Concentrations of AFP in fetal serum (FS), maternal serum (MS), and amniotic fluid (AF). The time course of fetal production (FP) of AFP is indicated in the top curve. (From Burtis CA, Ashwood ER. *Tietz textbook of clinical chemistry*. 2nd ed. Philadelphia: WB Saunders Company, 1994.)

by the fetal liver as the yolk sac degenerates. Alpha-fetoprotein is present in the fetal serum, excreted in the fetal urine, and appears in the AF.

Maximum concentration of AFP in the fetal serum is reached at about 16 weeks' gestation; the concentration then decreases steadily to term (Fig. 13-4). AFP concentration in fetal serum is much higher than its concentration in AF. However, with various congenital anomalies, the concentration in AF increases considerably above normal. The most common of these anomalies is an open NTD, in which there is direct leakage of AFP from the cerebrospinal fluid into the AF. Maternal serum AFP is also elevated with NTD (85–95% of cases). Radioimmunoassay, enzyme-labeled immunoassay, and fluorescence polarization immunoassay are the methods of choice for measuring AFP in AF.

Acetylcholinesterase (AChE) is used as an adjunct in the diagnosis of NTD and is measured by polyacrylamide gel electrophoresis. AFP from normal pregnancies contains a single AChE that migrates relatively slowly in electrophoresis. Pregnancies with NTD have a second AChE that migrates more rapidly. This enzyme appears to be relatively specific for neural tissue. Note that because AChE is present in RBCs, AF contaminated with blood is not suitable for this test. Testing AF for AFP and for AChE can predict open NTD more accurately than screening maternal serum. Any elevation of AFP in AF should lead to AChE analysis.[5]

Respiratory Distress Syndrome

Of the fetal organs, the lungs are among the last to mature. Fetal pulmonary maturation is associated with the production of a detergent-like substance, "surfactant," which decreases the work of breathing air by lowering the surface tension within the alveoli. This reduces the resistance to expansion during inspiration and also prevents alveolar collapse during expiration. Infants with insufficient or ineffective surfactant suffer from respiratory distress syndrome (RDS) and must be provided with supplemental oxygen and mechanical ventilation. RDS is the most common critical problem encountered in clinical management of premature newborns.

The most common situation in which a fetal lung maturity test is ordered is before performing a cesarean section when the age of gestation is somewhat uncertain. Another reason for a fetal lung maturity test would be an anticipated early delivery because of some medical or obstetric indication such as premature labor, premature rupture of the membranes, worsening maternal hypertension, severe renal disease, intrauterine growth retardation, or fetal distress.

Pulmonary surfactant is a complex mixture of lipids and proteins with less than 5% carbohydrates. Most of the lipid is phospholipid, and most of that is lecithin (phosphatidylcholine). Other lipids present are phosphatidylglycerol (PG), phosphatidylinositol (PI), and sphingomyelin (S). The major surface active phospholipid is lecithin (L). Sphingomyelin does not appear to have any major surface active properties, but its concentration in AF remains constant during the third trimester and it is used as an "internal standard" in the reference lecithin:sphingomyelin (L:S) ratio test for pulmonary maturity. Before delivery, breathing movements by the fetus cause the surfactant to diffuse from the unexpanded lung tissues, through the bronchial tree, and out into the AF.

THE LECITHIN:SPHINGOMYELIN RATIO

The first laboratory test for estimating fetal lung maturity was the L:S ratio in AF. The rationale was the large increase in the amount of lecithin between the 32nd week of gestation and term, together with the essentially unchanged (or slightly decreased) amount of sphingomyelin during that same period. It is assumed that the changes in lecithin observed in AF reflect those taking place in the lungs.

The procedure involves extraction of the AF lipids, partial purification of the phospholipids by acetone precipitation, separation by thin-layer chromatography (TLC), color development, and quantitation of the phospholipid spots by densitometry. An L:S ratio of 2 is the critical value usually accepted as the indicator for fetal lung maturity.

PHOSPHATIDYLGLYCEROL AND PHOSPHATIDYLINOSITOL

The concentration of PG in AF is usually too low to measure until about the 35th week of gestation. The levels then increase rapidly until term. In contrast, PI is detectable in AF before the 28th week of gestation. It increases slowly to a maximum around the 36th week (when PG begins to increase sharply) and then slowly decreases to term.

Measuring PG and PI provides a means for cross-checking the results of the L:S ratio in making a decision regarding fetal maturity. TLC techniques can be used to determine PG and PI, just as for the L:S ratio. A lung profile, or two-dimensional lung profile, can also be developed by using two-dimensional TLC to determine simultaneously the levels of L, S, PG, and PI in a specimen of AF.

THE FOAM STABILITY INDEX

The foam stability index (FSI) is based on the principle that more surfactant activity is necessary to support a stable foam as the fraction of ethanol in the mixture is increased. A fixed amount of undiluted AF is mixed with increasing volumes of 95% ethanol. The mixture is shaken vigorously for 30 seconds, and the contents are allowed to settle for 15 seconds. The meniscus is then examined for a ring of foam.

The largest fraction of ethanol in which the AF is still capable of supporting an uninterrupted ring of foam is the FSI. A value of 0.47 or greater for the FSI is taken to indicate fetal lung maturity. A commercial kit, Lumadex-FSI Test (Beckman Instruments) that avoids some of the problems with the "shake test," is available.

FLUORESCENCE POLARIZATION

Fluorescence polarization (P) measures the rotational diffusion of a fluorophore relative to its fluorescent half-life. If the half-life is short compared with the rate of rotational diffusion, P is high. If molecular rotation is faster than the excited state decay, P is low.

A fluorescent dye is added to a specimen of AF that binds to albumin and to surfactant. The resulting polarization is a function of the surfactant:albumin ratio. Because the amount of albumin in AF during the third trimester of pregnancy is relatively constant, albumin serves as an internal standard against which the sur-

factant content is compared. P is high in AF containing low levels of surfactants.

One fluorescent compound that has been used is 1-palmitoyl-2{6-[(7-nitro-2,1,3-benzoxadizol-4-yl)amino]caproyl}phosphatidylcholine (NBD-PC); the instrument used is the Abbott TDX. The NBD-PC compound is added to the AF, and the fluorescence polarization intensity is measured. The degree of fluorescence polarization is inversely proportional to the quantity of pulmonary surfactant present.

Hemolytic Disease of the Newborn

Prenatal testing of AF is used to estimate the degree of fetal danger in isoimmune hemolytic disease, also known as hemolytic disease of the newborn, or erythroblastosis fetalis. Isoimmune hemolytic disease is caused by maternal antibodies directed against antigen on fetal erythrocytes. The immunoglobulins produced are usually of the IgG class, which are able to cross the placenta and then react with and destroy fetal RBCs. Hemolysis may be detected as early as 16 weeks' gestation and may progress at an increasing rate until term. The risk is great for an RhD-positive fetus in an Rh-negative mother who is already sensitized to the D antigen.

In normal pregnancies, the destruction of senescent RBCs in the fetus produces unconjugated bilirubin, which is rapidly removed into the maternal circulation through the placenta. With a hemolytic disease process, the increased concentration of unconjugated bilirubin in the fetal circulation induces fetal hepatic glucuronyl transferase activity earlier than usual, so that conjugated bilirubin can be produced as early as 28 weeks.[11] The conjugated form of bilirubin is not cleared by the placenta, and variable amounts are found in the AF. In a fetus affected by severe disease, marked anemia and hypoproteinemia are often accompanied by antenatal hydrops and death, unless intrauterine transfusion is carried out.

Liley noted that the degree of hemolysis in sensitized pregnancies could be assessed by measuring the absorbance of bilirubinoid pigments in the AF and classifying the results into three zones based on gestational age.[5] The determination can be done directly by means of recording spectrophotometry. Bilirubin absorbs maximally at 450 nm; in the absence of significant amounts of bilirubin, the absorbance spectrum for AF between 365 and 550 nm is as shown in Figure 13-5. The degree to which the curve deviates from a straight line at 450 nm (the ΔA_{450}) is linearly proportional to the concentration of bilirubin in the AF.

The major contaminant of concern is oxyhemoglobin, with an absorbance peak at 410 nm. There-

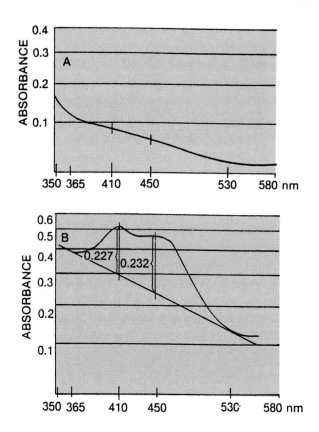

FIGURE 13-5 A, Normal amniotic fluid. Note near linearity of the curve when plotted on log-linear graph. B, Amniotic fluid showing the bilirubin peak at 450 nm and the oxyhemoglobin peak at approximately 410 nm. Note the baseline drawn between linear parts of the curve, from 550 and 365 nm. (From Burtis CA, Ashwood ER. *Tietz textbook of clinical chemistry*. 2nd ed. Philadelphia: WB Saunders Company, 1994.)

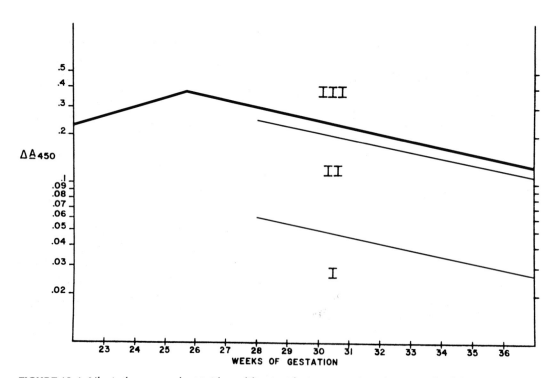

FIGURE 13-6 Liley's three zone chart (with modification) for interpretation of amniotic fluid ΔA_{450}. Note that the original three zones (divided by the two *lighter lines*) extended only to 28 weeks of gestation. The *uppermost* (heavy) *line* is the upward revision of the "danger line" defined by Dr. Irving Umansky. For further explanation, see the chapter text. (From Burtis CA, Ashwood ER. *Tietz textbook of clinical chemistry*. 2nd ed. Philadelphia: WB Saunders Company, 1994.)

fore, if blood is observed in a specimen of AF, it should be centrifuged immediately to remove any intact RBCs before hemolysis occurs.

Figure 13-6 is Liley's prediction graph that relates bilirubin concentration, fetal risk, and gestational age. Because there is normally a small amount of bilirubin in AF (which changes with gestational age), it is necessary to know the gestational age to interpret the graph. Values in Liley's bottom zone represent an unaffected

or very mildly affected fetus. As values in the middle zone rise, it is increasingly likely that a fetus is suffering moderate to marked hemolysis. Intervention may be recommended when the ΔA_{450} has reached the zone just below the heavy line marking the beginning of zone III. Values in zone III indicate severe disease. Without intervention, a fetus with AF bilirubin values in that region of the graph most likely will die.[5]

REFERENCES

1. Burtis CA, Ashwood ER. *Tietz textbook of clinical chemistry*. 2nd ed. Philadelphia: WB Saunders, 1994.
2. Kjeldsberg CR, Knight JA. *Body fluids*. 3rd ed. Chicago: ASCP Press, 1993.
3. Wenk RE, Rosenbaum JM. Analyses of amniotic fluid. In: Henry JB, ed. *Clinical diagnosis and management by laboratory methods*. 18th ed. Philadelphia: WB Saunders, 1991: 482–496.

BIBLIOGRAPHY

Bishop ML, Duben-Engelkirk JL, Fody, EP. *Clinical chemistry*. 3rd ed. Philadelphia: Lippincott–Raven Publishers, 1996.
Bennington JL, ed. *Saunders' dictionary and encyclopedia of laboratory medicine and technology*. Philadelphia: WB Saunders, 1984.
Brunzel NA. *Fundamentals of urine and body fluid analysis*. Philadelphia: WB Saunders, 1994.
Bullock BL, Rosendahl PP. *Pathophysiology*. 3rd ed. Philadelphia: JB Lippincott, 1992.
Kjeldsberg CR, Knight JA. *Body fluids*. Chicago: ASCP Press, 1983.
Ringsrud KM, Linné JJ. *Urinalysis and body fluids: A color text and atlas*. St. Louis: Mosby–Year Book, 1995.
Strasinger SK. *Urinalysis and body fluids*. 3rd ed. Philadelphia: FA Davis, 1994.
Tortora GJ, Anagnostakos NP. *Principles of anatomy and physiology*. New York: Harper & Row, 1981.

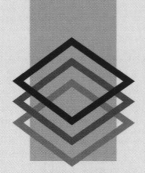

14 *Synovial Fluid Analysis*

ABBREVIATIONS USED IN THIS CHAPTER

C&S = culture and sensitivity

CPPD = calcium pyrophosphate dihydrate

EDTA = ethylenediaminetetra acetic acid

ER = emergency room

LE = lupus erythematosus

MSU = monosodium urate

RA = rheumatoid arthritis

RBC = red blood cell

SF = synovial fluid

SLE = systemic lupus erythematosus

WBC = white blood cell

Introductory Case Study

This patient, a 55-year-old woman, was seen in the ER for swelling on both her knees. She had had multiple attacks of gout over the last 15 years involving both knees, arms, back, toes, and ankles, and she was on allopurinol.

An arthrocentesis was performed on the right knee with the following results (tube 1): color pinkish red; appearance cloudy; supernatant yellow and clear; total nucleated cells/mm³ 1772; RBCs/mm³ 8250; lymphocytes 1%; neutrophils 95%; monocytes 4%. The appearance of the fluid sediment is illustrated in Figures 14-1 and 14-2. The axis of slow vibration of the red compensator is in the direction of the yellow crystal in both Figures. Microscopic examination of the crystals in the synovial fluid demonstrates monosodium urate and is positive for gout.

FIGURE 14-1 Synovial fluid showing monosodium urate crystals in polarized light, with a secondary red compensator; ×400.

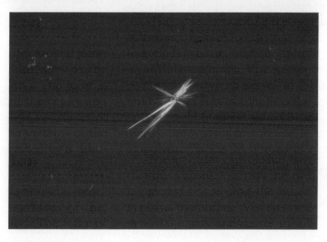

FIGURE 14-2 Synovial fluid showing monosodium urate crystals in polarized light, with a secondary red compensator; ×400.

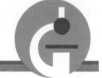

Physiology and Composition

Figure 14-3 illustrates an articulated diarthroidal joint. The space between the articulating surfaces of the bones is the joint cavity (synovial cavity). The joint is freely movable (diarthrotic) because of the cavity and the lack of tissue between the articulating surfaces of the bones. Articular cartilage covers the surfaces of the abutting bones, and the joint is surrounded by a tubular articular capsule that encloses the joint cavity.

The articular capsule has two layers, the outer layer (fibrous capsule), consisting of dense connective (collagenous) tissue, and the inner layer, formed by the synovial membrane. Viscous synovial fluid (SF) fills the synovial cavity and serves to lubricate the joint space and to transport nutrients to the articular cartilage.

Synovial fluid is formed by ultrafiltration of plasma across the synovial membrane; it is combined with a mucopolysaccharide (hyaluronate) synthesized by the synovial cells (synoviocytes) that line the surface of the syn-

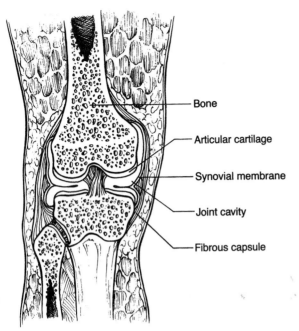

Bone

Articular cartilage

Synovial membrane

Joint cavity

Fibrous capsule

FIGURE 14-3 Schematic drawing showing anatomic relationship of parts in a diarthrodial joint. Cutaway view. (From Kjeldsberg CR, Knight JA: *Body fluids*. 3rd ed. Chicago: ASCP Press, 1993.)

ovial membrane surrounding the joint. Hyaluronate is a polymer composed of repeating disaccharide units (glucuronic acid–glucosamine) with a molecular weight between 5 to 10 million daltons, depending on the degree of polymerization. The hyaluronate is combined with about 2% protein. Concentrations of total protein and immunoglobulins in SF are about one third to one half that of plasma, whereas concentrations of glucose and uric acid are comparable to those of plasma (Table 14-1).

Classification of Joint Disorders

Mechanical, chemical, or bacteriologic damage to the joint may alter the permeability of the membranes and capillaries to produce varying degrees of inflammatory response. Changes in the chemical constituents of the joint fluid and in the types of cells present are associated with various disorders. Joint disorders can be divided into five categories (Table 14-2): group I, noninflammatory; group II, inflammatory; group III, infectious; group IV, crystal associated; and group V, hemorrhagic.

Specimen Collection

The aspiration of joint fluid (arthrocentesis) is carried out with a sterile, disposable plastic syringe to avoid contamination with exogenous birefringent material

from glass syringes. The patient should be fasting for 6 hours or more before arthrocentesis to allow equilibration of glucose between plasma and SF.

Although normal SF lacks fibrinogen and does not clot, the syringe can be moistened with sodium heparin to avoid possible clotting. Oxalate, powdered ethylenediaminetetraacetic acid (EDTA), and lithium heparin are not recommended because they can produce crystalline structures resembling monosodium urate (MSU) crystals.

In the ideal situation, when adequate fluid is available, the specimen may be divided into three samples: 5 to 10 mL in a sterile tube for microbiologic examination, 2 to 5 mL in an anticoagulated tube (heparin or liquid EDTA) for microscopic examination, and approximately 5 mL in a plain (no anticoagulant) red-top tube for additional studies as needed. To avoid the lysis of cells, altered chemical composition, and attenuation of microorganisms, SF—along with other body fluids—should be processed and tested as soon as possible after collection.

Gross Examination

Table 14-3 gives SF findings by disease category. Resembling uncooked egg white, normal SF is crystal clear, viscous, and colorless. SF from group I patients is usually clear, viscous, and pale yellow. With inflammatory arthritides (group II), the fluid is cloudy, turbid, and yellow. Clotting occurs because of the pres-

TABLE 14-1
Adult Reference Values for Synovial Fluid

	Conventional Units	SI Units
Leukocyte	<150/µL	<0.15 × 10⁹/L
Differential white blood cell count		
PMNs*	<25%	<0.25
Lymphocytes	<75%	<0.75
Monocytes	<70%	<0.70
Glucose level (blood–synovial fluid difference)	<10 mg/dL	<0.55 mmol/L
Hyaluronate	0.30–0.41 g/dL	3.0–4.1 g/L
Lactate	<25 mg/dL	<2.8 mmol/L
Protein	1–3 g/dL	10–30 g/L
Uric acid		
Male	<8.0 mg/dL	<476 µmol/L
Female	<6.0 mg/dL	<357 µmol/L

* PMNs, polymorphonuclear neutrophils.

(From Kjeldsberg CR, Knight JA. *Body fluids*. 3rd ed. Chicago: ASCP Press, 1993.)

TABLE 14-2
Classification of Arthritides

Group I (Noninflammatory)
Osteoarthritis
Traumatic arthritis
Osteochondritis dissecans
Osteochondromatosis
Neuropathic osteoarthropathy
Pigmented villonodular synovitis
Early rheumatoid arthritis
Paget's disease
Acromegaly
Ochronosis
Hyperparathyroidism

Group II (Inflammatory)
Rheumatoid arthritis
Lupus erythematosus
Reiter's syndrome
Rheumatic fever
Ankylosing spondylitis
Regional enteritis
Ulcerative colitis
Psoriatic arthritis
Fat droplet synovitis
Sarcoidosis
Scleroderma
Polymyalgia rheumatica
Erythema multiforme

Group III (Infectious)
Bacterial
Mycobacterial
Fungal
Viral
Spirochetal

Group IV (Crystal Induced)
Gout
CPPD crystal deposition disease
Apatite-associated arthropathy

Group V (Hemorrhagic)
Traumatic arthritis
Hemophiliac arthropathy
Anticoagulation
Pigmented villonodular synovitis
Neuropathic osteoarthropathy
Synovial hemangioma
Hemangioma
Thrombocytopenia

CPPD, calcium pyrophosphate dihydrate.

Used with permission from Rippey JH.

(From Kjeldsberg CR, Knight JA. *Body fluids.* 3rd ed. Chicago: ASCP Press, 1993.)

ence of fibrinogen and other coagulation factors as a result of the inflammatory condition.

Fluid from group III patients (infectious disease) often appears grossly purulent with a color dependent on the chromogen produced by the invading bacteria. SF from group V patients (hemorrhagic) is homogeneously bloody, whereas streaks of blood are seen in a traumatic aspirate. A yellow (xanthochromic) color suggests that blood has been present in the SF for some time and bilirubin has been produced. A purulent or white-opaque fluid may be observed with group IV patients (crystal-induced synovitis).

Although tests for viscosity are mentioned later under Chemical Examination, Kjeldsberg and Knight suggest that such tests are not considered reliable or useful in the classification of synovial effusions.[3]

Cell Counts and Microscopic Examination

Only a few WBCs are found in normal SF (0–150/μL), and these are primarily lymphocytes, with neutrophils rarely seen.[3] The ranges of leukocyte counts associated with the various diagnostic groups are shown in Table 14-3.

Usually the WBC count is performed with a standard hemacytometer, although electronic counting equipment may also be used (see Chapter 5, IRIS). If the leukocyte count is more than 50,000/μL, physiologic saline may be used to dilute the fluid before counting. Phase contrast or brightfield microscopy may be used for the cell count. With brightfield, adding methylene blue stain to the specimen is helpful in identifying the leukocytes. A diluent such as hypotonic saline may be used to lyse RBCs present in a fluid heavily contaminated with blood.

The differential count and cytologic examination should be performed within 1 hour of arthrocentesis.[3] After centrifuging the SF, a Wright-stained smear is made from the pellet. Cytocentrifuged specimens may also be prepared and stained with Wright's stain.

Cells observed in abnormal SF include neutrophils, lymphocytes, plasma cells, monocytes, eosinophils, mononuclear phagocytes (monocytes, macrophages, and histiocytes), synovial lining cells, and lupus erythematosus (LE) cells. Neutrophils may contain vacuoles, fat droplets, bacteria, or crystals; the nuclei commonly show pyknosis and karyorrhexis. A high percentage of neutrophils (>80%) strongly suggests septic arthritis, and a Gram stain should be performed.[3]

In the early stages of rheumatoid arthritis (RA),

TABLE 14-3
Synovial Fluid Findings by Disease Category*

Finding	Normal	Group I (Noninflammatory)	Group II (Inflammatory)	Group III (Infectious)	Group IV (Crystal Induced)	Group V (Hemorrhagic)
Appearance	Clear to straw colored	Yellow transparent	Yellow, cloudy, turbid, or bloody	Yellow, purulent	Cloudy, turbid, or white-opaque	Red-brown or xanthochromic
White blood cells/μL	0–150 ($0–0.15 \times 10^9$/L)	<3000 ($0–3 \times 10^9$/L)	3000–75,000 ($3–75 \times 10^9$/L)	50,000–200,000 ($50–200 \times 10^9$/L)	500–200,000 ($0.5–200 \times 10^9$/L)	50–10,000 ($0.05–10 \times 10^9$/L)
Polymorphonuclear leukocytes (%)	<25	<30	>50	>90	<90	<50
Crystals present	No	No	No	No	Yes	No
Red blood cells present	No	No	No	Yes	No	Yes
Blood glucose to synovial fluid glucose ratio (mg/dL)	0–10 (0–0.56 mmol/L)	0–10 (0–0.56 mmol/L)	0–4 (0–2.22 mmol/L)	20–100 (1.11–5.55 mmol/L)	0–80 (0–4.44 mmol/L)	0–20 (0–1.11 mmol/L)
Culture	Negative	Negative	Negative	Often positive	Negative	Negative

* Values in parentheses are SI units.Used with permission from Krieg AF and Rippey JH.
(From Kjeldsberg CR, Knight JA. *Body fluids*. 3rd ed. Chicago: ASCP Press, 1993.)

lymphocytes predominate, although neutrophils may be more numerous later on. Monocytes may predominate in arthritis associated with serum sickness and certain viral infections (hepatitis and rubella), and are occasionally observed with crystal-induced arthritis.

Synovial lining cells, which resemble the mesothelial cells in pleural and peritoneal fluids, may be observed in SF but seem not to have any specific diagnostic significance.

LE cells occur in approximately 10% of effusions from patients with systemic lupus erythematosus (SLE). In some patients, LE cells may initially be present in SF and not in the peripheral blood. LE cells also have been described in SF samples from patients with RA.[3]

An important laboratory test routinely performed on SF is the microscopic examination for crystals. As mentioned in Chapter 8, MSU crystals are birefringent and rotate the plane of polarized light; with crossed polarizers, the crystals appear as bright, needle-like objects with pointed ends against a black background. The use of polarized light and a red compensator plate permits the identification and differentiation both of positively birefringent substances and of negatively birefringent materials, on the basis of the colors observed.

MSU crystals in SF are diagnostic for gout (gouty arthritis). When viewed with polarized light and a red compensator, the crystals aligned along the compensator's axis of slow vibration appear yellow. MSUe crystals appear blue when their long axes are perpendicular to the axis of the compensator. These aspects are illustrated in the Introductory Case Study for this chapter.

Calcium pyrophosphate dihydrate (CPPD) crystals appear in SF in conditions termed "pseudogout." These crystals are smaller than MSU crystals, and are rodlike or rhomboid, not pointed and sharp. Polarized light and the red compensator are diagnostic: the CPPD crystals appear blue when their longitudinal axes are parallel to the compensator's axis of slow vibration, and yellow when perpendicular to the compensator axis. In other words, they appear just the opposite of MSU crystals.

Chemical Examination

Chemical analysis of SF is most useful when applied to the diagnosis of the infectious and crystal-induced arthritides. It usually consists of measuring glucose and total protein. Other tests still occasionally performed include the measurement of viscosity and the evaluation of the mucin and fibrin clot.

A measure of viscosity can be performed at the time of fluid aspiration by manually stringing the SF from the syringe tip after removing the needle. A string longer than 4 to 5 cm is formed by normal and noninflammatory fluids; inflammatory or septic fluids form a much shorter string.

The condition of the hyaluronic acid–protein complex also is related to viscosity and can be determined by the mucin clot test. Normal hyaluronate integrity is associated with good mucin, while poor mucin indicates hyaluronate destruction and dilution. Inflammatory conditions usually decrease both the mucin clot formation and hyaluronic acid concentration.

The test is performed by mixing two parts SF with one part 3% acetic acid and evaluating the clot, which is formed after 2 hours. A good result is a firm, ropy clot with clear, overlying fluid. A soft clot with slightly cloudy supernatant is fair; a small, friable clot with turbid supernatant is poor; and flecks of precipitate with cloudy supernatant is very poor.

Normally SF does not clot because it lacks fibrinogen and other clotting factors; however, with both inflammatory and bloody fluids, there may be spontaneous clotting. This is evaluated by observing the specimen for spontaneous clotting after placing the fluid in a red-stoppered tube (i.e., no anticoagulant is present).

Although normal SF contains essentially all plasma proteins, some high–molecular-weight proteins (e.g., fibrinogen, beta$_2$-macroglobulin, alpha$_2$-macroglobulin) are either absent or present in only trace amounts.[3] The same methods used for quantitating total serum protein may be used for measuring protein in SF. Increased levels are commonly seen in RA, gout, septic arthritis, SLE, the inflammatory arthropathies accompanying Crohn's disease, Reiter's syndrome, ankylosing spondylitis, psoriasis, and ulcerative colitis. Although local immunoglobulin synthesis occurs, most of the proteins are derived from the plasma because of increased vascular permeability related to an inflammatory process.

Even though the measurement of SF glucose may be of clinical value, abnormal levels do not indicate any specific disease process. Just as with cerebrospinal fluid glucose, levels of glucose in SF need to be interpreted along with serum values. To ensure that equilibrium has been reached, the synovial and serum levels should be obtained 6 to 8 hours postprandially. In general, noninflammatory joint disorders have SF glucose levels less than 25 mg/dL below the simultaneously measured serum levels (see Table 14-3). In cases of septic arthritis, the level of the SF glucose is frequently lower than the serum concentration by more than 40 mg/dL (see Table 14-3). However, there is considerable overlap of glucose levels in noninflammatory and inflammatory joint disorders and septic arthritis.[3]

Because the preferred laboratory diagnosis of gout is made by SF crystal identification, quantitation of SF uric acid is seldom recommended. If the laboratory does not have the proper polarizing equipment, the quantitative measurement of SF uric acid may be of help in the diagnosis of gout.

Lactic acid levels in SF are only slightly increased in most cases of nonseptic monoarticular arthritis.[3] However, lactate levels are usually markedly elevated in septic arthritis, as much as 40 times the upper reference level. Thus, lactate measurement in SF appears to be useful for the rapid diagnosis of septic arthritis.

Microbiologic Examination

Septic arthritis is usually acquired from the bloodstream and is the most rapidly destructive joint disease. Bacteria are the most common infectious agents, although viruses, *Mycobacterium tuberculosis*, and fungi are also possible causative agents. Certain bacteria present in the bloodstream are particularly likely to infect a joint, such as *Neisseria gonorrhoeae* and *Staphylococcus aureus*. Bacteria may also enter a joint by way of a deep penetrating wound, intraarticular steroid injections, arthroscopy, prosthetic joint surgery, or by contiguous rupture of osteomyelitis into the joint.

It is recommended that the routine examination of SF include a Gram's stain together with both aerobic and anaerobic culture for microorganisms, even if the Gram stain is negative.[3] Because positive smears are not always obtained, measurement of lactate in the fluid may also be helpful. Because *N. gonorrhoeae* is such an important causative agent, it is important that the proper media be inoculated immediately after fluid aspiration. Even with careful microbiologic techniques, *N. gonorrhoeae* is recovered in less than 50% of infected joints in patients with disseminated gonococcal infections.

Quality Control

At present, apparently no commercial controls are available to monitor the analysis of SF, although research and development on such materials is being undertaken. Many laboratories prepare permanent slides for positive controls of MSU crystals from gout patients for quality control of this particular test.

Illustrative Case Studies

CASE STUDY 14-1

This patient, a 35-year-old man, came in through the ER in a wheelchair, unable to walk because of the pain in his neck and back. He had been seen the previous week, treated, and released for pain he thought was due to his young son jumping on his neck.

On admission the patient was feverish but had no petechiae, no purpuric rash, no diarrhea or vomiting, but some nausea. The assessment was acute viral meningitis, total body myalgia, leuko-cytosis, and hyperpyrexia with dehydration. His right elbow was swollen, and an arthrocentesis was performed. The SF showed: color pale yellow; appearance cloudy; supernatant pale yellow and hazy; total nucleated cells/mm^3 = 79,000; RBCs/mm^3 = 2,000; lymphocytes 1%; neutrophils 95%; and macrophages 4%. C&S on the fluid was positive for *Neisseria meningitidis*. Discharge diagnosis was *N. meningitidis* meningitis, septic arthritis, and myalgias. The appearance of the SF is illustrated in Figures 14-4 and 14-5.

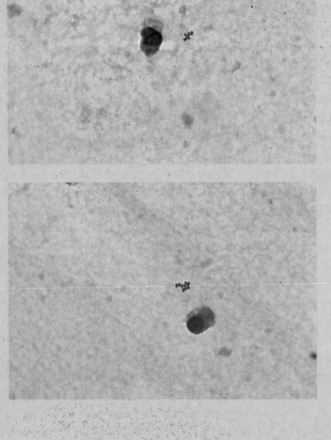

FIGURE 14-4 Gram's stain of synovial fluid showing gram-negative diplococci (*Neisseria meningitidis*); ×1000.

FIGURE 14-5 Gram's stain of synovial fluid showing gram-negative diplococci (*Neisseria meningitidis*); ×1000.

continued

CASE STUDY 14-2

This 18-year-old woman was admitted directly though the Rheumatology Clinic complaining of a swollen left elbow (sudden onset) with pain and limited range of motion. Arthrocentesis was performed and the SF showed: color white; appearance milky; supernatant pale yellow and slightly hazy with a large fibrin clot; total nucleated cells/mm^3 = 275,000; RBCs/mm^3 = 3000; lymphocytes 2%; neutrophils 94%; eosinophils 1%; "mononuclear phagocyte" (= macrophage) 3%. She was placed on IV Ancef (cefazolin) for a total of 6 days, and her condition improved steadily.

Although the C&S on the SF was consistently negative, the WBC count decreased, the range of motion improved, and the pain decreased. Discharge diagnosis was infected left elbow with a sterile tap, and a secondary diagnosis was juvenile RA. The appearance of the SF sediment is shown in Figure 14-6.

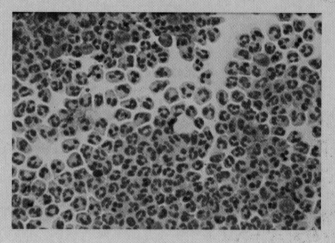

FIGURE 14-6 Wright-stained Cytospin preparation of synovial fluid showing inflammatory reaction (mostly neutrophils); ×400.

REFERENCES

1. Kjeldsberg CR, Knight JA. *Body fluids*. 3rd ed. Chicago: ASCP Press, 1993.

BIBLIOGRAPHY

Brunzel NA. *Fundamentals of urine and body fluid analysis*. Philadelphia: WB Saunders, 1994.
Kjeldsberg CR, Knight JA. *Body fluids*. Chicago: ASCP Press, 1983.
Krieg AF, Kjeldsberg CR. Cerebrospinal fluid and other body fluids. In: Henry JB, ed. *Clinical diagnosis and management by laboratory methods*. 18th ed. Philadelphia: WB Saunders, 1991: 445–473.
Ringsrud KM, Linné JJ. *Urinalysis and body fluids: A color text and atlas*. St. Louis: Mosby–Year Book, 1995.
Strasinger SK. *Urinalysis and body fluids*. 3rd ed. Philadelphia: FA Davis, 1994.

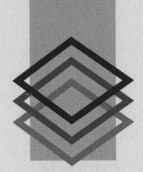

15

Serous Fluid Analysis (Pleural, Pericardial, and Peritoneal Fluids)

ABBREVIATIONS USED IN THIS CHAPTER

2° = secondary

AFB = acid-fast bacilli

ALD = alcoholic liver disease

ALP = alkaline phosphatase

BP = blood pressure

C&S = culture and sensitivity

COPD = chronic obstructive pulmonary disease

ER = emergency room

H&E = hematoxylin and eosin

IV = intravenous

LDH = lactate dehydrogenase

PMN = polymorphonuclear neutrophil

R/O = rule out

RBC = red blood cell

SBP = spontaneous bacterial peritonitis

SOB = shortness of breath

WBC = white blood cell

Introductory Case Study

Previously seen for an infection in the umbilicus with purulent discharge (patient was given dicloxacillin), this 45-year-old woman was admitted with a temperature of 102°F, BP 97/57, pulse 126, and respirations 42. She was complaining of fever and chills, diarrhea, and abdominal distention and pain, and was feeling very ill. She was diaphoretic and appeared to be in a very toxic state. The admission diagnosis was alcoholic liver disease (ALD); possible sepsis, unknown focus; dehydration; possible bowel obstruction; R/O gastroenteritis vs. constipation.

Paracentesis was performed, and about 20 mL of thick, serosanguineous fluid was obtained for analysis. The fluid analysis showed color dark amber; appearance cloudy; supernatant yellow and hazy; total nucleated cells/mm^3 29,550; RBCs/mm^3 23,100; lymphocytes 30%; neutrophils 65%;

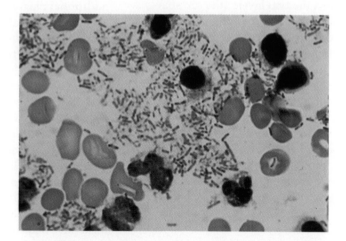

FIGURE 15-1 Bacteria in cytospin preparation of peritoneal fluid, identified by C&S as *Escherichia coli*. Wright's stain; ×1000.

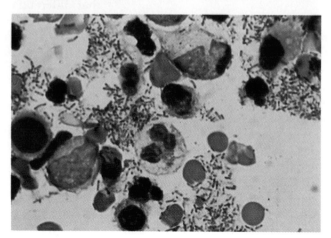

FIGURE 15-2 Bacteria in cytospin preparation of peritoneal fluid, identified by C&S as *Escherichia coli*. Wright's stain; ×1000.

eosinophils 1%; monocytes 1%; mesothelial cells 1%. Comment: many bacteria seen (later identified as *Escherichia coli*).

The patient was started on vancomycin and ceftazidime IV. She required intubation and ventilatory assistance as well as fluids and supplemental dopamine to maintain BP. She continued to be hemodynamically unstable and continued to require dopamine and epinephrine to support BP. She had episodes of asystole and bradycardia, became progressively bradycardic, and finally epinephrine boluses did not restore BP. The day after admission she went into asystole and died.

Final diagnosis was gram-negative septic shock, disseminated intravascular coagulation, and alcoholic liver disease. The appearance of the peritoneal fluid sediment is shown in Figures 15-1 and 15-2.

Classification of Fluids

The body cavities that do not open to the exterior are lined by serous membranes, which cover the organs that lie within the cavities. The membranes are thin layers of loose connective tissue covered by a layer of mesothelium; they are in the form of double-walled sacs. The part of the membrane that covers the organs inside the cavities is called the visceral portion. The part attached to the cavity wall is the parietal portion.

The space between the two layers (the sac space) is filled with serous fluid formed by the parietal layer. The fluid is termed "serous" because it is similar to serum in composition. The serous fluid serves as a lubricant between the membranes, permitting free movement of the enclosed organ. The membrane lining the thoracic cavity and covering the lungs is called the pleura, and it gives rise to pleural fluid; that lining the heart cavity and covering the heart is the pericardium, and it produces pericardial fluid. The serous membrane lining the abdominal cavity and covering the abdominal organs, as well as some pelvic organs, is called the peritoneum; it gives rise to the peritoneal or ascitic fluid.

Terminology—Transudates and Exudates

Serous fluid is formed by the parietal membranes and absorbed by the visceral membranes. Formation is by ultrafiltration of plasma through the capillary endothelium. This process depends on hydrostatic pressure in the capillaries, oncotic pressure of the plasma, and the permeability of the capillaries. The accumulation of fluid within a cavity is called an effusion. Fluids that accumulate in pleural, pericardial, and peritoneal cavities are referred to as serous effusions.

Historically, pleural, pericardial, and peritoneal effusions have been divided into *transudates* and *exudates*. In general, transudates are effusions that have accumulated because of a systemic disease such as congestive heart failure or cirrhosis of the liver. Exudates usually form in association with a localized process involving the membranes, such as inflammation, malignancy, or infection. Characterizing an effusion as a transudate or exudate is useful in making a decision concerning the need for further laboratory evaluation and testing. If the effusion is a transudate, usually no additional diagnostic work is needed. If it is an exudate, more extensive diagnostic procedures are required to determine the cause of the effusion.

Differences in color, appearance, and cell count are often observed for transudates and exudates. Historically, however, these effusions have been differentiated by measuring specific gravity and total protein content. Defined in this way, a transudate is an effusion with a specific gravity of less than 1.015 and a total protein level of 3.0 g/dL or lower. An exudate is an effusion with a specific gravity of greater than 1.015 and a total protein level greater than 3.0 g/dL. Unfortunately, these criteria based on specific gravity and total protein do not hold in all cases. As discussed later, additional criteria have been added to the definitions. It also appears that differentiating pericardial effusions into transudates and exudates may not be as meaningful as it is for pleural and peritoneal fluids. At present, no single set of criteria separates all transudates from all exudates for all patients.[5]

Classification and Characterization of Effusions

PLEURAL EFFUSIONS

Table 15-1 lists the causes of pleural effusions. Table 15-2 gives information on the laboratory differentiation of pleural fluid transudates and exudates.

TABLE 15-1
Causes of Pleural Effusions

Transudates
Acute atelectasis
Congestive heart failure
Cirrhosis with ascites
Hypoproteinemia with nephrotic syndrome
Postoperative abdominal surgery
Postpartum effusion
Peritoneal dialysis
Superior vena cava obstruction

Exudates
Infectious diseases
   Bacterial pneumonia (parapneumonic effusion)
   Tuberculosis
   Viral infection
   Fungal infection
   Parasitic infection
   Lung abscess
Neoplastic disease
   Metastatic carcinoma
   Lung carcinoma
   Mesothelioma
   Lymphoma and leukemia
Pulmonary embolization or infarction
Collagen vascular disease
   Rheumatoid arthritis
   Systemic lupus erythematosus
Gastrointestinal disease
   Pancreatitis
   Esophageal rupture
   Subphrenic abscess
   Hepatic abscess
Postmyocardial infarction
Trauma
   Hemothorax
   Chylothorax
Chylous effusion
   Trauma
   Lymphoma
   Carcinoma
   Tuberculosis

(From Kjeldsberg CR, Knight JA. *Body fluids*. 3rd ed. Chicago: ASCP Press, 1993.)

TABLE 15-2
Pleural Fluid Laboratory Differentiation of Transudates and Exudates

	Transudate	Exudate
Appearance	Clear, pale yellow	Cloudy, turbid, purulent or bloody
Pleural fluid: serum protein ratio	<0.5	>0.5
Pleural fluid: serum lactate dehydrogenase ratio	<0.6	>0.6
Pleural fluid: serum bilirubin ratio	<0.6	>0.6
Pleural fluid: cholesterol	<60 mg/dL	>60 mg/dL
Pleural fluid: serum cholesterol ratio	<0.3	>0.3

(From Kjeldsberg CR, Knight JA. *Body fluids*. 3rd ed. Chicago: ASCP Press, 1993.)

TABLE 15-3
Causes of Pericardial Effusions

Infections
   Bacterial pericarditis
   Viral or mycoplasma pericarditis
   Tuberculosis
   Fungal pericarditis
Cardiovascular disease
   Myocardial infarction
   Postinfarction syndrome
   Cardiac rupture
   Aortic dissection
   Congestive heart failure
Neoplastic disease
   Metastatic carcinoma
   Mesothelioma
   Lymphoma, leukemia
Trauma
Metabolic disorders
   Uremia
   Myxedema
Collagen vascular disorder
Coagulation disorder, anticoagulant therapy

(From Kjeldsberg CR, Knight JA. *Body fluids*. 3rd ed. Chicago: ASCP Press, 1993.)

PERICARDIAL EFFUSIONS

Table 15-3 indicates the causes of pericardial effusions. Classifying pericardial effusions as transudates or exudates is of doubtful value because most pericardial effusions appear to fit the definition of exudates, since they are caused by damage to mesothelial linings rather than by mechanical factors.

PERITONEAL EFFUSIONS

Table 15-4 suggests the laboratory tests to be done on peritoneal effusions. Table 15-5 gives the causes of peritoneal effusions. As with pleural fluid, peritoneal effusions can be divided into transudates and exudates, although the laboratory criteria may be less clearly defined.

For peritoneal lavage (see Table 15-4), a perforated peritoneal dialysis catheter is inserted into the peritoneal cavity through a small, midline, infraumbilical incision.[4] First, a small amount of fluid is aspirated. If gross blood is not observed, then 1 L of Ringer's lactate solution is infused. The lavage fluid is immediately retrieved by gravity and analyzed. Peritoneal lavage may be used to evaluate patients with blunt or penetrating trauma to the abdomen, acute pancreatitis (amylase and lipase), and suspected acute peritonitis. If the result is "indeterminate," the catheter may be left in place and the procedure repeated within 1 to 2 hours.

TABLE 15-4
Laboratory Tests in Peritoneal Effusions

Useful in most patients
  Gross examination
  Cytology
  Stains and culture for organisms
  Serum–ascites albumin concentration gradient
Useful in selected patients
  Tumor markers
  Immunocytochemistry/flow cytometry
  Leukocyte count and differential count
  Red blood cell count (lavage)
  Alkaline phosphatase
  Cholesterol (malignancy-related ascites)
  Amylase
  Lipase
Useful in few patients
  Glucose
  Lactate dehydrogenase

(From Kjeldsberg CR, Knight JA. *Body fluids*. 3rd ed. Chicago: ASCP Press, 1993.)

TABLE 15-5
Causes of Peritoneal Effusions

Transudates (increased hydrostatic pressure or decreased plasma oncotic pressure)
Congestive heart failure
Hepatic cirrhosis
Hypoproteinemia (e.g., nephrotic syndrome)

Exudates (increased capillary permeability or decreased lymphatic resorption)
Infections
  Tuberculosis
  Primary bacterial peritonitis
  Secondary bacterial peritonitis (e.g., appendicitis)
Neoplasms
  Hepatoma
  Metastatic carcinoma
  Lymphoma
  Mesothelioma
Trauma
Pancreatitis
Bile peritonitis (e.g., ruptured gallbladder)

Chylous Effusion

(From Krieg AF, Kjeldsberb CR. *Cerebrospinal fluid and other body fluids*. In Henry JB, ed. *Clinical diagnosis and management by laboratory methods*. 18th ed. Philadelphia: WB Saunders Company, 1991.)

Specimen Collection

The general term for the puncture of a body cavity to aspirate fluid is "paracentesis." Sometimes the term "paracentesis" is also used to mean the collection of peritoneal fluid. Thoracentesis (thoracocentesis, pleurocentesis) is the puncture of the pleural cavity to collect pleural fluid; pericardiocentesis is the puncture of the pericardium for the collection of pericardial fluid; and peritoneocentesis (abdominal paracentesis or paracentesis) is the puncture of the peritoneal cavity to aspirate peritoneal fluid. To avoid chemical and cellular changes in the specimen, serous fluids obtained from body cavities should be transported to the laboratory as soon as possible after their collection.

Serous fluids are collected by a physician under strictly sterile conditions by using a needle inserted into the serous cavity and by aspirating the fluid in a syringe. This collection is done for diagnostic purposes as well as to relieve the patient of symptoms, such as difficult breathing due to excess fluid accumulating around the lungs or from massive ascites in the abdomen.

Kjeldsberg and Knight provide useful advice on the requirements for laboratory evaluation of serous fluid

---

TABLE 15-6
Requirements for Laboratory Evaluation of Serous Fluid Specimens*

Volume (mL)†	Anticoagulant Tube	Tests
3–7	EDTA	Hematology (WBC and RBC counts, differential cell count, and smear evaluation)
8–10	Heparin	Chemistry (total protein, lactate dehydrogenase, cholesterol, bilirubin, and amylase determinations)
8–10	Heparin (sterile)	Microbiology (Gram's stain, acid-fast bacilli stain, culture, counterimmunoelectrophoresis)
>25	Heparin container	Cytology (Papanicolaou's stain, cell block, immunocytologic techniques)

* A blood specimen should be obtained simultaneously for serum total protein, lactate dehydrogenase, cholesterol, bilirubin, and amylase when indicated.

† Smaller amounts of fluid may be adequate, depending on the instruments available and the type of tests requested.

(From Kjeldsberg CR, Knight JA. *Body fluids.* 3rd ed. Chicago: ASCP Press, 1993.)

---

specimens (Table 15-6). For comparative studies in chemistry, a serum sample should also be obtained at the same time the serous fluid is aspirated.

Gross Examination

Pleural Fluid

Table 15-7 summarizes the pleural fluid gross appearance and clinical significance. It is necessary to differentiate a traumatic tap from a hemorrhagic effusion. For a typical traumatic tap, the blood is not distributed uniformly in the specimen but gradually clears as aspiration continues. Also, small blood clots may form. In contrast, with hemothorax or hemorrhagic effusions, blood is distributed evenly in the specimen and clots are not formed (i.e., fibrinogen is rapidly removed from the pleural space). Large numbers of leukocytes associated with septic or nonseptic inflammation (e.g., bacterial infection, tuberculosis, rheumatoid disease, or rheumatic fever) may result in a cloudy or turbid specimen.

A turbid, milky, or bloody pleural fluid should be centrifuged and the supernatant examined.[4] Turbidity that is cleared by centrifugation is most likely due to debris or an increased number of cells; turbidity that remains after centrifugation is most likely caused by chylothorax or pseudochylothorax.

Pericardial Fluid

The pericardial cavity normally contains only a small amount of clear, pale yellow fluid. With an infection or malignancy, the pericardial effusion is usually turbid.

Tumors or tuberculosis may be associated with a blood-streaked, cloudy fluid. Cardiac rupture or puncture gives rise to a bloody effusion. A clear, straw-colored fluid usually indicates renal failure with uremia. When the lymphatic system has been damaged, a milky fluid may be observed.

TABLE 15-7
Pleural Fluid Gross Appearance and Clinical Significance

Appearance	Significance
Transudates	
Clear, straw colored	Further analysis usually not necessary
Exudates*	
Cloudy, purulent	Infectious process, empyema
Red tinge to bloody	If not traumatic tap: malignancy, pulmonary infarction, trauma
Green-white, turbid	Rheumatoid pleuritis
Milky white or yellow bloody	Chylous effusion
Milky or green, metallic sheen	Pseudochylous (chyliform) effusion
Viscous, hemorrhagic, or clear	Mesothelioma
Anchovy-paste color ("chocolate sauce")	Rupture of amebic liver abscess

* Some exudates may also appear clear and straw colored.

(From Kjeldsberg CR, Knight JA. *Body fluids.* 3rd ed. Chicago: ASCP Press, 1993.)

TABLE 15-8
Gross Appearance of Peritoneal Fluid and Associated Disorders

Appearance	Disorder
Clear, pale yellow	Cirrhosis
Cloudy, turbid	Bacterial peritonitis, pancreatitis, malignant condition
Green-brown	Biliary tract disease, ruptured bowel
Bloody	Trauma, malignant disorder, pancreatitis, intestinal infarction
Milky	Chylous or pseudochylous ascites

(From Kjeldsberg CR, Knight JA. *Body fluids*. 3rd ed. Chicago: ASCP Press, 1993.)

Peritoneal Fluid

Table 15-8 summarizes the gross appearance of peritoneal fluid along with associated disorders. Peritoneal fluid is normally clear and pale yellow, and the volume is less than 50 mL. Blood in a traumatic tap clears as aspiration proceeds, in contrast to a grossly bloody aspirate or blood-tinged fluid.

A cloudy or turbid fluid may be associated with conditions like appendicitis, pancreatitis, ruptured bowel after trauma, or primary bacterial peritonitis. Fluid with a greenish color may be observed with perforated duodenal ulcer, perforated intestine, cholecystitis, perforated gallbladder, and acute pancreatitis. A chylous or pseudochylous effusion may produce a milky fluid. A damaged or blocked thoracic duct due to lymphoma, carcinoma, tuberculosis, parasitic infestation, adhesion, or hepatic cirrhosis may give rise to true chylous effusions.

Cell Counts and Microscopic Examination

The cell types encountered in pleural, pericardial, and peritoneal fluids are neutrophils, eosinophils, basophils, lymphocytes, plasma cells, mononuclear phagocytes (monocytes, histiocytes, and macrophages), mesothelial cells, and malignant cells. Total cell counts may be performed manually using a hemacytometer or by an automated cell counter (IRIS; see Chapter 5). Cytocentrifugation followed by staining is a good way to prepare the smear for differential counts. Although most of the cells may be readily identified, some difficulty may be encountered in identifying mesothelial cells and malignant cells found in the effusions.

Mesothelial cells line the serous membranes and are routinely found in specimens after being sloughed off in the fluid. They are large and can measure up to 25 μm in diameter. Their appearance may vary because of reactive or degenerative changes. They may occur singly, in flat sheets, or occasionally in three-dimensional clusters. The cytoplasm is usually abundant and is light gray to deep blue. The nuclear outline is usually smooth and the chromatin is fine and evenly distributed. The round or oval nucleus occupies from one third to one half of the cell diameter and may be eccentric. The nuclear:cytoplasmic ratio is usually not increased. In some cases, mesothelial cells may resemble large plasma cells. One to three spherical nucleoli are present and are usually small. Mesothelial cells in pleural fluid are shown in Figs. 15-5 and 15-6; and in peritoneal fluid, Figs. 15-14 and 15-15.

In contrast to mesothelial cells, malignant cells commonly occur in clumps or in three-dimensional clusters. Nuclei of malignant cells often have an irregular or jagged outline, an uneven distribution of chromatin, and several prominent, large, irregular nucleoli. The cells usually exhibit an increased nuclear:cytoplasmic ratio.

It is of paramount importance that malignant cells in effusions be properly identified. Identification is carried out by the pathology staff.

Pleural Fluid

Total WBC counts in pleural fluid have been used to distinguish transudates from exudates, but there is overlap.[5] For differential counts, neutrophils predominate in about 90% of effusions caused by acute inflammation due to pneumonia, pulmonary infarct, and pancreatitis. However, a high proportion of neutrophils has been observed for transudates about 10% of the time. Lymphocytes predominate in approximately 80% to 90% of pleural effusions associated with tuberculosis and other conditions (e.g., lymphoma, rheumatoid pleuritis, systemic lupus erythematosus), but lymphocytes may also be present in high numbers in about 10% of transudates. Conversely, neutrophilic rather than lymphocytic reactions have been reported for about 10% of tuberculous effusions.[5]

Pleural eosinophilia (greater than 10% eosinophils) is a nonspecific reaction to pleural injury and may be associated with pneumothorax, ventriculopleural shunt, fungal and parasitic infections, and many other conditions.[5]

Pericardial Fluid

Total WBC and RBC counts are of limited value in the differential diagnosis of pericardial effusions.[4] Although there is overlap, WBC counts of less than $1000/\mu$L usually are associated with transudates, whereas WBC counts of more than $1000/\mu$L are seen with exudates.

Peritoneal Fluid

Ascites may be due to uncomplicated cirrhosis but may also be related to spontaneous bacterial peritonitis (SBP)—the passage of bacteria from the blood to ascitic fluid. To distinguish between these two conditions, the total WBC count may be useful.

For SBP, about 90% of the patients have an ascitic fluid WBC count over $500/\mu$L (with more than 50% neutrophils), with an estimated specificity of approximately 90%. For a diagnosis of SBP, absolute neutrophil counts with a cutoff level of 240 to 500 neutrophils/μL have been used with sensitivity and specificity, in the range of about 90%.

Shifts in extracellular fluid may result in marked changes in the ascitic fluid WBC count. For example, during diuresis, the ascitic fluid WBC count may change from under $300/\mu$L to over $1000/\mu$L. Although uncommon, peritoneal fluid eosinophilia has been observed with congestive heart failure, chronic peritoneal dialysis, vasculitis, abdominal lymphoma, and ruptured hydatid cyst.[5]

Fever and ascites (with no infection) have been observed several weeks after surgery associated with the introduction of powder from surgical gloves into the peritoneum. Abdominal paracentesis and the use of polarized light to demonstrate birefringent particles in the fluid provides the diagnosis.

Chemical Examination
. . . .

Total Protein and Lactate Dehydrogenase

As suggested by Kjeldsberg and Knight, two of the most reliable tests to differentiate between transudates and exudates are the simultaneous analyses of total protein and lactate dehydrogenase (LDH) levels in serous fluid and in serum.[4] For transudates, the ratio of serous fluid total protein to serum total protein is less than 0.5, whereas the corresponding LDH ratio is less than 0.6. For exudates, the total protein ratio is higher than 0.5 and the LDH ratio higher than 0.6. However, for peri-

toneal fluid, the serum–ascites albumin concentration gradient is an even more reliable procedure in differentiating transudates from exudates.[4] This gradient is calculated by subtracting the ascitic fluid albumin concentration from the corresponding serum albumin concentration.

The serum–ascites albumin gradient is significantly greater in transudates (1.6 ± 0.5 g/dL) than in exudates (0.6 ± 0.4 g/dL). However, no single criterion separates all transudates from all exudates in every patient. For example, diuresis can cause significant changes in this gradient and make interpretation difficult.

In the case of pleural fluid, a pleural fluid:serum protein ratio greater then 0.5 and a pleural fluid:serum LDH ratio greater than 0.6 would define the effusion as an exudate. Additional tests improve the specificity. For example, a pleural fluid cholesterol greater than 60 mg/dL, a pleural fluid:serum cholesterol ratio greater than 0.3, and a pleural fluid:serum bilirubin ratio greater than 0.6, all are characteristic for a pleural exudate.

Glucose

A decreased level of glucose (<60 mg/dL) in pleural fluid is characteristic for rheumatoid pleuritis and grossly purulent parapneumonic exudates.[8] In a few cases, low glucose levels may occur with effusions due to malignancy, tuberculosis, nonpurulent bacterial infections, lupus erythematosus, and rupture of the esophagus. Changes in glucose levels in pericardial and in peritoneal effusions do not appear to offer much diagnostic help.

Lipids

Cholesterol and triglyceride levels, along with lipoprotein electrophoresis, may be helpful in the differential diagnosis of chylous vs. pseudochylous effusions (Table 15-9). Chylous effusions characteristically show elevated triglycerides with chylomicrons on lipoprotein electrophoresis, whereas pseudochylous fluids usually have triglyceride levels under 50 mg/dL and no chylomicrons. As mentioned earlier, a pleural fluid cholesterol greater than 60 mg/dL and a pleural fluid:serum cholesterol ratio greater than 0.3 are consistent with a pleural exudate.

Enzymes

Table 15-10 provides a listing of the most useful enzymes to measure, along with clinical correlations. As already mentioned, LDH activity in serous fluid has

TABLE 15-9
Chylous and Pseudochylous Effusions

	Chylous Effusion	Pseudochylous Effusion
Appearance	Milky; may form creamy top layer on standing	Milky, greenish, or "gold paint" appearance
Microscopic examination	Lymphocytes plus fine fat droplets	Mixed cellular reaction with cholesterol crystals
Triglycerides	2–8 × serum triglycerides	Lower than serum triglycerides
Cholesterol		Often higher than serum cholesterol
Lipoprotein electrophoresis	Chylomicrons prominent	Chylomicrons scanty or absent
Ingestion of lipophilic dye	Dye appears in effusion	Dye does not appear in effusion
Culture	Always sterile	Usually sterile (check for tuberculosis, fungi)
Etiology	Damage or obstruction to thoracic duct	Chronic effusion of any cause (e.g., cyst fluid, rheumatoid disease, tuberculosis, myxedema)

(From Krieg AF, Kjeldsberb CR. Cerebrospinal fluid and other body fluids. In Henry JB, ed. *Clinical diagnosis and management by laboratory methods.* 18th ed. Philadelphia: WB Saunders Company, 1991.)

some value in the differential diagnosis of transudates vs. exudates. With acute pancreatitis, pancreatic pseudocyst, and esophageal rupture, pleural fluid amylase activity is elevated to about two times the serum level. For patients with SBP, the LDH activity in ascitic fluid is often elevated, resulting in an ascitic fluid:serum LDH ratio greater than 0.4.

Elevated ascitic fluid amylase activity is observed more than 90% of the time with acute pancreatitis, pancreatic trauma, or pancreatic pseudocyst. In these cases, the ratio of ascitic fluid:serum amylase is usually well above 2.0.[5] Elevated ascitic fluid amylase also may occur with other conditions (e.g., gastroduodenal perforation and intestinal strangulation).

The measurement of ascitic fluid lipase activity is another reliable test for the diagnosis of pancreatic ascites. For patients with pancreatic disease, lipase activity was significantly increased over normal serum levels and appeared to fluctuate less than amylase activity.[4]

Patients with intestinal obstruction (both simple and ischemic), strangulation, intestinal perforation, or traumatic hemoperitoneum may all have greatly elevated peritoneal fluid alkaline phosphatase (ALP) levels in comparison with reference serum values. It is noteworthy that serum ALP levels are usually normal in these patients.

Few biochemical tests have been carried out on pericardial fluid to diagnose specific disorders of the heart or pericardium.

TABLE 15-10
Selectively Measured Pleural Fluid Enzymes

Enzyme	Associated Clinical Disorder
Adenosine deaminase	Tuberculosis
Amylase	Pancreatitis
Amylase isoenzymes	Pancreatitis, esophageal fistula, tumor marker
Creatine kinase	Tumor marker (e.g., prostatic carcinoma)
LDH	Transudate vs. exudate
LDH isoenzymes	Differentiate several clinical disorders
Lysozyme	Tuberculosis
Neuron-specific enolase	Tumor marker

LDH, lactate dehydrogenase.
(From Kjeldsberg CR, Knight JA. *Body fluids.* 3rd ed. Chicago: ASCP Press, 1993.)

pH

For parapneumonic effusions (pneumonia), pH may be valuable in predicting the course of the effusion. If the exudate has a pH greater than 7.20 to 7.30, it usually resolves completely with appropriate antibiotic therapy and without a drainage tube. On the other hand, an exudate with a pH below 7.20 tends to loculate and not completely resolve unless drainage is provided.[4]

The pH of ascitic fluid may help in the diagnosis of SBP in cases of cirrhotic ascites, particularly when used together with WBC counts. A fluid pH of less than 7.32 or a pH difference greater than 0.1 between the blood and ascitic fluid indicates a diagnosis for SBP with a sensitivity and specificity of about 90%.[5]

Specimens of serous fluid for pH measurement should be collected and measured with the same care as that used for arterial blood gas determinations: anaerobic collection in a heparinized syringe; placement of the specimen on ice; and prompt transportation to the laboratory for analysis.

Ammonia

Compared to simultaneously measured levels in plasma, ammonia levels in peritoneal fluid are increased in cases of ruptured appendix, perforated peptic ulcer, bowel strangulation with or without perforation, and ruptured urinary bladder with extravasation of urine. For patients with pancreatitis, ammonia values are normal.

Microbiologic Examination

Pleural Fluid

Staphylococcus aureus and coliform species are the most common bacteria observed in parapneumonic effusions. Anaerobic as well as aerobic cultures should be set up because the bacteria found in 35% to 40% of the effusions may be anaerobic. Combining pleural biopsy and acid-fast stain with culture to diagnose tuberculosis can increase the sensitivity of diagnosis to the range of 95% from only about 30% for culture alone.[8]

Pericardial Fluid

Infections of the pericardium are occasionally seen (e.g., *Hamophilus influenzae* pericarditis in children). Tuberculous pericarditis is an increasingly important problem because of the resurgence of tuberculosis (due to acquired immunodeficiency syndrome) in many countries.

Peritoneal Fluid

Infection of the peritoneal cavity may occur spontaneously in patients with chronic ascites (e.g., in cases of cirrhosis). It may also occur as a result of leakage or rupture of the gastrointestinal tract, during chronic continuous peritoneal dialysis, or as a complication of a surgical procedure. In cases of rupture or leakage from hollow organs or after surgery, infection is often evident as a localized abscess or as generalized peritonitis. Cultures usually grow a mixture of aerobic and anaerobic microorganisms.

Spontaneous bacterial peritonitis is relatively common in patients with hepatic cirrhosis, and the mortality rate is usually high. The ascitic fluid is cloudy, and the WBC count (predominantly PMNs) usually exceeds 1000/μL. For SBP, culture of ascitic fluid is positive for about 90% of cases, whereas the Gram stain has a sensitivity of only 25% to 50%.[5]

Spontaneous bacterial peritonitis is usually caused by a single organism that generally seeds the peritoneal fluid from the bloodstream. In about two thirds of cases, gram-negative bacilli (*E. coli*) are present; pneumococci account for most of the remaining cases. In contrast to tuberculous peritonitis, the protein content in ascitic fluid specimens from patients with SBP is unusually low—less than 2.0 g/dL in most cases, and in some cases less than 1.0 g/dL.

Sensitivity of the acid-fast stain for tuberculous peritonitis is only about 20% to 30%; therefore, it may be advisable to begin treatment before a positive culture is available if the clinical picture points to a tuberculous involvement.

Quality Control

At present, it appears that no commercial controls are available to monitor the analysis of pleural, pericardial, or peritoneal fluids, although research and development on such materials are being undertaken.

CASE STUDY 15-1

This patient, a 60-year-old woman with a history of metastatic breast carcinoma (14 years earlier) and double modified radical mastectomies, was admitted for increasing weakness and SOB. She said she was unable to walk more than 8 to 10 feet without SOB. There was no complaint of fever, chills, nausea, vomiting, chest pain, or edema. Medications on admission were Ativan (for anxi-

continued

ety), Tylenol, and codeine. Her admission diagnosis was recurrent, acute, malignant pleural effusion, anemia, and pneumothorax.

She was given 3 units of packed cells for her anemia, and a therapeutic thoracentesis was performed. About 650 mL of orange-colored, cloudy pleural fluid was obtained from the right pleural cavity. After centrifugation, the supernatant was yellow and clear. The microscopic examination of the pleural fluid showed 12,000 RBCs/mm and 95 nucleated cells/mm^3. The differential was 97% lymphocytes and 3% monocytes. The appearance of a Cytospin preparation of the fluid is shown in Figures 15-3 and 15-4.

Smears and cell block sections on the pleural fluid were prepared for H&E and mucicarmine stains. The microscopic evaluation was similar for both specimens: proteinaceous fluid containing necrotic inflammatory cell infiltrate consisting largely of lymphocytes and scattered plasma cells. Occasional reactive mesothelial cells were noted. The mucicarmine stain showed no mucicarmine-positive tumor cells.

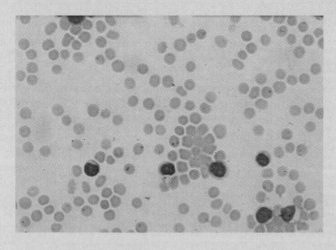

FIGURE 15-3 Cytospin preparation of pleural fluid illustrating "inflammatory cells." Wright's stain; ×400.

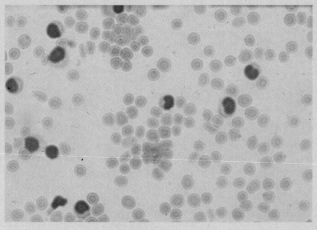

FIGURE 15-4 Cytospin preparation of pleural fluid illustrating "inflammatory cells." Wright's stain; ×400.

CASE STUDY 15-2

This patient, a 53-year-old man, was admitted for SOB and feelings of pressure in the right side of his chest. He had a history of pneumonia. Admitting diagnosis was right pleural effusion. Pleural fluid was withdrawn that showed color red; appearance cloudy; supernatant pink and clear; total nucleated 4250 cells/mm^3; 134,666 RBCs/mm^3; lymphocytes 3%; monocytes 3%; neutrophils 93%; and eosinophils 1%.

Figures 15-5 and 15-6 illustrate the appearance of the Cytospin preparation. Cell blocks (for H&E stain) and smears (for Papanicolaou' stain) were also prepared from the pleural fluid speci-

continued

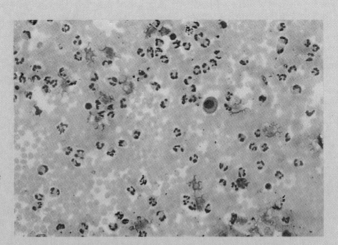

FIGURE 15-5 Cytospin preparation of pleural fluid illustrating "an acute inflammatory exudate." Mesothelial cell with mixed cell background. Wright's stain; ×200.

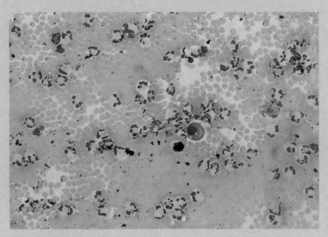

FIGURE 15-6 Cytospin preparation of pleural fluid illustrating "an acute inflammatory exudate." Mesothelial cell with mixed cell background. Wright's stain; ×200.

men. The assessment was acute inflammatory exudate; no malignant cells identified; sheets of inflammatory cells seen; proteinaceous fluid and debris observed. No infectious agents were isolated from the fluid.

A chest tube was placed to drain the pleural fluid continuously, and the patient was eventually discharged in stable condition. A follow-up visit to remove the single suture in the right side of the chest (from the tube) provided a discharge diagnosis of pneumonia resolved.

CASE STUDY 15-3

This patient, a 57-year-old woman, with a history of SOB, asthma, and COPD, was admitted complaining of increasing cough, green sputum, pleuritic left-sided chest pain, and fever for the preceding 4 days. Her diagnosis was left lower lobe pneumonia with hypoxia. A pleural fluid specimen showed: light amber color and a "purulent" appearance; supernatant was light amber and cloudy; 80,250 total nucleated cells/mm^3; 18,250 RBCs/mm^3; and the differential was lymphocytes 1%; neutrophils 98%; and monocytes 1%. Comment: many bacteria resembling *Pseudomonas*. A Gram stain of the pleural fluid confirmed the presence of many gram-negative rods, and the C&S indicated an infection with P. *aeruginosa*. The final diagnosis was *Pseudomonas* empyema and pneumothorax. Figures 15-7 to 15-9 illustrate the pleural fluid microscopic analysis (Cytospin).

continued

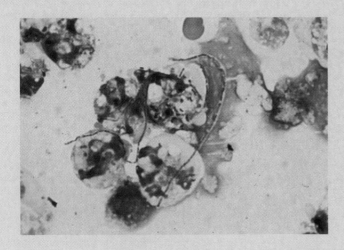

FIGURE 15-7 Cytospin preparation of pleural fluid showing bacteria identified by C&S as *Pseudomonas aeruginosa*. It appears that some of the bacteria are intracellular. Wright's stain; ×1000.

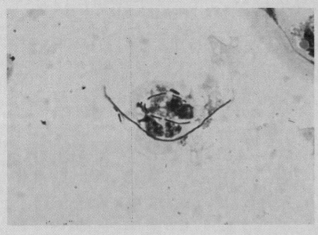

FIGURE 15-8 Cytospin preparation of pleural fluid showing bacteria identified by C&S as *Pseudomonas aeruginosa*. It appears that some of the bacteria are intracellular. Wright's stain; ×1000.

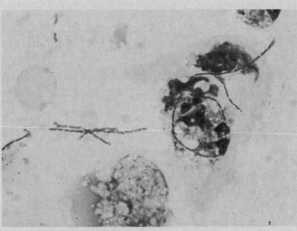

FIGURE 15-9 Cytospin preparation of pleural fluid showing bacteria identified by C&S as *Pseudomonas aeruginosa*. It appears that some of the bacteria are intracellular. Wright's stain; ×1000.

CASE STUDY 15-4

This patient came to the ER by ambulance because of altered mental status, unresponsiveness, shaking of the extremities, eyes rolling backward, and seizures. The patient, a 55-year-old man, had a long history of IV drug abuse and noncompliance with medications. According to his wife, he

continued

had used at least 1 g of heroin per day for the previous 2 years and had consumed about one half pint of whiskey per day as well.

His admission diagnosis was hepatic encephalopathy (2° to alcoholism), right lower lobe pneumonia, seizures, and malnutrition. Throughout his hospital stay of 2 months, he showed signs of hepatic encephalopathy (blood ammonia = 54) and multiple complications: ascites, empyema of lungs, esophagopleural fistula, respiratory failure, and esophageal varices. He died in the hospital 2° to esophageal bleeding from varices.

Shortly before his death, a pleural fluid specimen was obtained that showed color light brown; appearance turbid; supernatant light amber and hazy; 101,850 total nucleated cells/mm³; 1610 RBCs/mm³; lymphocytes 4%; neutrophils 92%; eosinophils 2%; mesothelials 1%; monocytes 1%. Comment: many bacteria seen. The Gram stain of this fluid showed gram-positive cocci resembling *Staphylococcus* and *Streptococcus*, many gram-variable rods, and yeast. C&S showed coag-negative *Staphylococcus*, *P. aeruginosa*, and *Candida glabrata*. The appearance of a smear prepared from this fluid is illustrated in Figures 15-10 and 15-11.

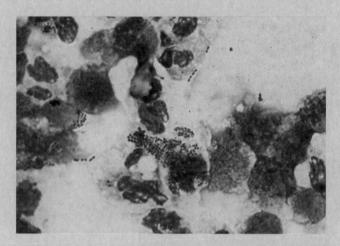

FIGURE 15-10 Smear of pleural fluid sediment showing bacteria. Wright's stain; ×1000.

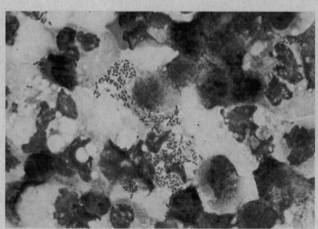

FIGURE 15-11 Smear of pleural fluid sediment showing bacteria. Wright's stain; ×1000.

CASE STUDY 15-5

This patient, a 54-year-old man, had been living in a rural community. His medical history included emphysema and peptic ulcer disease. After 4 days of increasing "pressure" on his chest, SOB, progressive fatigue, and abdominal discomfort, he decided to seek medical treatment. He walked a considerable distance to the rural hospital in his area because a bridge was closed to

continued

vehicular traffic. Because of the cold weather he became hypothermic and dyspneic. At the hospital, he was rewarmed and examined; it was thought that pneumonia was complicating his COPD, and he was transferred to the county facility.

His admission diagnosis was hepatitis with hepatic failure, pericardial effusion with symptoms of tamponade, coagulopathy, cervical adenopathy, hyperkalemia, lactic acidosis, hyponatremia, thrombocytopenia, possible chest mass, and leukocytosis with hypothermia. Operative procedures included pericardiocentesis, pericardial drainage catheter, and anterior pericardiectomy with sternotomy. His chest x-ray study showed a large left pleural effusion and a small right pleural effusion with an enlarged heart and questionable right hilar mass. The ER ultrasound showed a large pericardial effusion.

In the intensive care unit, pericardiocentesis yielded 230 mL of serosanguineous fluid. After this fluid was withdrawn, the patient experienced an immediate improvement in cardiopulmonary, renal, and hepatic function. The pericardial fluid contained malignant cells consistent with adenocarcinoma. The pathology report was metastatic adenocarcinoma. Later his condition worsened, and he underwent an anterior pericardiectomy because of clot formation. Because of the advanced stage of his malignancy, it was decided not to treat it aggressively. The patient died in the hospital.

The pericardial fluid on admission showed color red; appearance cloudy; supernatant amber and hazy; 5110 total nucleated cells/mm^3; 67,500 RBCs/mm^3; lymphocytes 63%; neutrophils 20%; eosinophils 1%; monocytes 10%; mesothelial cells 2%. Comment: 4 atypical mesothelial cells observed. Figures 15-12 and 15-13 illustrate the microscopic on this pericardial fluid (Cytospin).

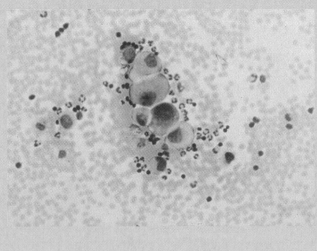

FIGURE 15-12 Cytospin preparation of pericardial fluid, with cells resembling adenocarcinoma. Wright's stain; ×200.

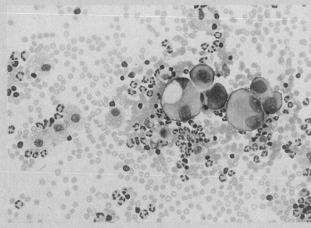

FIGURE 15-13 Cytospin preparation of pericardial fluid, with cells resembling adenocarcinoma. Wright's stain; ×200.

continued

CASE STUDY 15-6

With a history of abusing alcohol for 15 years, this 44-year-old woman was admitted complaining of a swollen abdomen and increasing SOB for the preceding 3 weeks. Her admission diagnosis was ALD with ascites, and a therapeutic abdominal paracentesis was performed. The volume of fluid drained from the peritoneal cavity was about 800 mL. Analysis of the fluid (tube 3) showed color pink; appearance cloudy; supernatant yellow and clear; 298 total nucleated cells/mm^3; 5950 RBCs/mm^3; lymphocytes 91%; plasma cells 1%; monocytes 8%; mesothelial cells 10%. Gram' stain and C&S on the fluid were negative. After the paracentesis, her SOB was markedly improved and she was discharged home in stable condition. The appearance of the peritoneal fluid sediment is shown in Figures 15-14 and 15-15.

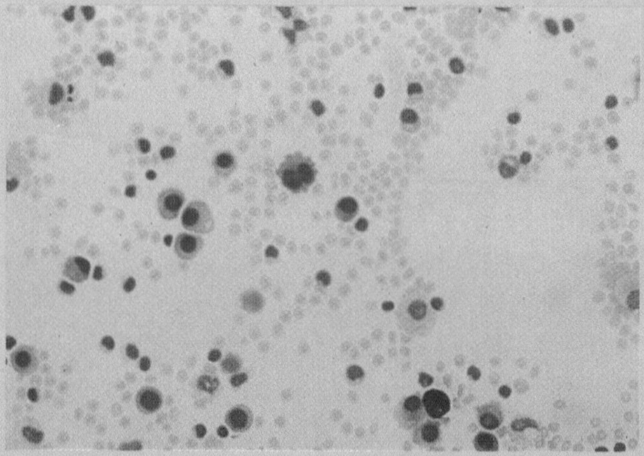

FIGURE 15-14 Cytospin preparation of peritoneal fluid showing occasional mesothelial cells, with RBCs and WBCs. Wright's stain; ×200.

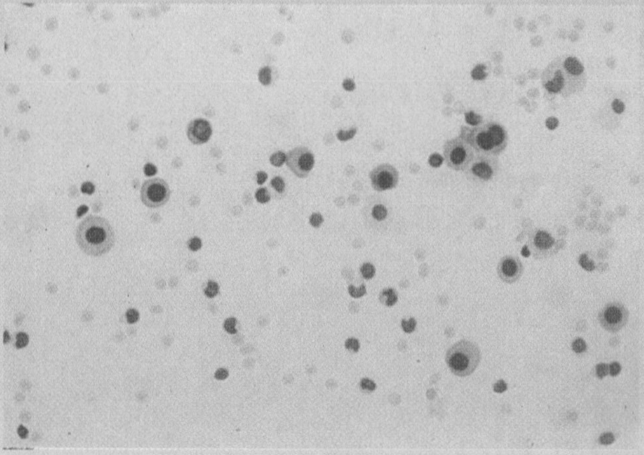

FIGURE 15-15 Cytospin preparation of peritoneal fluid showing occasional mesothelial cells; with RBCs and WBCs. Wright's stain; ×200.

Case Histories With Study Questions

CASE HISTORY 15-1

This patient, a morbidly obese 17-year-old boy (310 pounds), was admitted complaining of chest pains and difficulty in breathing. His temperature was 97.3°F, pulse 109, BP 183/106, respiration 32. Lungs were clear with no rhonchi or rales. Radiology showed an

Continued

infiltrate in the right lobe, and his admission diagnosis was right lobe pneumonia with empyema and respiratory failure.

Thoracentesis was performed, and right lobe pleural fluid was obtained (tube 1) that showed color yellow; appearance cloudy; supernatant yellow and clear; 22,750 total nucleated cells/mm^3; 2750 RBCs/mm^3; lymphocytes 1%; neutrophils 94%; monocytes 5%. Tests on the pleural fluid included AFB culture and smear (negative); Gram's stain for organisms (negative); aerobic C&S negative; culture for fungus negative; total protein 5.4 g/dL (serum was 7.2 g/dL)); LDH 1160 U/L (serum was 150 U/L); and glucose 6 mg/dL (serum was 80 mg/dL). Figures 15-16 through 15-18 show the appearance of the Cytospin preparation of the fluid.

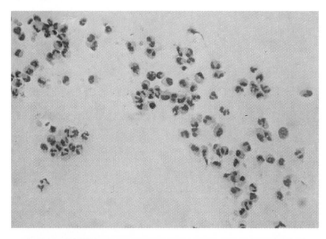

FIGURE 15-16 Cytospin preparation of pleural fluid. Wright's stain; ×200.

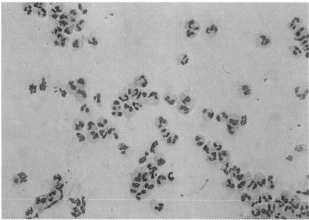

FIGURE 15-17 Cytospin preparation of pleural fluid. Wright's stain; ×200.

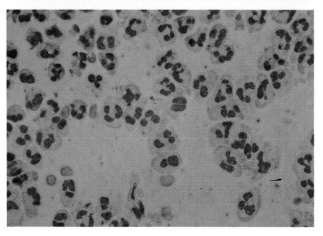

FIGURE 15-18 Cytospin preparation of pleural fluid. Wright's stain; ×400.

continued

Study Questions for Case History 15-1

1. What does the cellularity of the Cytospin preparation suggest given the negative microbiologic results? Explain.

2. A transudate would have a glucose concentration equal to the serum, total protein < 50% of serum, and LDH < 60% of serum. An exudate would have a glucose concentration ≤serum, total protein > 50% of serum, and LDH > 60% of serum. What do the results for this pleural fluid suggest it is—a transudate or an exudate? Does your conclusion agree with the clinical history and your answer for question 1? Explain.

CASE HISTORY 15-2

With a history of alcoholic cirrhosis and chronic ascites, this patient, a 61-year-old man, was admitted through the ER for orthopnea, SOB, and pain in the lower abdomen and suprapubic areas. This condition had been progressively getting worse over the preceding 2 weeks.

The abdominal paracentesis (tube 1) showed color pale yellow; appearance slightly hazy; supernatant pale yellow and slightly hazy; 243 total nucleated cells/mm^3; 115 RBCs/mm^3; lymphocytes 88%; monocytes 7%; neutrophils 3%; eosinophils 1%; and basophils 1%. A Gram stain on this fluid indicated gram-positive cocci resembling *Staphylococcus* or *Streptococcus* species. The C&S resulted in coag-negative *Staphylococcus*. The appearance of this fluid is illustrated in Figures 15-19 through 15-21.

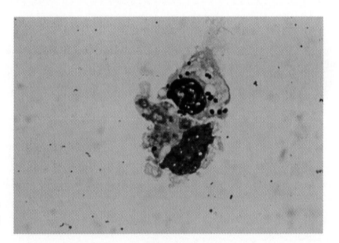

FIGURE 15-19 Cytospin preparation of peritoneal fluid. Wright's stain; ×1000.

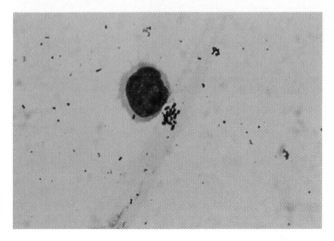

FIGURE 15-20 Cytospin preparation of peritoneal fluid. Wright's stain; ×1000.

continued

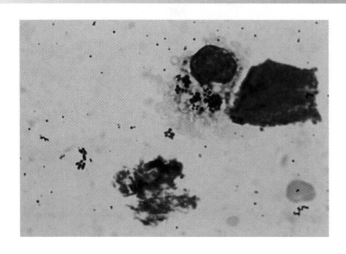

FIGURE 15-21 Cytospin preparation of peritoneal fluid. Wright's stain; ×1000.

Study Questions for Case History 15-2

1. There was a comment recorded on the differential report that was not included in the case history. What do you think it might have been? Explain.
2. What diagnosis would you give this case? Does the elevated lymphocyte count add or detract from your diagnosis? Explain.

REFERENCES

1. Kjeldsberg CR, Knight JA. *Body fluids*. 3rd ed. Chicago: ASCP Press, 1993.
2. Krieg AF, Kjeldsberg CR. Cerebrospinal fluid and other body fluids. In: Henry JB, ed. *Clinical diagnosis and management by laboratory methods*. 18th ed. Philadelphia: WB Saunders, 1991: 445–473.
3. Strasinger SK. *Urinalysis and body fluids*. 3rd ed. Philadelphia: FA Davis, 1994.

BIBLIOGRAPHY

Brunzel NA. *Fundamentals of urine and body fluid analysis*. Philadelphia: WB Saunders, 1994.
International Remote Imaging Systems. *Technical literature*. Chatsworth, CA: IRIS, 1996.
Kjeldsberg CR, Knight JA. *Body fluids*. Chicago: ASCP Press, 1983.
Ringsrud KM, Linné JJ. *Urinalysis and body fluids: A color text and atlas*. St. Louis: Mosby–Year Book, 1995.
Smith GP, Kjeldsberg CR. Cerebrospinal, synovial, and serous body fluids. In: Henry JB, ed. *Clinical diagnosis and management by laboratory methods*. 19th ed. Philadelphia: WB Saunders, 1996: 457–482.

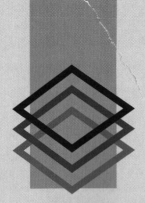

16

Bronchial Washings and Bronchoalveolar Lavage

ABBREVIATIONS USED IN THIS CHAPTER

ANA = antinuclear antibody

BAL = bronchoalveolar
  lavage

CAD = coronary artery
  disease

CHF = congestive heart
  failure

GMS-P = Gomori
  methenamine silver
  stain—P*neumocystis*
  modification

LE = lupus erythematosus

PAP = Papanicolaou

Introductory Case Study

This case is presented because of the interesting specimens involved, even though it was not fully resolved before the patient died. The patient, a 71-year-old man residing in a convalescent hospital, was seen in the emergency room complaining of fever, increasing shortness of breath, and respiratory distress. He claimed he had lost 12 lbs in the previous week. The assessment was right and left lower lobe pulmonary infiltrate, increased dyspnea and respiratory failure, CHF, and anemia. He was taken to the intensive care unit and placed on a ventilator.

Part of his diagnostic workup included a BAL (bronchoalveolar lavage), which gave the following results: color light pink; appearance slightly bloody; supernatant colorless and clear; 690 total nucleated cells/mm^3; 1010 RBCs/mm^3; lymphocytes 6%; neutrophils 86%; monocytes 8%; some "LE-like" cells present. Cytology on the fluid indicated no malignancy, numerous inflammatory cells (primarily neutrophils), several macrophages (occasionally multinucleate), and LE cells. Before further studies could be initiated, the patient died, final diagnosis: cardiac arrest secondary to poor cardiovascular status, CHF, chronic obstructive pulmonary disease, and CAD.

The appearance of the Cytospin preparation of the BAL is shown in Figures 16-1 to 16-4. The appearance of the sediment (Cytospin) from a urine specimen collected the same day as the BAL is shown in Figures 16-5 and 16-6. Is it possible that this patient died from the effects of systemic LE: pneumonitis/chronic interstitial lung disease, myocarditis/ischemic heart disease, and interstitial nephritis?

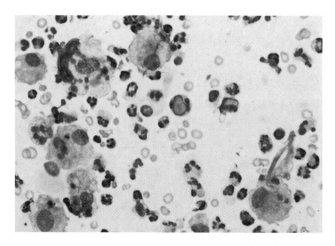

FIGURE 16-1 Cytospin preparation of BAL showing LE cell. Wright's stain; ×400.

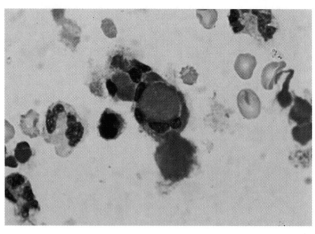

FIGURE 16-2 Cytospin preparation of BAL showing LE cell. Wright's stain; ×1000.

continued

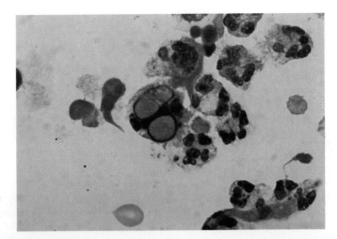

FIGURE 16-3 Cytospin preparation of BAL showing LE cell. Wright's stain; ×1000.

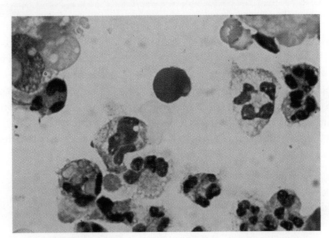

FIGURE 16-4 Cytospin preparation of BAL showing an unphagocytized nucleus degraded by ANA. Wright's stain; ×1000.

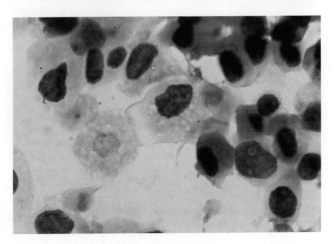

FIGURE 16-5 Cytospin preparation of urine sediment showing unidentified mononuclear cells. Wright's stain; ×1000.

continued

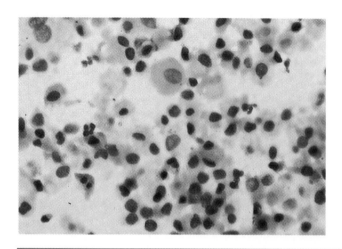

FIGURE 16-6 Cytospin preparation of urine sediment showing unidentified mononuclear cells. Wright's stain; ×400.

Specimen Collection and Clinical Correlations

The trachea (or windpipe) is a tubular airway about 12 cm in length and 2.5 cm in diameter. It is located in front of the esophagus and extends from the larynx down to the fifth thoracic vertebra, where it divides into the right and left primary bronchi (Fig. 16-7). In the lungs, the primary bronchi divide to form smaller bronchi, the secondary or lobar bronchi, one for each lobe of the lung. The secondary bronchi continue to branch, forming still smaller bronchi (tertiary or segmental bronchi), which divide into bronchioles which, in turn, branch into even smaller tubes called terminal bronchioles.

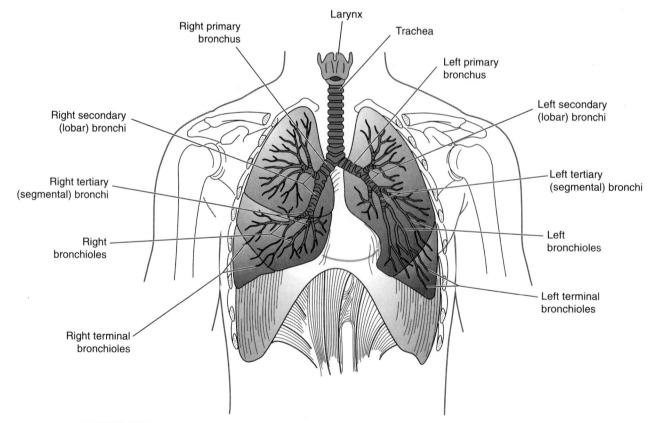

FIGURE 16-7 Air passageways to the lungs. Diagram of the bronchial tree in relationship to the lungs. (From Tortura GJ, Anagnostakos NP. *Principles of anatomy and physiology*. 3rd ed. New York: Harper & Row Publishers, 1981.)

A bronchoscope, a lighted optical instrument used for clinical examination of the lumen of the tracheobronchial tree, can help diagnose bronchial obstructions, unresolved pneumonia, unexplained hemoptysis, suspected carcinoma, foreign bodies, abscesses, and aspiration pneumonia. Originally the bronchoscope was a rigid, hollow metal tube with an illumination system at the distal end. Rigid-tube bronchoscopy is now preferred only for retrieval of large biopsy specimens and for management of tracheal stenosis.

The preferred and more recent design is the fiberoptic bronchoscope, a flexible tube using specialized glass fibers that form a bidirectional light system that conducts light to the interior of the bronchi and returns a magnified image. Either instrument can be equipped with suction catheters, bronchial brushes, and various types of biopsy and forceps attachments that permit the recovery of washings and other specimens for bacterial or fungal culture and cytologic examination. The fiberoptic instrument has a smaller diameter. Because of its flexibility, it is more easily manipulated into upper lobe bronchi and can reach to the subsegmental bronchi level.[1]

In general, the bronchoscope is advanced into a bronchial segment until it occludes the lumen. Aliquots of 20 to 60 mL of saline are infused and then retrieved by aspiration. The first aliquot usually has the largest number of cells and is best for cytologic studies. Additional aliquots can be used for chemical analyses and microbiologic workup. A bronchial washing obtains specimens from the more proximal portions of the bronchoalveolar tree. The bronchoalveolar lavage (BAL) is conducted at a more distal level to retrieve material more characteristic of the alveoli and to produce a greater yield of cellular material.

The BAL is a relatively new technique and is particularly useful in evaluating immunocompromised patients, interstitial lung disease, and airway diseases.[2] Bronchoalveolar procedures, as well as methods of processing and analyzing the specimens, are not standardized and differ widely among laboratories. Studies have shown that the sensitivity of BAL for detecting infectious organisms such as *Pneumocystis carinii* or *Aspergillus* species approaches or exceeds the sensitivity of traditional biopsy procedures.[2] Bronchial washings are less likely to contain material from the alveoli, where *Pneumocystis* exudate is found, and are therefore less effective in recovering the organism, compared with BAL.

In the laboratory, the fluid volume of each specimen is measured and analyses conducted. Cell counts are performed manually with a hemacytometer. Cytocentrifugation using routine procedures and staining may be used to prepare slides for the differential count. Cells seen in BAL fluid include macrophages, lymphocytes, neutrophils, eosinophils, ciliated columnar bronchial epithelial cells, and squamous epithelial cells. Macrophages, often containing a variety of phagocytized material, are the cells most frequently seen, with proportions ranging from 56% to 79%.[4]

Figures 16-8 to 16-10 illustrate alveolar macrophages containing blue-black carbon particles often seen from the lungs of people who inhale smoke. Figures 16-11 and 16-12 show macrophages containing lipid particles from a patient who aspirated milk. Lymphocytes, usually 1% to 10% of the cell population, are increased in interstitial lung disease, drug reactions, pulmonary lymphoma, and nonbacterial infections. Neutrophils (normally 2–21%) are increased with cigarette smokers, bronchopneumonia, exposure to toxins, and diffuse alveolar damage. Eosinophils are usually less than 1% of the total cells, and their numbers are elevated in asthma, hypersensitivity, pneumonitis, and eosinophilic pneumonia.

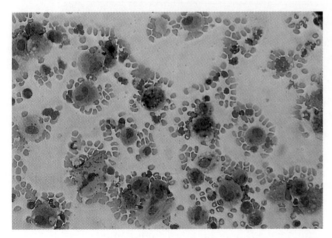

FIGURE 16-8 Cytospin preparation of BAL showing alveolar macrophages with intracellular carbon particles. Wright's stain; ×400.

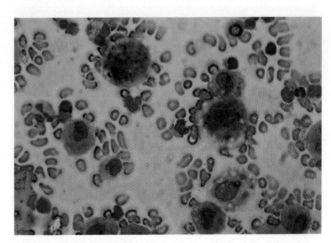

FIGURE 16-9 Cytospin preparation of BAL showing alveolar macrophages with intracellular carbon particles. Wright's stain; ×400.

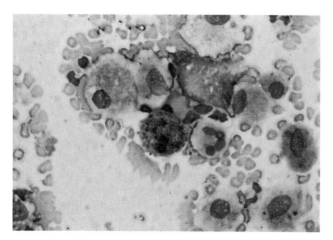

FIGURE 16-10 Cytospin preparation of BAL showing alveolar macrophages with intracellular carbon particles. Wright's stain; ×400.

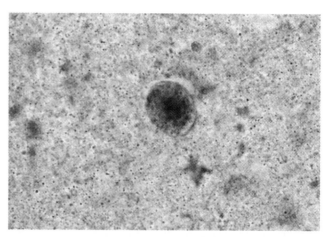

FIGURE 16-12 Cytospin preparation of BAL showing alveolar macrophages with intracellular lipid droplets caused by aspiration of milk. (Patient tried to counteract a drug OD by ingesting milk.) Oil Red O stain; × 1000.

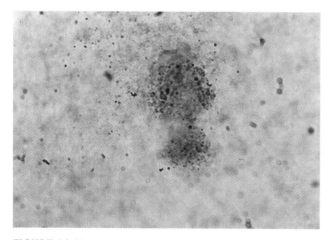

FIGURE 16-11 Cytospin preparation of BAL showing alveolar macrophages with intracellular lipid droplets caused by aspiration of milk. (Patient tried to counteract a drug OD by ingesting milk.) Oil Red O stain; ×1000.

Illustrative Case Studies

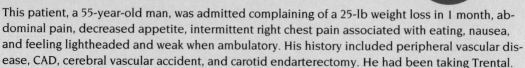

CASE STUDY 16-1

This patient, a 55-year-old man, was admitted complaining of a 25-lb weight loss in 1 month, abdominal pain, decreased appetite, intermittent right chest pain associated with eating, nausea, and feeling lightheaded and weak when ambulatory. His history included peripheral vascular disease, CAD, cerebral vascular accident, and carotid endarterectomy. He had been taking Trental.

In the course of his diagnostic workup, a bronchial washing was performed. The cytology report was significant for intracellular encapsulated yeast forms suggestive of *Histoplasma* species. A culture of the fluid grew out H. *capsulatum*. The appearance of the bronchial washing sediment is illustrated in Figures 16-13 to 16-15.

CASE STUDY 16-2

This 31-year-old man, with a long history of Wegener's granulomatosis, was admitted complaining of fever, cough, headaches, and nausea for the preceding 3 weeks. There was no vomiting, diar-

continued

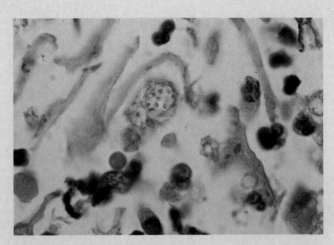

FIGURE 16-13 Cell-block preparation of bronch washing showing intracellular encapsulated yeast forms suggestive of *Histoplasma* sp. H&E stain; ×1000.

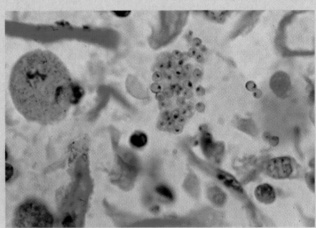

FIGURE 16-14 Cell-block preparation of bronch washing showing encapsulated yeast forms suggestive of *Histoplasma* sp. GMS-C stain; ×1000.

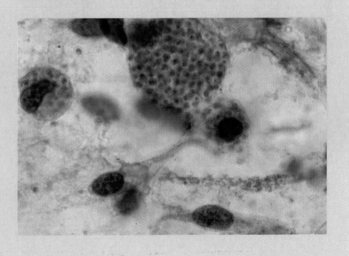

FIGURE 16-15 Cell-block preparation of bronch washing showing intracellular encapsulated yeast forms suggestive of *Histoplasma* sp. PAP stain; ×1000.

rhea, or abdominal pain. A BAL (right middle lobe) was performed that was positive for *Pneumocystis carinii*, negative for *Coccidioides immitis*, and negative for acid-fast bacilli. A sputum specimen grew out *Candida* species. The appearances of the variously stained preparations from sputum, and the BAL are shown in Figures 16-16 to 16-19.

continued

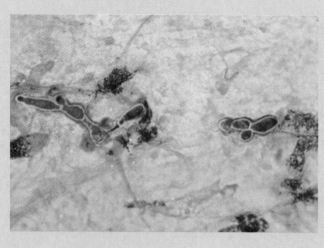

FIGURE 16-16 Smear from sputum showing hyphal forms, probably *Candida* sp. PAP stain; ×1000.

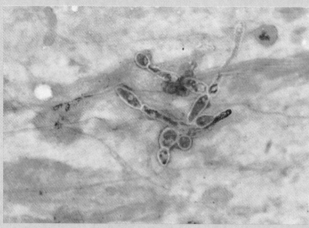

FIGURE 16-17 Smear from sputum showing hyphal forms, probably *Candida* sp. PAP stain; ×1000.

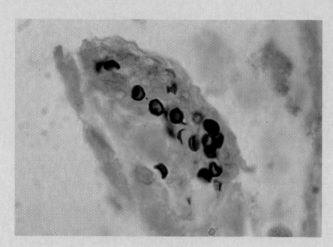

FIGURE 16-18 Cell block preparation of BAL showing cysts of *Pneumocystis carinii.* GMS-P stain; ×1000.

continued

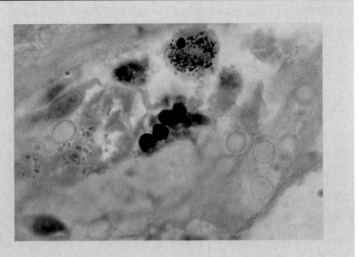

FIGURE 16-19 Cell block preparation of BAL showing cysts of *Pneumocystis carinii*. GMS-P stain; ×1000.

REFERENCES

1. Bennington JL, ed. *Saunder's dictionary and encyclopedia of laboratory medicine and technology*. Philadelphia: WB Saunders, 1984.
2. Niejadlik DC. Sputum. In: Henry JB, ed. *Clinical diagnosis and management by laboratory methods*. 18th ed. Philadelphia: WB Saunders, 1991:504–518.
3. Strasinger SK. *Urinalysis and body fluids*. 3rd ed. Philadelphia: FA Davis, 1994.

BIBLIOGRAPHY

Ringsrud KM, Linné JJ. *Urinalysis and body fluids: A color text and atlas*. St. Louis: Mosby–Year Book, 1995.

Tortora JT, Anagnostakos NP. *Principles of anatomy and physiology*. 3rd ed. New York: Harper and Row, 1981.

APPENDIX A: Relative Centrifugal Force Nomograph

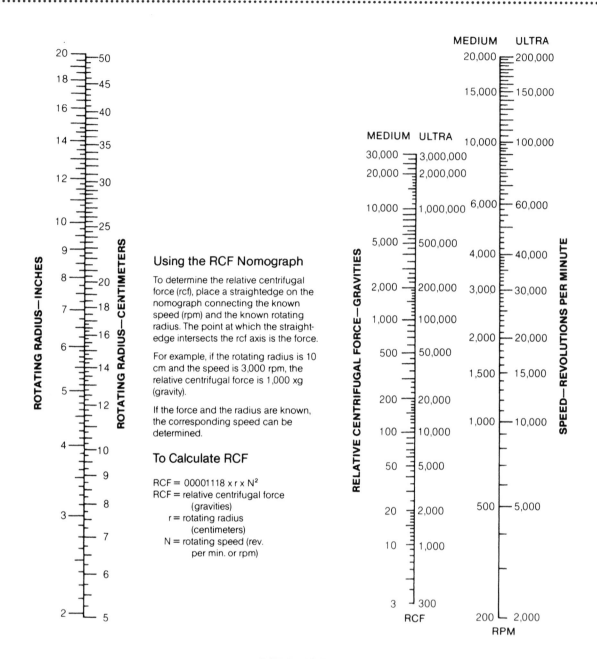

Using the RCF Nomograph

To determine the relative centrifugal force (rcf), place a straightedge on the nomograph connecting the known speed (rpm) and the known rotating radius. The point at which the straightedge intersects the rcf axis is the force.

For example, if the rotating radius is 10 cm and the speed is 3,000 rpm, the relative centrifugal force is 1,000 xg (gravity).

If the force and the radius are known, the corresponding speed can be determined.

To Calculate RCF

$$RCF = 00001118 \times r \times N^2$$
RCF = relative centrifugal force (gravities)
r = rotating radius (centimeters)
N = rotating speed (rev. per min. or rpm)

ROTATING TIP RADIUS

The distance measured from the rotor axis to the tip of the liquid inside the tubes at the greatest horizontal distance from the rotor axis is the rotating tip radius.

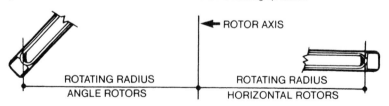

(Reprinted by permission from International Equipment Co., Damon Corporation)

APPENDIX B: Nomogram for the Determination of Body Surface Area

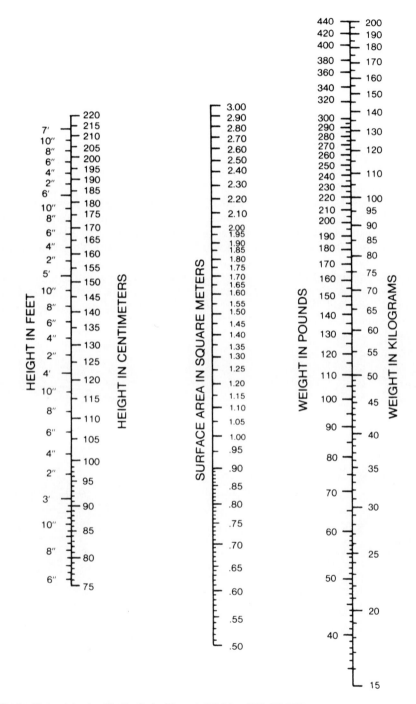

(Reprinted by permission from The New England Journal of Medicine, 1921; 185:337.)

APPENDIX C: Cell Counts Using a Hemacytometer

A hemacytometer or counting chamber is used to perform manual cell counts. Dilutions may be made with a micropipette and small test tubes or a self-contained diluting device such as the Unopette (Becton-Dickinson, Rutherford, NJ). The principle for performing cell counts is essentially the same for all cells except for variations in the dilution factor, the diluting fluid, and the area of the chamber to be counted.

The most commonly used hemacytometer is the Levy chamber with improved Neubauer ruling (Figure C-1). The device has two raised area each in the shape of a 3 × 3 mm square area (total area 9 mm²). As shown in Figure C-1, each 9 mm² area is made up of nine 1 × 1 mm² areas. The center square is subdivided into 25 squares, and each of these is further divided into 16 squares. The distance between the surface of the counting areas and the cover slip is 0.1 mm. The areas for the standard WBC count are labeled "W" and those for the RBC count "R". The usual protocol for counting cells which touch the lines of the counting areas is illustrated in Figure C-2.

For CSF, a disposable Pasteur pipette is used to load both sides of the chamber with fluid. With the 40 × objective, red blood cells are counted in a total area of 10 mm² (five 1 mm² squares each side). If the number of RBCs is fairly high (more than 200 cells/10 squares), fewer squares are counted and the calculations are adjusted accordingly. It may be necessary to dilute an extremely bloody fluid volumetrically with saline. If the cells in 10 squares are enumerated, the volume of fluid examined is 1 μL (10 mm² X 0.1 mm). If there was no dilution, the number of cells counted in the 10 squares is therefore equal to the number of cells per μL. WBCs are counted in a similar fashion except that for a bloody fluid the RBCs must first be lysed with glacial acetic acid. This also serves to increase the contrast between the WBC nuclei and cytoplasm.

For synovial fluid, WBCs and RBCs are counted in a similar fashion except that acetic acid is not used to lyse the RBCs prior to counting WBCs in a bloody fluid. Since the acetic acid precipitates the hyaluronic acid (producing cell clumping), the RBCs may be lysed with hypotonic saline (0.3 g/dL). Very viscous fluid may be difficult to pipette and may be pretreated with buffered hyaluronidase before loading into the hemacytometer.

Cell counts on the serous fluids (pleural, pericardial, and peritoneal) are carried out in a fashion similar to that for CSF.

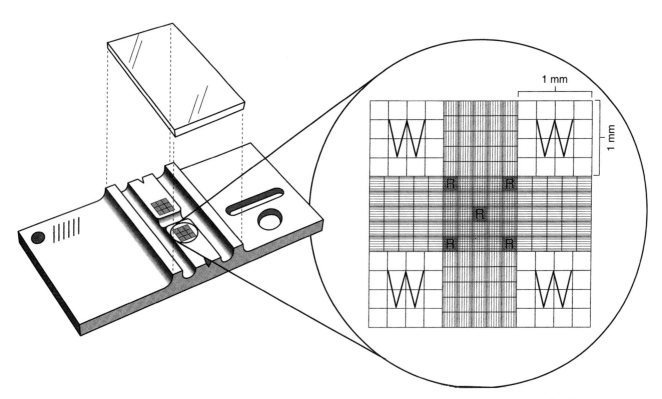

APPENDIX FIGURE C-1 A hemacytometer and a close-up view of the counting areas as seen under the microscope. The areas for the standard WBC are labeled by W, and those for RBC, by R. (In Rodak FB. *Diagnostic hematology.* Philadelphia: WB Saunders, 1995.)

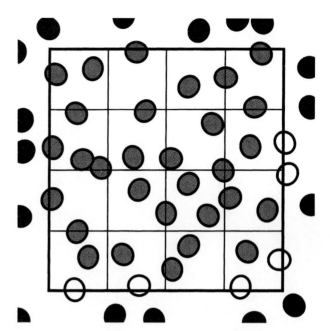

APPENDIX FIGURE C-2 One square of hemacyometer indicating which cells to count. Cells touching the left and top lines (solid circles) are counted. Cells touching bottom and right (open circles) are not counted. (In Rodak BF. *Diagnostic hematology*. Philadelphia: WB Saunders, 1995.)

For semen, a well-mixed liquefied sample is diluted 1:20 with a staining solution unless phase-contrast microscopy is used, in which case the stain can be omitted. Plain distilled water may be used as a diluent. Using the $40 \times$ objective, sperm are counted in the central square millimeter of the hemacytometer grid (where RBCs are counted) on each side of the chamber. This 1 mm² area contains 25 1/25 mm squares. If the sample contains fewer than 10 spermatozoa in each 1/25 mm square, the sperm in the entire 1 mm² area should be counted. For samples with 10 to 40 sperm in each 1/25 mm square, those in 10 1/25 mm squares should be enumerated and for a specimen with more than 40 sperm in each 1/25 mm square, counts in five squares may be carried out.

Answers to the Case History Questions

CASE HISTORY 7-1

1. The urinalysis results that correlate with the diagnosis of diabetic ketoacidosis (DKA) are glucose >1000 mg/dL and ketones >80 mg/dL. Uncontrolled diabetes mellitus results in elevated blood glucose which, in turn, results in glucosuria. Because of incomplete fat metabolism, ketone bodies are produced resulting in ketonuria.
2. The blood analyses that correlate with uncontrolled DKA include a low CO_2 (as well as a low arterial blood pCO_2), which results from Kussmaul breathing (hyperventilation) in response to the metabolic acidosis; elevated blood glucose; acidosis (ABG pH of 7.28); and low bicarbonate as a result of losing buffer base (correlating with negative base excess) as part of excreting ketoacids in the urine.

CASE HISTORY 7-2

1. Renal insufficiency (ischemia) is suggested by proteinuria and renal epithelial cells.
2. The blood work correlates with renal insufficiency because of the elevated creatinine and BUN.
3. The pathophysiology of the renal insufficiency is suggested to be decreased renal perfusion related to the acute exacerbation of the patient's CHF.

CASE HISTORY 7-3

1. The urine results correlating with severe obstructive jaundice include the large bilirubin; amber color; and positive Ictotest. A positive urinary bilirubin is due to increased amounts of conjugated bilirubin in the blood regurgitating back into the liver and then to the blood because of bile flow blockage.
2. The blood analyses that correlate with the above-mentioned results include the elevated total and conjugated bilirubin; the elevated ALP and AST; the decreased total protein and albumin; and the elevated LD. The elevated enzymes, particularly the ALP, correlate with the hepatic toxicity caused by the regurgitated bile (due to the obstruction in the biliary tree), and the decreased total protein and albumin are associated with depressed liver function due to the same toxicity.

CASE HISTORY 9-1

1. Significant urinalysis findings include ketones 40 mg/dL; protein 30 mg/dL; leukocyte esterase trace; color orange; WBCs 5-10/HPF; bacteria 1+; and 1-5 granular casts/LPF.
2. The photomicrographs of the urine sediment (Figs. 93–97) illustrate some of the casts observed, mostly mixed cellular/granular.
3. The ketones, protein, and granular casts suggest a response to the stresses of pregnancy and the surgery procedures (the C-section and appendectomy). The 1+ bacteria correlates with the trace of leukocyte esterase and the slight elevation in WBCs, suggesting a mild UTI. The orange color may have been due to medications. The casts illustrated in Figs. 93–97 are not the granular type reported in the urinalysis but are mixed cellular/granular. The cells incorporated in the casts are the same as those observed throughout the sediment, and their presence in the casts suggests some renal involvement in the UTI.

CASE HISTORY 9-2

1. The significant aspects of the urine sediment are the bacteria (rods) and WBCs.
2. The diagnosis is a urinary tract infection.
3. The treatment would be antibiotics for the *E. coli* UTI.

CASE HISTORY 9-3

1. The significant urinalysis results include glucose 250 mg/dL; blood small; protein 100 mg/dL; appearance hazy; WBCs 20-50/HPF; bacteria 1+; and TNTC granular casts.
2. The casts observed in Figures 9-100 to 9-102 are granular with some cellularity.
3. The pathophysiology of the case most closely related to the urinary sediment findings is interpreted to be the respiratory arrest and acute pulmonary edema leading to an episode of diminished oxygen supply and renal hypoxia.

CASE HISTORY 9-4

1. Although there is a slight amount of protein, the urinalysis is not remarkable.
2. The casts are of mixed cellularity, and the casts as well as the sediment appear to contain renal tubular epithelial cells (collecting duct).
3. The presence of renal tubular epithelial cells in the sediment suggests a toxic and/or hypoxic insult to the renal system—in this case the most likely association is narcotic abuse together with the distinct possibility of side effects from the many medications the patient was using.

CASE HISTORY 10-1

1. The significant aspects of the urinalysis include ketones 15 mg.dL; blood moderate; protein 100 mg/dL; leukocyte esterase small; WBCs 20-50/HPF; RBCs 20-50/HPF;and epithelial cells rare RTE/HPF.
2. The significant pathophysiology here is the observation of a proximal renal tubular cell in Figure 10-58 and reactive transitional cells in Figure 10-59. The interpretation is a toxic insult to the renal system due to drug abuse.

CASE HISTORY 10-2

1. The significant aspects of the urinalysis include slight protein; small leukocyte esterase; increased WBCs; renal tubular epithelials; and casts containing renal tubular epithelials.
2. The pathophysiology of this case is the well-documented renal toxicity of Myochrisine which is seen here with the finding of RTEs in the sediment and in the casts.

CASE HISTORY 10-3

1. The significant aspects of the UA include moderate blood; protein 30 mg/dL; positive nitrite; small leukocyte esterase; hazy appearance; TNTC WBCs; RBCs TNTC; and 4+ bacteria.
2. The urine sediment illustrated in Figures 10-64 and 10-65 suggests an inflammatory response, including the finding of histiocytes.
3. The diagnosis is an acute UTI—*Klebsiella pneumoniae.*

CASE HISTORY 10-4

1. The urinalysis is unremarkable except for small leukocyte esterase; increased WBCs in clumps; and few bacteria.
2. The urine sediment illustrated in Figs. 10-66 and 10-67 suggests an inflammatory response (the increased numbers of WBCs in clumps).
3. The UA, the WBCs in clumps, and the positive C&S suggest the diagnosis of an E. *coli* UTI.

CASE HISTORY 11-1

1. The cellular objects are characteristic for yeast forms of a fungus.
2. The organism shown in the Figures is *Cryptococcus neoformans*.
3. The cell count and differential on the CSF is unusual because there are no leukocytes. Although not stated in the medical records, the implied problem is AIDS (severe immunodeficiency with a CD4 count of 20 and AZT therapy).

CASE HISTORY 11-2

1. The Figures illustrate diplococci (as seen with Wright's stain) leading to the diagnosis of bacterial meningitis.
2. From the choice of answers offered in the question, the most likely organism is *Streptococcus pneumoniae*.

CASE HISTORY 11-3

1. The phenomenon illustrated in the Cytospin preparations of the CSF is termed erythrophagocytosis.
2. The most likely cause for the erythrophagocytosis is a subarachnoid hemorrhage.

CASE HISTORY 15-1

1. The cellularity of the Cytospin preparation of the pleural fluid is a neutrophilia. Since the microbiological tests were all negative, the impression is that the observed condition is an inflammatory reaction.
2. If the fluid is an exudate (the product of an inflammatory reaction), several parameters could be looked at to decide if this is in fact the case. Three good possibilities are the glucose, total protein, and LD (lactic dehydrogenase) levels. If the fluid is an exudate, the glucose level should be {≤} the serum value; the total protein should be >50% of the serum value; and the LD level should be >60% of the serum value. These tests were actually done on this fluid with the following results (reference values in parentheses): glucose, 6 mg/dL (70-110); total protein 5400 mg/dL (6.4-8.2); and LD 1160 U/L (100-190). The evidence favors the diagnosis of an inflammatory exudate.

CASE HISTORY 15-2

1. The comment on the differential report was "intracellular bacteria, seen". Several of the leukocytes have ingested the bacteria, which are visible with the Wright's stain.
2. The Gram stain results indicated gram-positive cocci resembling *Staphylococcus* or *Streptococcus*, and the C&S results were coag-negative *Staphylococcus*. Both the intracellular bacteria and extracellular bacteria seen in the Cytospin preparations agree with the C&S results, *Staphylococcus*.

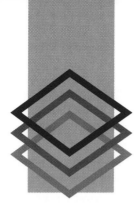

Index

Page numbers followed by *f* indicate figures; those followed by *t* indicate tables.